Plasticity in the human nervous system

Investigations with transcranial magnetic stimulation

It is now well known that the functional organization of the cerebral cortex is plastic, and that changes in organization occur throughout life in response to normal and abnormal experience. Transcranial magnetic stimulation (TMS) is a non-invasive and painless technique that has opened up completely new and fascinating avenues to study neural plasticity. First, TMS can be used to detect changes in excitability or connectivity of the stimulated cortex which may have occurred through processes such as learning or recovery from a lesion. Second, repeated TMS by itself can induce changes in excitability and connectivity of the stimulated cortex which may be used therapeutically in neurological and psychiatric disease. Third, TMS can induce short-lasting 'virtual lesions' which may directly test the functional relevance of brain plasticity.

Current knowledge of all these exciting possibilities is brought together in this book, written by the world's leading experts in the field. The book is an essential compendium on plasticity of the human brain in health and disease, for clinical neurophysiologists, neurologists, psychiatrists and neuroscientists.

Simon Boniface is Consultant Neurophysiologist and Director of Neurophysiology, Addenbrooke's Hospital and Wolfson Brain Imaging Centre, Cambridge, UK.

Ulf Ziemann is Assistant Professor of Neurology, Clinic of Neurology, Johann Wolfgang Goethe-University of Frankfurt, Germany.

Plasticity in the Human Nervous System

Investigations with Transcranial
Magnetic Stimulation

Edited by

Simon Boniface

Department of Clinical Neurophysiology
Addenbrooke's Hospital Wolfson Brain Imaging Centre
University of Cambridge
UK

and

Ulf Ziemann

Clinic of Neurology
Johann Wolfgang Goethe-University of Frankfurt
Germany

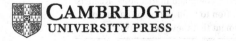
CAMBRIDGE
UNIVERSITY PRESS

CAMBRIDGE UNIVERSITY PRESS
Cambridge, New York, Melbourne, Madrid, Cape Town, Singapore, São Paulo, Delhi

Cambridge University Press
The Edinburgh Building, Cambridge CB2 8RU, UK

Published in the United States of America by Cambridge University Press, New York

www.cambridge.org
Information on this title: www.cambridge.org/9780521114462

First published 2003
This digitally printed version 2009

A catalogue record for this publication is available from the British Library

Library of Congress Cataloguing in Publication data

Motor plasticity and TMS : basic science and clinical applications / edited by Simon J. Boniface and
Ulf Ziemann.
   p. cm.
  Includes bibliographical references and index.
  ISBN 0 521 80727 1
  1. Neuroplasticity. 2. Magnetic brain stimulation.   I. Boniface, Simon J., 1964– II. Ziemann, Ulf.
  QP363.3 .M685 2003
  612.8 – dc21   2002031559

ISBN 978-0-521-80727-2 hardback
ISBN 978-0-521-11446-2 paperback

Additional resources for this publication at www.cambridge.org/9780521114462

Contents

Contributors

Editors

Simon Boniface
Department of Clinical Neurophysiology
Addenbrooke's Hospital
 and the Wolfson Brain Imaging Centre
Cambridge CB2 2QQ, UK

Ulf Ziemann
Neurologische Klinik
Johann Wolfgang Goethe-Universität
 Frankfurt
Theodor-Stern-Kai 7
60590 Frankfurt am Main
Germany

Contributors

Michael J. Angel
Toronto Western Hospital
5W 445, 399 Bathurst Street
Toronto, Ontario,
M5T 2S8, Canada

Pablo A. Celnik
Department of Physical Medicine and
 Rehabilitation
Johns Hopkins University
136 West Lanvale Street
Baltimore
MD 21217, USA

Robert Chen
Toronto Western Hospital
5W 445, 399 Bathurst Street

Toronto, Ontario,
M5T 2S8, Canada

Joseph Classen
Department of Neurology
University of Würzburg
Josef-Schneider-Str 11
D-97080 Würzburg, Germany

Leonardo G. Cohen
Human Cortical Physiology Section
NINDS
National Institutes of Health
Building 10, Room 5N 234
10 Center Drive, MSC 1428
Bethesda
MD 20892-1428, USA

Nicholas J. Davey
Department of Sensorimotor Systems
   (Room 10L09)
Division of Neuroscience and
Psychological Medicine
Imperial College School of Medicine,
Charing Cross Hospital
Fulham Palace Road
London W6 8RF, UK

John P. Donoghue
Department of Neuroscience
Brown University
Box 1953
Providence
RI 02912, USA

Peter H. Ellaway
Department of Sensorimotor Systems
   (Room 10L09)
Division of Neuroscience and
   Psychological Medicine
Imperial College School of Medicine,
Charing Cross Hospital
Fulham Palace Road
London W6 8RF, UK

Chip M. Epstein
Department of Neurology
Emory Clinic
1365 Clifton Road NE
Atlanta
GA 30322, USA

Janet A. Eyre
Department of Child Health
The Royal Victoria Infirmary
Queen Victoria Road
Newcastle upon Tyne
NE1 4LP, UK

Chris Fraser
Department of Medicine
Royal Bolton Hospital
Farnworth
Bolton BL4 0JR, UK

David Gow
Department of G.I. Sciences and
   Medicine
University of Manchester
Hope Hospital
Eccles Old Road
Salford M6 8HD, UK

Mark Hallett
Human Motor Control Section
NINDS
National Institutes of Health
Building 10, Room 5N 226
10 Center Drive, MSC 1428
Bethesda
MD 20892-1428, USA

Shaheen Hamdy
Department of Gastroenterology
University of Manchester
Hope Hospital
Eccles Old Road
Salford M6 8HD, UK

Joachim Liepert
Clinic of Neurology
University of Hamburg
Hamburg
52 20246, Germany

Alvaro Pascual-Leone
Laboratory for Magnetic Brain
   Stimulation
Behavioral Neurology Unit

Beth Israel Deaconess Medical
 Center
330 Brookline Avenue, Kirstein
 Building KS 452
Boston
MA 02215, USA

Mengia-S. Rioult-Pedotti
Department of Neuroscience
Brown University
Box 193
Providence
RI 02912, USA

Edwin M. Robertson
Laboratory for Magnetic Brain
 Stimulation
Behavioral Neurology Unit
Beth Israel Deaconess Medical
 Center
330 Brookline Avenue, Kirstein
 Building KS 452
Boston
MA 02215, USA

Paolo M. Rossini
Department of Neuroscience
Ospedale Fatebenefratelli
Isola Tiberina 39
00186 Rome, Italy

John C. Rothwell
Sobell Department
Institute of Neurology (Box 146)
Queen Square
London WC1N 3BG, UK

Hugo Theoret
Laboratory for Magnetic Brain Stimulation
Behavioral Neurology Unit
Beth Israel Deaconess Medical Center
330 Brookline Avenue, Kirstein Building
 KS 452
Boston
MA 02215, USA

Eric M. Wassermann
NINDS
National Institutes of Health
Building 10, Room 5N 226
10 Center Drive, MSC 1428
Bethesda
MD 20892-1428, USA

Ulf Ziemann
Neurologische Klinik
Johann Wolfgang Goethe-Universität
 Frankfurt
Theodor-Stern-Kai 7
60590 Frankfurt am Main
Germany

Preface

Plasticity of the brain is an increasingly important topic in many areas of neuroscience including development, learning and repair. It is still a challenge to study plasticity directly in the human nervous system. Transcranial magnetic stimulation (TMS), however, has become a suitable non-invasive and painless technique, which can be applied to detect changes in cortical excitability or connectivity as indicators of plasticity. Further, TMS can be used to induce short-lasting virtual lesions in order to test the functional relevance of brain plasticity. Finally, TMS can induce plasticity itself. In this book, we utilize TMS in these ways to investigate and manipulate plasticity in the human nervous system. In so doing, we have been fortunate to gather many of the world's leading contributors in this field.

The basic nature and mechanisms of plasticity are tackled in the introductory chapter, with particular reference to the animal primary motor cortex. This is followed in the next chapter by an introduction to the technique and physiological effects of human TMS.

In the next section we then apply this background to TMS studies of plasticity in healthy subjects. Chapter 3 is about developmental plasticity of the human corticospinal tract. The next two chapters demonstrate the maintained capability of the adult human brain for plastic change by looking into TMS studies of use-dependent plasticity and learning of motor skills. Finally, the induction of plasticity by TMS itself is the focus of Chapter 6.

The next section is more clinically orientated and examines functional deficits and the principles of recovery of function after cortical lesions, stroke in particular, and lesions of the periphery and spinal cord. This is followed by a demonstration of the functional relevance of cortical plasticity. The concluding two chapters of this section provide a survey of TMS as a potential therapeutic tool for promoting beneficial plasticity in various neurological and psychiatric disorders, and the applications of TMS in the process of neurological rehabilitation. The book closes with a look towards the future, speculating on novel and farther reaching avenues for the study and influence of human brain plasticity with TMS.

We would like to thank the contributors for all their time and effort, and chiefly we would like to thank our families for their support, past and future.

Simon Boniface and Ulf Ziemann
Cambridge and Frankfurt, September 2002

1

The nature and mechanisms of plasticity

Mengia-S. Rioult-Pedotti and John P. Donoghue

Department of Neuroscience, Brown University, Providence, RI, USA

Cortical map plasticity

It is now well established that the functional organization of the cerebral cortex is plastic, that is, changes in organization occur throughout life in response to normal as well as abnormal experience. The potential for reorganization has been demonstrated in both sensory and motor areas of adult cortex, either as a consequence of trauma, pathological changes, manipulation of sensory experience, or learning. These changes can only be evaluated with reference to an extensive experimental base that has identified a repeatable representation pattern (e.g. somatotopy, tonotopy, or retinotopy), for which change can be detected. While the scope of changes are often at the edge of our technical capabilities to assess, there are striking examples of significant and rapid change (for reviews, see Sanes & Donoghue, 2000; Buonomano & Merzenich, 1998). There is an overwhelming belief that modifications in cortical organization emerge through changes in synaptic efficacy within the cortex and elsewhere in the nervous system. Further, these changes are have been closely linked to the phenomena called long-term potentiation (LTP) and long-term depression (LTD). This review deals mainly with the changes that have been detected in the motor cortex and their link to synaptic modification. Some of the most convincing evidence that learning and practice influences cortical organization and that learning operates through LTP/D-mediated mechanisms has come through work in the motor cortex. This work is also of profound significance to the medical community because it implies that the impaired or damaged motor cortex can be restructured through appropriate physical rehabilitation schemes or through pharmacological means that alter mechanisms accounting for LTP/D.

Functional topography of the primary motor cortex (MI) can be modified by peripheral or central injury, electrical stimulation, pharmacological
manipulations, or experience. Behaviourally or experimentally induced reorganization of MI output maps are characterized by shifts in borders between
different motor representations. For example, MI representations undergo
rapid reorganization within hours of peripheral nerve lesions (Sanes et al.,
1988, 1990; Donoghue et al., 1990). Following transection of the peripheral
facial motor nerve to the whiskers in rats, movements of the forelimb can be
evoked by stimulation of the former MI whisker representation (Donoghue
et al., 1990; Fig. 1.1, see colour plate at www.cambridge.org/9780521114462),
indicating that cortex dedicated to the control of one set of muscles can be
switched rapidly to process information for another set. It is further evident
that sensory nerve damage can alter motor maps (Huntley, 1997; Keller et al.,
1996). In these cases, the cortical territories adjacent to the functionally silent
areas expanded into the cortical zone that previously represented output to
the vibrissa as a result of the nerve lesion. Similar changes in cortical output
maps can be induced with prolonged changes in limb positions (Sanes et al.,
1992; Sanes & Donoghue, 1997), supporting the conclusion that sensory
feedback is important in shaping MI representations. Very recently, a
doubling of forelimb motor representation has been shown as a result of
repeated seizure activity that is also accompanied by increased synaptic strength within adult rat MI (Teskey et al., 2002), indicating that activity drives
the form of representations. The expanded areas do not have to represent new
areas of forelimb motor cortex; rather they have undergone some functional
changes that lead to facilitated induction of forelimb movement in areas in
which they could not be induced previously.

MI is also a site where reorganization occurs during the acquisition or
practice of motor skills. In monkeys, skilled finger use expanded the digit
representation in MI (Nudo et al., 1996), and learning a new visuomotor
task altered the output representation of wrist muscles (Sanes & Donoghue,
1997). Skill learning-induced changes in MI were also detected on the single
cell level in primates (Gandolfo et al., 2000). Monkeys learned to adapt their
reaching movements to externally applied force fields. The firing rate and
the tuning of individually recorded cells in MI changed during the adaptation period to the new force field. A group of these cells (the memory
cells) retained the newly acquired activity pattern even after the force field

was turned off and the monkey's hand trajectory returned to control condition. Other memory cells that normally were untuned became tuned with acquisition of the new skill and remained tuned after turning off the force-field. These data provide evidence for single-cell plasticity in MI. In humans, MI representations also appear to enlarge or rearrange during motor learning (Grafton et al., 1992; Pascual-Leone et al., 1994; Karni et al., 1995; Muellbacher et al., 2001). Further, a role of MI in early motor consolidation (Muellbacher et al., 2002) and in motor memory (Karni et al., 1995) has been demonstrated in humans.

In rats, learning a skilled but not an unskilled reaching task leads to a significant increase in the mean area of the wrist and digit representations at the expense of the size of the shoulder representation, demonstrating that training-induced map reorganization is characterized by an expansion of 'trained' into 'untrained' representations without an overall increase in map size (Kleim et al., 1998). These results indicate that representational map plasticity is driven by skill acquisition, learning, or practice of a newly acquired action, but not by simple repetitive motor activity (Plautz et al., 2000; Classen et al., 1998), which suggests that only specific patterns of activity are capable of producing functional MI plasticity.

Plasticity substrate

Cortical networks appear to contain an anatomical substrate that is well suited to provide a flexible framework for a multitude of representations. Horizontal (also called lateral) fibres form a dense network of short- and long-range connections within the cortex. They spread tangentially along cortical layers and form a diffuse, but extensive, intrinsic pathway that provide excitatory connections across wide areas of cortex. In primary visual cortex these fibres have precisely patterned terminations, but in motor cortex they appear to be largely unpatterned. This diffuse organization could make it possible to couple wide extents of cortex; synaptic plasticity would allow for the functional patterning of these connections. The most extensive intracortical pathways travel through layer II/III and form a broad projection system. The functions of these horizontal projections in MI have remained obscure until recently. Evidence for a role of horizontal connections in shaping the properties of adult cortical neurons originated from a series of experiments in the visual cortex, which linked horizontal connections to receptive field dynamics (Gilbert et al., 1996).

Experimental studies in the rat support the conclusion that intrinsic horizontal connections spanning MI are a substrate for motor cortical map plasticity (Donoghue et al., 1996). Motor representations can be modified by pharmacological adjustments of the balance between excitation and inhibition within MI, suggesting that occult representations can be revealed by unmasking existing horizontal pathways (Jacobs & Donoghue, 1991). The role of horizontal connections in supporting MI representations is also suggested by the patterns of reorganization that occur after nerve lesions. Facial nerve lesions result in rapid MI reorganization at sites with strong horizontal connections between forelimb and whisker representation, while reorganization is not evident at sites with sparse horizontal connections (Huntley, 1997). The masking of horizontal excitatory connections by feed-forward inhibition has been demonstrated even more directly in vitro using cortical slice preparations containing MI. Local application of bicuculline enhances excitatory responses of horizontal connections in MI (Hess & Donoghue, 1994); in these preparations concerns about localization of drug application or stimulation site are reduced by much better control than in the in vivo situation. Most convincingly, these effects can be observed in slices in which subcortical and deep layer connections have been cut away. This evidence strongly supports the idea that intrinsic horizontal pathways form a substrate for motor cortex plasticity. However, MI plasticity also requires a mechanism inherent to horizontal connections in order to modify maps.

Plasticity mechanisms

Evidence for candidate mechanisms to support cortical plasticity on the population level as well as on the cellular level have been proposed and evaluated. Mechanisms that support rapid plasticity are uncovering latent or existing connections, activating existing but silent synapses, activity-dependent synaptic plasticity, or generalized excitability changes in postsynaptic neurons. Morphological changes such as neurogenesis, synaptogenesis or synaptic remodelling require time for full expression and therefore, might rather be involved in providing new space for further changes. Evidence exists for the operation of most of these mechanisms during development, with learning or response to injury. Moreover, these mechanisms are not mutually exclusive; different mechanisms could operate simultaneously or in some serial order.

Uncovering or unmasking of pre-existing connections in MI (Jacobs & Donoghue, 1991; Huntley, 1997) could serve as a mechanism for rapid (early) plasticity as a response to manipulations of sensory inputs (Kaas, 1991; Merzenich & Shameshima, 1993) or motor outputs (Sanes et al., 1990; Donoghue et al., 1996) of cortical representational maps. As discussed above, a change in the balance between excitation and inhibition can also lead to rapid map plasticity, if such changes persist (Jacobs & Donoghue, 1991). An alternative or additional mechanism for rapid plasticity is the activation of existing but silent synapses. Silent synapses are connections between neurons displaying no AMPA-mediated glutamate responses (e.g. Liao et al., 1995; Isaac et al., 1995); presynaptic transmitter release would not result in a rapid potential shift in the target neuron. The 'awakening' of silent synapses by insertion of postsynaptic AMPA receptors (Liao et al., 1999; Gomperts et al., 1998; Nusser et al., 1998; Petralia et al., 1999) is a proposed mechanism to account for rapid increases in synaptic efficacy that have been observed experimentally. Silent synapses have been implicated in brain plasticity of both young and mature animals (Atwood & Wojtowicz, 1999). There is convincing evidence for the occurrence of silent synapses in the developing nervous system (e.g. Durand et al., 1996; Wu et al., 1996; Liao et al., 1995; Isaac et al., 1995, 1997; Malenka & Nicoll, 1997, 1999; Malenka, 1998; Malinow, 1998; Rumpel et al., 1998), but as maturation progresses, silent synapses become rare (Nusser et al., 1998; He et al., 1998) and are presumably replaced by active ones. Although there is little evidence for the existence of silent synapses in the mature nervous system, their presence remains an open question. If present, the unmasking of silent synapses could support functional reorganization.

The most widely studied mechanism to support representational plasticity is long-term potentiation (LTP) (Bliss & Lomo, 1973), but it remains controversial (Shors & Matzel, 1997, for an extensive review), especially as a critical link between behavioural change and synaptic function. In the hippocampal cortex, neocortex and amygdala evidence for a possible role of LTP in learning and memory has accumulated over the past 30 years; population measures indicate that LTP and LTD operate during learning to modify synaptic efficacy (Martin et al., 2000). Certain forms of learning lead to an enhancement of synaptic responses in a variety of brain structures (Moser et al., 1993; Rogan et al., 1997; McKernan & Shinnick-Gallagher, 1997; Rioult-Pedotti et al., 1998). Recently, LTP has been demonstrated to be involved in learning new motor skills (Rioult-Pedotti et al., 2000) and provides compelling evidence for LTP to be a mechanism involved in natural learning. A great deal of effort has been devoted to the question as to whether LTP is a mechanism of memory storage (Miller & Mayford, 1999). Long-lasting LTP in the hippocampus decays within weeks of its induction and can parallel memory loss (Thompson et al., 1996; Castro et al., 1989; Villareal et al., 2002). If this were true for the motor cortex, one would expect that discontinuing skill training would lead to synaptic weakening and possibly declining skill performance. Results, however, indicate that increased synaptic efficacy with initial skill learning as well as skill performance is maintained (Rioult-Pedotti & Donoghue, 2002). Learning effects seem to persist for a longer time in MI than in the hippocampus, which is consistent with results from Trepel & Racine (1998), indicating that neocortical LTP lasts longer than hippocampal LTP. The appeal of LTP as a mechanism of learning and memory is that it is activity dependent and specific to the active synapses and their target neurons.

Excitability changes represent another way to change coupling between neurons, but this is less specific than LTP-like mechanisms. A generalized long-lasting increase in excitability of postsynaptic neurons in MI has been demonstrated to be involved in classical conditioning (Brons & Woody, 1980; Baranyi et al., 1991; Woody, 1986; Aou et al., 1992). In the hippocampus, trace eye blink conditioning leads to a transient increase in CAI excitability within a time window of 1 hour to 7 days with a peak effect at 24 hours and therefore might represent a mechanism that enables consolidation of a learned behaviour (Moyer et al., 1996). A change in postsynaptic excitability would be less specific than LTP/D because it alters the effectiveness of all synapses to a neuron.

The mechanisms described up to this point rely on modifications of existing synapses that are readily available within the substantial horizontal intracortical plexus. Experience could also produce new connections through synaptogenesis or neurogenesis. Such processes, however, require more time for full expression and therefore might be involved in creating new space for subsequent learning rather than being involved in ongoing information encoding.

The traditional view of adult primate neocortex was the structural stability and inability of neurogenesis and synapse formation that seemed to occur only during development. Such structural plasticity, however, is found in adult lower vertebrates (Alvarez-Buylla & Lois, 1995), in the olfactory bulb (Rousselot et al., 1995; Doetsch et al., 1997), and in the hippocampus, even in primates (Altman & Das, 1965; Gould et al., 1997, 1999a–c; Kornack & Rakic, 1999), and in humans (Eriksson et al., 1998). The traditional view of a structurally stable neocortex has recently been challenged by Gould et al., (1999d). Newly generated neurons were detected in neocortex of adult primates that were exposed to the DNA marker BrdU (bromodeoxyuridine). New neurons were added in regions of the association cortex, areas that are involved in learning and memory (Miller et al., 1996). Adult neurogenesis in the hippocampus is increased by training on associative learning tasks that require the hippocampus (Gould et al., 1999c), indicating that hippocampus-dependent learning may affect adult-generated neurons.

The formation of new synapses or the remodelling of existing synapses has long been believed to be involved in cellular mechanisms of learning and memory (for review, see Geinisman, 2000; Klintsova & Greenough, 1999; Bailey & Kandel, 1993). Motor skill learning has been shown to increase the number of synapses per neuron in the motor cortex (Kleim et al., 1996) and the cerebellum (Black et al., 1990; Kleim et al., 1997, 1998). Like learning, exposure to a complex environment results in a larger number of synapses per neuron (Turner & Greenough, 1985), increases in spine density (Moser et al., 1997) and changes in spine morphology (Comery et al., 1996; Jones et al., 1997). However, Bourgeois et al. (1999) found no ultrastructural changes in synaptic density despite continuous acquisition of long-term memories over the entire period of adulthood in macaque monkeys, indicating that the formation of long-term memories following learning may not necessarily involve a net synaptogenesis.

Whether the induction of LTP, the most viable current memory model, induces synaptogenesis or synaptic remodelling also remains controversial. Using stereological techniques Sorra & Harris (1998) could not show any change in synapse number. In contrast to these results, new synapses were detected 30–60 minutes following LTP induction in hippocampal slice cultures using the two photon imaging technique (Engert & Bonhoeffer, 1999; Maletic-Savatic et al., 1999; Toni et al., 1999) indicating that synaptogenesis might be involved in synaptic modification. It remains to be proven that such processes also take place during acquisition of new behaviours.

Plasticity of MI horizontal connections (in vitro)

Mechanisms of synaptic modification are more easily studied in slice preparations than in intact animals. An in vitro approach allows local connections to be evaluated directly under controlled conditions using intracellular- as well as extracellular population measures. Extracellular field potentials (FP), which reflect the concerted synaptic activity of groups of fibres, can be readily evoked in MI horizontal connections (Hess & Donoghue, 1994) (Fig. 1.2(c)). In neocortex, the amplitude of FPs reflects a monosynaptic current sink, which can be used to measure the strength of excitatory synaptic responses for a population of neurons (Aroniadou & Keller, 1995). Thus the FP amplitude correlates with intracellular excitatory postsynaptic potentials (EPSP) (Fig. 1.2(c); Hess et al., 1996). Pharmacological manipulations revealed that horizontal excitatory connections are mainly glutamatergic (Keller, 1993; Hess & Donoghue, 1994), with larger, fast AMPA and slower, low amplitude NMDA components. The strength of excitation is also regulated by feed-forward inhibition. The MI slice preparation is useful in that the same region can be repeatedly localized. To study horizontal connections in MI, stimulation and recording electrodes are placed on the surface of coronal slices containing MI (Fig. 1.2(a), see colour plate at www.cambridge.org/9780521114462). Most in vitro studies in MI have examined layer II/III horizontal connections within the region of the MI forelimb area. Stimulation of the superficial layers is more restricted to horizontal connections than in deeper layers, which contain a more complex mix of vertical, extrinsic connections as well as other intrinsic connections. The placement of stimulation and recording electrodes in the MI forelimb region has been verified by labelling layer V corticospinal neurons using fast blue injections into the cervical spinal cord. (Fig. 1.2(b), see colour plate at www.cambridge.org/9780521114462).

Using slice preparations it has been possible to test for the ability of horizontal connections to be modified and to search for the mechanisms that support modification. Studies in the hippocampus and in other cortical areas suggested that activity-dependent processes leading to long-term potentiation (LTP) and long-term depression (LTD) are likely candidates for plasticity in MI. LTP, discovered in the hippocampus (Bliss & Lomo, 1973) a structure known to be critical for learning, is rapidly induced, and shows long-lasting increases in synaptic strength as a response to short bursts of coinciding activity at specific synapses, all useful features for a natural memory mechanism (Hebb, 1949). Classical forms of LTP, and variants, have also been documented in the amygdala (Clugnet & LeDoux, 1990; Marren, 1999; Martin et al., 2000) and neocortex (Artola & Singer, 1987; Iriki et al., 1989; Kirkwood et al., 1996; Trepel & Racine, 1998) and specifically in MI (Baranyi & Feher, 1978, 1981; Baranyi et al., 1991; Aroniadou & Keller, 1995; Castro-Alamancos et al., 1995; Hess et al., 1996; Rioult-Pedotti et al., 1998). Most forms of LTP are glutamatergic and depend on the activation of voltage-dependent NMDA receptors.

The potential for LTP of layer II/III intrinsic horizontal pathways in MI has been established (Castro-Alamancos et al., 1995; Hess & Donoghue, 1996; Hess et al., 1996). This activity-dependent synaptic modification is NMDA receptor dependent, pathway specific and long lasting (Hess et al., 1996) and thus resembles classical LTP. LTP is normally induced by high frequency stimulation or theta burst stimulation where several high frequency bursts are delivered in short succession. In the adult MI, similar stimulation patterns alone did not lead to an increase in synaptic strength as in the hippocampus and other cortical areas. LTP was only induced when inhibition was reduced transiently by local application of bicuculline, a GABA antagonist, prior to theta burst stimulation (Chen et al., 1994; Hess et al., 1996) or by concomitant stimulation of vertical and horizontal inputs (Hess et al., 1996). These findings suggest that local, GABA-mediated inhibition plays a critical role in cortex in regulating the potential for LTP induction, though maintenance of LTP does not require the sustained reduction of inhibition.

Partially because of theoretical considerations, it has been recognized that, if there is a mechanism for activity-dependent increases in synaptic strength, there should also be a mechanism to decrease synaptic strength in order to keep synaptic weights constant and to prevent runaway potentiation leading to synapse saturation. Therefore, individual synapses need to be capable of bidirectional modification, a strengthening and weakening, to avoid saturation effects. Mild but repetitive stimulation of synaptic inputs leads to long-term depression (LTD), a lasting activity-dependent decrease in synaptic efficacy. LTD was first discovered in the hippocampus by Lynch et al. (1977; e.g. Levi & Steward, 1979; Thiels et al., 1994; Dudek & Bear, 1992) and later in other brain structures including the amygdala (Li et al., 1998) and neocortex (Artola et al., 1990; Kirkwood & Bear, 1994). As its LTP counterpart, LTD is long lasting and may be NMDA receptor dependent or independent. In MI, LTD depends on the activation of NMDA receptors, and, unlike LTP, LTD is readily induced in MI horizontal pathways by low frequency stimulation without additional manipulations (Hess et al., 1996).

In summary, then, MI horizontal connections meet important conditions for reorganizing motor representation patterns: they strengthen and weaken, based on established activity-dependent synaptic modification processes, and they interconnect widespread sets of neurons through their lateral-spreading connections.

MI's direct role in motor learning and memory

Motor skill learning and its trace in MI

The presence of this connectional substrate and activity-dependent synaptic modification mechanism provides strong support for the conclusion that operations within motor cortical circuitry are important for learning. Learning enhances synaptic responses in the hippocampus (Moser et al., 1993; Power et al., 1997), the amygdala (Rogan et al., 1997; McKernan & Shinnick-Gallagher, 1997), and the piriform cortex (Roman et al., 1999; Saar et al., 1999). Does motor learning lead to a similar enhancement in MI? There is now compelling evidence that motor skill learning involves LTP-mediated synaptic plasticity in MI, providing an important link between behavioural change, synaptic modification and LTP. In this novel model, evidence for synaptic change and mechanisms of change were examined in motor cortex slices (Rioult-Pedotti et al., 1998). Rats learned to reach, with their preferred forelimb, through a small aperture in a food box and grasp single food pellets (Fig. 1.3 left, see colour plate at www.cambridge.org/9780521114462). The rats acquired the skill and improved performance over 5 training days (Fig. 1.3 right, see colour plate at www.cambridge.org/9780521114462).

Because the reach and grasp task is quantifiable, improvement in behaviour can be directly associated with changes in synaptic strength observed in slices prepared after learning (Fig. 1.4, see colour plate at www.cambridge.org/9780521114462). Layer II/III intracortical connections were markedly enhanced only in the trained MI that related to the forelimb used in the task. The opposite (ipsilateral) MI for each animal showed no change and served as an important control for global, motivational, or state effects. Further, the changes appeared to be topographically specific because modifications were not present in the MI hindlimb area. These results are consistent with results of learning-induced functional reorganization of MI following skill learning in rats (Kleim et al., 1998) and primates (Nudo et al., 1996).

Mechanisms of learning-induced increases in synaptic efficacy
The LTP-learning controversy

The relationship between synaptic strengthening as produced by electrical stimulation (LTP) and learning and memory (the learning-synaptic plasticity-LTP hypothesis) has been extensively examined in the hippocampus in relation to spatial learning and memory, as in water maze learning. The hypothesis that LTP is required for learning has been evaluated either by occlusion of learning by prior pathway saturation, or by blockade of LTP mechanisms by pharmacological and genetic interventions. Both approaches are expected to lead to an impairment of learning (for review see Martin et al., 2000).

The concept of saturation of LTP has often been used to study the involvement of LTP in learning and memory. According to the LTP-learning hypothesis saturation of synaptic efficacy achieved by repeated LTP induction until no further LTP occurs should block further learning. Saturation of LTP in the hippocampal perforant path induced a reversible occlusion of subsequent spatial learning (McNaughton et al., 1986; Castro et al., 1989; Barnes et al., 1994; Moser et al., 1998; but see Cain et al., 1993; Jeffrey & Morris, 1993; Korol et al., 1993; Sutherland et al., 1993). While this finding shows that synapse saturation blocks learning, it does not demonstrate that this modification mechanism is used during natural learning.

In the early 1980s Collindridge et al. (1983) discovered that NMDA receptor activation is necessary for the induction of LTP. NMDA receptors act as coincidence detectors because the channels open only with concomitant pre- (glutamate release) and postsynaptic (depolarization which releases the Mg^{2+} block) activity (Nowak et al., 1984; Mayer et al., 1984; McBain & Mayer, 1994). This finding led to many behavioural studies in which NMDA receptor antagonists were used to block LTP and LTD in order to test the hypothesis that LTP blockade will interfere with learning. An initial and intriguing study by Morris (1986) demonstrated that the NMDA receptor antagonist APV impaired hippocampus-dependent spatial learning. Many similar studies using systemic or local application of NMDA receptor antagonists followed with results strongly supporting a role of LTP in learning and memory (Morris, 1989; Bannerman et al., 1995; Kentros et al., 1998; but Saucier & Cain, 1995). Interpretation was often difficult because of problems associated with drug application, drug diffusion, and side effects of the drug (discussed by Martin et al., 2000).

An alternative approach to investigate LTP's role in learning and memory is gene targeting, which includes deletion or overexpression of specific genes (Mayford et al., 1997; Chen & Tonegawa, 1997; Elgersma & Silva, 1999), and the effects were tested for LTP and learning. Grant et al. (1992) and Silva et al. (1992) were the first to demonstrate a correlation between LTP and hippocampus-dependent learning using the gene knockout technique. Later, Sakimura et al. (1995) demonstrated reduced hippocampal LTP and spatial learning in mice lacking the NMDA receptor subunit 1 (NR1, part of all NMDA receptors). The second generation knockout technique made it possible to restrict the gene deletion to one area of the brain. Tsien et al. (1996) produced a mouse strain with NMDAR1 (NR1 is essential for channel function) gene deletion that was specific to CA1 pyramidal cells of the hippocampus. These mutants lacked NMDA receptor-mediated responses and LTP in the CA1, and exhibited impaired spatial but unimpaired non-spatial memory, strongly suggesting a role of NMDA receptor dependent LTP in the acquisition of spatial memory. Further, mice with NR2B subunit (longer excitatory postsynaptic potentials) overexpression had a greater ability to learn and memorize various behavioural tasks and showed enhanced potentiation (Tang et al., 1999). A third-generation knockout technique was used to produce inducible, reversible, and CA1 specific knockout mice that allowed NMDA receptors (NR1) to switch off and on by adding tetracycline to their drinking water (Shimazu et al., 2000). This technique, like the pharmacological approach (McGaugh & Izquierdo, 2000) made it possible to study memory encoding, consolidation and retrieval in isolation. Using this technique, Shimazu et al. (2000) found evidence for a crucial role of NMDA receptors in memory consolidation. These results, however, contradict established findings from pharmacological studies, showing that NMDA receptors are necessary for induction but not consolidation or retrieval of memories (Day & Morris, 2001). Taken together, these gene manipulation studies strongly support the involvement of NMDA receptors in learning and memory, most plausibly through synaptic strength changes.

Nevertheless, the links between learning and synaptic plasticity and LTP still remain unproven (Stevens, 1998; Bliss, 1998; Goda & Stevens, 1996; Miller & Mayford, 1999).

The connection between learning, synaptic plasticity and LTP in MI

The large base of work on MI structure and function, its ability to modify representations, as well as the existence of a substrate and mechanism for synaptic modification presents a powerful system to explore the relationship between LTP/D mechanisms, synaptic plasticity and learning (Donoghue, 1995; Sanes & Donoghue, 2000). Motor skill learning leads to enhanced responses unilaterally in the MI forelimb area that can be recorded in vitro after learning has occurred (Rioult-Pedotti et al., 1998). This model makes it possible to test whether the synaptic plasticity that accompanies learning actually requires the participation of the LTP-process.

Rioult-Pedotti et al. (2000) showed that learning placed synapses near the top of their modification range (i.e. saturation) and occluded further LTP in vitro. To evaluate this result, one must consider that synapse populations have a range of operation, termed the synaptic modification range. That is, they have a finite ceiling and a finite floor over which they operate (Fig. 1.5, see colour plate at www.cambridge.org/9780521114462). This range can be defined experimentally in control or experimental animals using saturating levels of electrically induced LTP and LTD (Rioult-Pedotti et al., 2000). Saturation effects were used as a tool to determine whether synaptic enhancement caused by skill learning utilized the same mechanism as LTP. Following 5 days of skill training maximum LTP (ceiling) and LTD (floor) capacity was determined. Maximum or minimum synaptic strength was assessed by repeated induction of LTP or LTD. Simultaneous recordings in sign-in both hemispheres revealed that repeated theta burst stimulation resulted ificantly less LTP in the trained, compared to the untrained, hemisphere (Fig. 1.5, left and right, see colour plate at www.cambridge.org/9780521114462). Repeated low frequency stimulation produced significantly more LTD in the trained compared to the untrained MI. Five days of motor skill training moved the baseline synaptic efficacy upwards within an unchanged synaptic modification range. Using the motor system as a model to study learning on the behavioural and cellular level provided compelling and direct evidence for the involvement of LTP in learning-induced synaptic strengthening (Rioult-Pedotti et al., 2000; Martin & Morris, 2001).

The LTP-learning hypothesis further suggests that blockade of LTP should interfere with learning. This can be tested by systemic application of CPP ([(±)-3-(2-carboxypiperazin-4-yl)-propyl-1-phosphonic acid]), a competitive NMDA receptor antagonist that crosses the blood–brain barrier. LTP in MI is NMDA receptor dependent (Hess et al., 1996), and skill learning occludes LTP in MI (Rioult-Pedotti et al., 2000). Therefore, inactivation of NMDA receptors during learning should impair learning and reduce or eliminate the learning-induced electrophysiological trace in MI. Rats given CPP 1 hour before each training session initially learned to reach through a hole and grasp food pellets, but showed no further improvement after the second training day, compared to controls that continue to improve over subsequent days. No synaptic strengthening occurred in MI horizontal connections of the CPP-treated animals, in contrast to normal or saline-injected rats that learned this task (Margolis et al., 2000). Therefore, these results indicate that NMDA-mediated LTP must operate within MI circuitry in order for normal motor skill learning to occur. These results reinforce the relationship between learning-synaptic strengthening and LTP.

In humans, Buetefisch et al. (2000) found results consistent with these studies in rats. Systemic administration of NMDA receptor blockers (dextrometorphan) or $GABA_A$ receptor enhancing drug (lorazepam) blocked use-dependent plasticity in the hand area of MI. That these manipulations can block LTP induction supports the conclusion that LTP is required for MI reorganization associated with motor learning.

Dynamics of the synaptic modification range

Is the capacity for learning equivalent to the capacity for LTP? If the hypothesis that skill learning parallels changes in synaptic strength holds true, learning should be impaired when LTP is saturated. As a consequence of pathway saturation, the cortex would seem to have a limited capacity to contribute to learning and, one might predict, that learning one skill would impair learning of another skill. One way to test this prediction is to train rats on a second different motor skill at the time of pathway saturation and stable skill performance and test whether learning of the second skill is impaired.

Another way to test the prediction is to train rats for an extended period of time and test for LTP recovery.

Whether the full potential for synaptic modification is reinstated over time, either by decay of potentiation or a change in the synaptic modification range, was examined by training rats on the reach and grasp skill for an extended period of time (23–105 successive days). Extended training maintained the enhanced synaptic strength of intrinsic MI connections and shifted the synaptic modification range, for a synapse population, upward (Rioult-Pedotti & Donoghue, 2003 submitted). This upward shift appears to place synaptic efficacy back to the middle of its operating range, allowing prelearning levels of LTP and LTD (Fig. 1.5, right, see colour plate at www.cambridge.org/9780521114462). Whether recovered LTP can be used for new learning remains to be examined.

Conclusions

Using cellular plasticity associated with cortical motor learning and memory as its focus, this chapter has introduced some current advanced concepts about cortical plasticity as it pertains to plasticity in the motor cortex and its role in motor skill learning as well as more general principles concerning synaptic plasticity and early brain development, learning and memory, and reorganization after lesions. These mechanisms are likely to be critical not only to normal development, motor system function, and skill learning, but also to understanding the neural responses to injury, disease and rehabilitation therapy. In humans, it is not possible to have the access to circuitry that is afforded by experimental animal models. However, TMS, provides a valuable method to explore cortical plasticity in humans. It promises to play a fundamental role especially in understanding plasticity in humans.

Acknowledgements

Supported by NIH grant US 27164.

REFERENCES

Altman, J. & Das, G.D. (1965). Autoradiographic and histological evidence of postnatal hippocampal neurogenesis in rats. *J. Comp. Neurol.*, **124**: 319–335.

Alvarez-Buylla, A. & Lois, C. (1995). Neuronal stem cells in the brain of adult vertebrates. *Stem Cells*, **13**: 263–272.

Aou, S., Oomura, Y., Woody, C.D. & Nishino, H. (1988). Effects of behaviorally rewarding hypothalamic electrical stimulation on intracellularly recorded neuronal activity in the motor cortex of awake monkeys. *Brain Res.*, **439**: 31–38.

Aou, S., Woody, C.D. & Birt, D. (1992). Changes in the activity of units of the cat motor cortex with rapid conditioning and extinction of a compound eye blink movement. *J. Neurosci.*, **12**: 549–559.

Aroniadou, V.A. & Keller, A. (1995). Mechanisms of LTP induction in rat motor cortex in vitro. *Cereb. Cortex*, **5**: 353–362.

Artola, A. & Singer, W. (1987). Long-term potentiation and NMDA receptors in rat visual cortex. *Nature*, **330**: 649–652.

Artola, A., Broecher, S. & Singer, W. (1990). Different voltage-dependent thresholds for inducing long-term depression and long-term potentiation in slices of rat visual cortex. *Nature*, **347**: 69–72.

Atwood, H.L. & Wojitowicz, J.M. (1999). Silent synapses in neural plasticity: current evidence. *Learn. Mem.*, **6**: 542–571.

Bailey, C.H. & Kandel, E.R. (1993). Structural changes accompanying memory storage. *Ann. Rev. Physiol.*, **55**: 397–426.

Bannerman, D.M., Good, M.A., Butcher, S.P., Ramsay, M. & Morris, R.G.M. (1995). Distinct components of spatial learning revealed by prior training and NMDA receptor blockade. *Nature*, **378**: 182–186.

Baranyi, A. & Feher, O. (1978). Conditioned changes of synaptic transmission in the motor cortex of the cat. *Exp. Brain Res.*, **33**: 283–289.

Baranyi, A. & Feher, O. (1981). Long-term facilitation of excitatory synaptic transmission in single motor cortical neurons of the cat produced by repetitive pairing of synaptic potentials and action potentials following intracellular stimulation. *Neurosci. Lett.*, **23**: 303–308.

Baranyi, A., Szente, M.B. & Woody, C.D. (1991). Properties of associative long lasting potentiation induced by cellular conditioning in the motor cortex of conscious cats. *Neuroscience*, **42**: 321–334.

Barnes, C.A., Jung, M.W., McNaughton, B.L., Korol, D.L., Andreasson, K. & Worley, P.F. (1994). LTP saturation and spatial learning disruption: effects of task variables and saturation levels. *J. Neurosci.*, **14**: 5793–5806.

Bliss, T.V.P. (1998). The saturation debate. *Science*, **281**: 1975–1976.

Bliss, T.V.P. & Lomo, T. (1973). Long-lasting potentiation of synaptic transmission in the dentate area of the anesthetized rabbit following stimulation of the perforant path. *J. Physiol.*, **232**: 331–356.

Black, J.E., Isaaks, K.R., Anderson, B.J., Alcantara, A.A. & Greenough, W.T. (1990). Learning causes synaptogenesis, whereas motor activity causes angiogenesis, in the cerebral cortex of adult rats. *PNAS*, **87**: 5568–5572.

Bourgeois, J-P., Goldman-Rakic, P. & Rakic, P. (1999). Formation, elimination, and stabilization of synapses in the primate cerebral cortex. In *Cognitive Neuroscience. A Handbook for the Field*, 2nd edn, ed. M.S. Gazzaniga, pp. 23–32. Cambridge, MA: MIT Press.

Brons, J. & Woody, C. (1980). Long-term changes in excitability of cortical neurons after Pavlovian conditioning and excitation. *J. Neurophysiol.*, **44**: 605–615.

Buetefisch, C.M., Davis, B.C., Wise, S.P. et al. (2000). Mechanisms of use dependent plasticity in the human motor cortex. *PNAS*, **97**: 3661–3665.

Buonomano, D.V. & Merzenich, M.M. (1998). Cortical plasticity: from synapses to maps. *Ann. Rev. Neurosci.*, **21**: 149–186.

Castro, C.A., Silbert, L.H., McNaughton, B.L. & Barnes, C.A. (1989). Recovery of spatial learning deficits after decay of electrically induced synaptic enhancement in the hippocampus. *Nature*, **342**: 545.

Cain, D.P., Hargreaves, E.L., Boon, F. & Dennison, Z. (1993). An examination of the relations between hioppocampal long-term potentiation, kindling, afterdischarge, and place learning in the water maze. *Hippocampus*, **3**: 153–163.

Castro-Alamancos, M.A., Donoghue, J.P. & Connors, B.W. (1995). Different forms of synaptic plasticity in the somatosensory and the motor areas of the neocortex. *J. Neurosci.*, **15**: 5324–5333

Chen, W., Hu, G.Y., Zhou, Y.D. & Wu, C.P. (1994). Two mechanisms underlying the induction of LTP in motor cortex of adult cat in vitro. *Exp. Brain Res.*, **100**: 149–154.

Chen, C. & Tonegawa, S. (1997). Molecular genetic analysis of synaptic plasticity, activity-dependent neural development, learning, and memory in the mammalian brain. *Annu. Rev. Neurosci.*, **20**: 157–184.

Classen, J., Lippert, J., Wise, S.P., Hallet, M. & Cohen, L.G. (1998). Rapid plasticity of human cortical movement representation induced by practice. *J. Neurophysiol.*, **79**: 1117–1123.

Clugnet, M-C. & LeDoux, J.E. (1990). Synaptic plasticity in fear conditioning circuits: induction of LTP in the lateral nucleus of the amygdala by stimulation of the medial geniculate body. *J. Neurosci.*, **10**: 2818–2824.

Collindridge, G.L., Kehl, S.J. & McLennan, H. (1983). Excitatory amino acids in synaptic transmission in the Schaffer collateral-commissural pathway of the rat hippocampus. *J. Physiol. (Lond.)*, **334**: 33–46.

Comery, T.A., Stamoudis, C.X., Irwin, S.A. & Greenough, W.T. (1996). Increased density of multiple-head dendritic spines on medium-sized spiny neurons of the striatum in rats reared in a complex environment. *Neurobiol. Learn. Mem.*, **66**: 93–96.

Day, M. & Morris, R.G.M. (2001). Memory consolidation and NMDA receptors: discrepancy between genetic and pharmacological approaches. *Science*, **293**: 755a.

Doetsch, F., Garcia-Verdugo, J.M. & Alvarez-Buylla, A. (1997). Cellular composition and three-dimensional organization of the subventricular germinal zone in the adult mammalian brain. *J. Neurosci.*, **17**: 5046–5061.

Donoghue, J.P. (1995). Plasticity of adult sensorimotor representations. *Curr. Opin. Neurobiol.*, **5**: 749–754.

Donoghue, J.P., Suner, S. & Sanes, J.N. (1990). Dynamic organization of primary motor cortex output to target muscles in adult rats. II. Rapid reorganization following motor nerve lesion. *Exp. Brain Res.*, **79**: 492–503.

Donoghue, J.P., Hess, G. & Sanes, J.N. (1996). Substrates and mechanisms for learning in motor cortex. In *Acquisition of Motor Behavior*, ed. J. Bloedel, T. Ebner & S.P. Wise. Cambridge, MA: MIT Press.

Dudek, S.M. & Bear, M.F. (1992). Homosynaptic long-term depression and effects of *N*-methyl-D-aspartate receptor blockade. *Proc. Natl Acad. Sci., USA*, **89**: 4363–4367.

Durand, G.M., Kovalchuk, Y. & Konnerth, A. (1996). LTP and functional synapse induction in developing hippocampus. *Nature*, **381**: 71–75.

Elgersma, Y. & Silva, A.J. (1999). Molecular mechanisms of synaptic plasticity and memory. *Curr. Opin. Neurobiol.*, **9**: 209–213.

Engert, F. & Bonhoeffer, T. (1999). Dendritic spine changes associated with hippocampal longterm synaptic plasticity. *Nature*, **399**: 66–70.

Eriksson, P.S., Perfilieva, E., Bjork-Eriksson, T., Nordborg, C., Peterson, D.A. & Gage, F.H. (1998). Neurogenesis in the adult human hippocampus. *Nat. Medicine*, **4**: 1207.

Gandolfo, F., Li, C-S.R., Benda, B.J., Padoa Scioppa, C. & Bizzi, E. (2000). Cortical correlates of learning in monkeys adapting to a new dynamical environment. *PNAS*, **97**: 2259–2263.

Geinisman, Y. (2000). Structural synaptic modifications associated with hippocampal LTP and behavioral learning. *Cereb. Cortex*, **10**: 952–962.

Gilbert C.D., Das, A., Ito, M., Kapadia, M. & Westheimer, G. (1996). Spatial integration and cortical dynamics. *PNAS*, **93**: 615–622.

Goda, Y. & Stevens, C.F. (1996). Synaptic plasticity: the basis of particular type of learning. *Curr. Biol.* **6**: 375–378.

Gomperts, S.N., Rao, A., Craig, A.M., Malenka, R.C. & Nicoll, R.A. (1998). Postsynaptically silent synapses in single neuron cultures. *Neuron*, **21**: 1443–1451.

Gould, E., McEven, B.S., Tanapat, P., Galea, L.A. & Fuchs, E. (1997). Neurogenesis in the dentate gyrus of the adult tree shrew is regulated by psychosocial stress and NMDA receptor activation. *J. Neurosci.*, **17**: 2492–2498.

Gould, E., Tanapat, P., Hastings, N.B. & Shors, T.J. (1999a). Neurogenesis in the adulthood: a possible role in learning. *Trends Cogn. Sci.*, **3**: 186–192.

Gould, E., Reeves, A.J., Fallah, M., Tanapat, P., Gross, C.G. & Fuchs, E. (1999b). Hippocampal neurogenesis in adult Old World primates. *PNAS*, **96**: 5263–5267.

Gould, E., Beylin, A., Tanapat, P., Reeves, A. & Shors, T.J. (1999c). Learning enhances adult neurogenesis in the hippocampal formation. *Nat. Neurosci.*, **2**: 203–205.

Gould, E., Reeves, A.J., Graziani, M.S.A. & Gross, C.G. (1999d). Neurogenesis in the neocortex of adult primates. *Science*, **286**: 548–552.

Grafton, S.T., Mazziotta, J.P., Presty, S., Friston, K.J., Frackowiak, R.S.J. & Phelps, M.E. (1992). Functional anatomy of human procedural learning determined with regional cerebral blood flow and PET. *J. Neurosci.*, **12**: 2542–2548.

Grant, S.G., O'Dell, T.J., Karl, K.A., Stein, P.L., Soriano, P. & Kandel, E.R. (1992). Impaired longterm potentiation, spatial learning, and hippocampal development in fyn mutant mice. *Science*, **258**: 1903–1910.

Hallett, M. (2001). Plasticity in the human motor cortex and recovery from stroke. *Brain Res. Rev.*, **36**: 169–174.

He, Y., Janssen, W.G.M. & Morrison, J.H. (1998). Synaptic coexistence of AMPA and NMDA receptors in the rat hippocampus: a postembedding immunogold study. *J. Neurosci. Res.*, **54**: 444–449.

Hebb, D.O. (1949). *Organization of Behavior.* New York: Wiley.

Hess, G. & Donoghue, J.P. (1994). Long-term potentiation of horizontal connections provides a mechanism to reorganize cortical motor maps. *J. Neurophysiol.*, **71**: 2543–2547.

Hess, G. & Donoghue, J.P. (1996). Long-term depression of horizontal connections in rat motor cortex. *Eur. J. Neurosci.*, **8**: 658–665.

Hess, G., Aizenman, C.D. & Donoghue, J.P. (1996). Conditions for the induction of long-term potentiation in layer II/III horizontal connections of the rat motor cortex. *J. Neurophysiol.*, **75**: 1765–1778.

Huntley, G.W. (1997). Correlations between patterns of horizontal connectivity and the extent of short-term representational plasticity in rat motor cortex. *Cereb. Cortex*, **7**: 143–156.

Iriki, A., Pavlides, C., Keller, A. & Asanuma, H. (1989). Long-term potentiation in the motor cortex. *Science*, **245**: 1385–1387.

Isaac, J.T., Nicoll, R.A. & Malenka, R.C. (1995). Evidence for silent synapses: implications for the expression of LTP. *Neuron*, **15**: 427–434.

Isaac, J.T., Crair, M.C., Nicoll, R.A. & Malenka, R.C. (1997). Silent synapses during development of thalamocortical inputs. *Neuron*, **18**: 269–280.

Jacobs, K.M. & Donoghue, J.P. (1991). Reshaping the cortical motor map by unmasking latent intracortical connection. *Science*, **251**: 944–947.

Jeffrey, K.J. & Morris, R.G.M. (1993). Cumulative LTP in the rat dentate gyrus correlates with, but does not modify, performance in the water maze. *Hippocampus*, **3**: 133–140.

Jones, T.A., Klintsova, A.Y., Kilman, V.L., Sirevaag, A.M. & Greenough, W.T. (1997). Induction of multiple synapses by experience in the visual cortex of adult rats. *Neurobiol. Learn. Mem.*, **68**: 13–20.

Kaas, J.H. (1991). Plasticity of sensory and motor maps in adult mammals. *Annu. Rev. Neurosci.*, **14**: 137–167.

Karni, A., Meyer, G., Jezzard, P., Adams, M.M., Turner, R. & Ungerleider, L.G. (1995). Functional MRI evidence for adult motor cortex plasticity during motor skill learning. *Nature*, **377**: 155–158.

Keller, A. (1993). Intrinsic synaptic organization of the motor cortex. *Cereb. Cortex*, **3**: 430–441.

Keller, A., Weintraub, N.D. & Miyashita, E. (1996). Tactile experience determines the organization of movement representations in rat motor cortex. *Neuroreport*, **7**: 2373–2378.

Kentros, C., Hargreaves, E., Hawkins, R.D., Kandel, E.R., Shapiro, M. & Muller, R.V. (1998). Abolition of long-term stability of new hippocampal place cell maps by NMDA receptor blockade. *Science*, **280**: 2121–2126.

Kirkwood, A. & Bear M.F. (1994). Homosynaptic long-term depression in the visual cortex. *J. Neurosci.*, **14**: 3404–3412.

Kirkwood, A., Rioult, M.G. & Bear, M.F. (1996). Experience-dependent modification of synaptic plasticity in visual cortex. *Nature*, **381**: 526–528.

Kleim, J.A., Lussing, E., Schwarz, E.R., Comery, T.A., & Greenough, W.T. (1996). Synaptogenesis and fos expression in the motor cortex of adult rat after motor skill learning. *J. Neurosci.*, **16**: 4529–4535.

Kleim, J.A., Vij, K., Ballard, D.H. & Greenough, W.T. (1997). Learning dependent synaptic modifications in the cerebellar cortex of the adult rat persist at least four weeks. *J. Neurosci.*, **17**: 717–721.

Kleim, J.A., Barbay, S. & Nudo, R.J. (1998a). Functional reorganization of the rat motor cortex following motor skill learning. *J. Neurophysiol.*, **80**: 3321–3325.

Kleim, J.A., Swain, R.A., Armstrong, K.E., Napper, R.M.A., Jones, T.A. & Greenough, W.T. (1998b). Selective synaptic plasticity within the cerebellar cortex following complex motor skill learning. *Neurobiol. Learn. Mem.*, **69**: 274–289.

Klintsova, A.Y. & Greenough, W.T. (1999). Synaptic plasticity in cortical systems. *Curr. Opin. Neurobiol.*, **9**: 203–208.

Kornack, D.R. & Racik, P. (1999). Continuation of neurogenesis in the hippocampus of the adult macaque monkey. *PNAS*, **96**: 5768–5773.

Korol, D.L., Abel, T.W., Church, L.T., Barnes, C.A. & McNaughton, B.L. (1993). Hippocampal synaptic enhancement and spatial learning in the Morris swim task. *Hippocampus*, **3**: 127–132.

Levy, W.B. & Steward, O. (1979). Synapses as associative memory elements in the hippocampal formation. *Brain Res.*, **175**: 233–245.

Li, H., Weiss, S.R.B., Chuang, D-M., Post, R.M. & Rogawski, M.A. (1998). Bidirectional synaptic plasticity in the rat basolateral amygdala: characterization of an activity–dependent switch sensitive to the presynaptic metabotropic glutamate receptor antagonist 2S-alpha-ethylglutamic acid. *J. Neurosci.*, **18**: 1662–1670.

Liao, D.N., Hessler, A. & Malinow, R. (1995). Activation of postsynaptically silent synapses during pairing-induced LTP in CA1 region of hippocampal slice. *Nature*, **375**: 400–404.

Liao, D., Zhang, X., O'Brien, R., Ehlers, M.D. & Huganir, R.L. (1999). Regulation of morphological postsynaptic silent synapses in developing hippocampal neurons. *Nat. Neurosci.*, **2**: 37–43.

Lynch, G.S., Dundwiddie, T. & Gribkoff, V. (1977). Heterosynaptic depression: a postsynaptic correlate of long-term potentiation. *Nature*, **266**: 737–739.

McBain, C. & Mayer, M. (1994). NMDA receptor structure and function. *Physiol. Rev.*, **74**: 723–760.

McGaugh, J.L. & Izquierdo, I. (2000). The contribution of pharmacology to research on the mechanisms of memory formation. *TIPS*, **21**: 208–210.

McKernan, M.G. & Shinnick-Gallagher, P. (1997). Fear conditioning induces a lasting potentiation of synaptic currents in vitro. *Nature*, **390**: 607–611.

McNaughton, B.L., Barnes, C.A., Rao, G., Baldwin, J. & Rasmussen, M. (1986). Long-term enhancement of hippocampal synaptic transmission and the acquisition of spatial information. *J. Neurosci.*, **6**: 563–571.

Malenka, R. (1998). Silent synapses in the hippocampus and cortex. In *Central Synapses: Quantal Mechanisms and Plasticity.*, ed. D.S. Faber, H. Korn, S.J. Redman, S.M. Thompson & J.S. Altman, pp. 207–214. Strasbourg, France: Human Frontier Science Program.

Malenka, R.C. & Nicoll, R.A. (1997). Silent synapses speak up. *Neuron*, **19**: 552–553.

Malenka, R.C. & Nicoll, R.A. (1999). Long-term potentiation – a decade of progress. *Science*, **285**: 1870–1874.

Maletic-Savatic, M. & Svoboda, K.S. (1999). Rapid dendritic morphogenesis in CA1 hippocampal dendrites induced by synaptic activity. *Science*, **283**: 1923–1927.

Malinow, R. (1998). Silent synapses in three forms of central plasticity. In *Central Synapses: Quantal Mechanisms and Plasticity*, ed. D.S. Faber, H. Korn, S.J. Redman, S.M. Thompson & J.S. Altman: pp. 226–234. Strasbourg, France: Human Frontier Science Program.

Margolis, D.J., Donoghue, J.P., Rioult, M.G. & Rioult-Pedotti, M.-S. (1999). Role of NMDA receptors in skill learning and learning-induced synaptic strengthening. *Soc. Neurosci. Abstr.*, **25**: 888.

Martin, S.J. & Morris, R.G.M. (2001). Cortical plasticity: it's all the range! *Curr. Biol.*, **11**: R57–R59.

Martin, S.J., Grimwood, P.D. & Morris, R.G.M. (2000). Synaptic plasticity and memory: an evaluation of the hypothesis. *Annu. Rev. Neurosci.*, **23**: 649–711.

Marren, S. (1999). Long-term potentiation in the amygdala: a mechanism for emotional learning and memory. *TINS*, **22**: 561–567.

Mayer, M.L., Westbrook, G.L. & Guthrie, P.B. (1984). Voltage-dependent block by Mg^{2+} of NMDA responses in spinal cord neurons. *Nature*, **309**: 261–263.

Mayford, M., Mansuy I.M., Muller, R.U. & Kandel, E.R. (1997). Memory and behavior: a second generation of genetically modified mice. *Curr. Biol.*, **7**: R580–R589.

Merzenich, M.M. & Shameshima, K. (1993). Cortical plasticity and memory. *Curr. Opin. Neurobiol.*, **2**: 187–196.

Miller, S. & Mayford, M. (1999). Cellular and molecular mechanisms of memory: the LTP connections. *Curr. Opin. Genet. Developm.*, **9**: 333–337.

Miller, E.K., Erikson, C.A. & Desimone, R. (1996). Neural mechanisms of visual working memory in prefrontal cortex of the macaque. *J. Neurosci.*, **16**: 5154–5167.

Morris, R.G.M. (1986). Selective impairment of learning and blockade of long-term potentiation by an NMDA receptor antagonist, AP5. *Nature*, **319**: 774–776.

Morris, R.G.M. (1989). Synaptic plasticity and learning: selective impairment of learning rats and blockade of long-term potentiation in vivo by the NMDA receptor antagonist AP5. *J. Neurosci.*, **9**: 3040–3057.

Moser, E., Moser, M.B. & Andersen, P. (1993). Synaptic potentiation in the rat dentate gyrus during exploratory learning. *Neuroreport*, **5**: 317–320.

Moser, M.B., Trommald, M., Egeland, T. & Andersen, P. (1997). Spatial training in a complex environment and isolation alter the spine distribution differently in rat CA1 pyramidal cells. *J. Comp. Neurol.*, **380**: 373–381.

Moser, E.L., Krobert, K.A., Moser, M.B. & Morris, R.G.M. (1998). Impaired spatial learning after saturation of LTP. *Science*, **281**: 2038–2042.

Moyer, J.R., Thompson, L.T. & Disterhoft, J.F. (1996). Trace eyeblink conditioning increase CA1 excitability in a transient and learning-specific manner. *J Neurosci.*, **16**: 5536–5546.

Muellbacher, W., Ziemann, U., Boroojerdi, B., Cohen, L. & Hallett, M. (2001). Role of the human motor cortex in rapid motor learning. *Exp. Brain Res.*, **136**: 431–438.

Muellbacher, W., Ziemann, U., Wissel, J. et al. (2002). Early consolidation in human primary motor cortex. *Nature*, **415**: 640–644.

Nowak, L., Bregestovski, P., Ascher, P., Herbert, A. & Prochiantz, A. (1984). Magnesium gates glutamate-activated channels in mouse central neurons. *Nature*, **307**: 462–465.

Nudo, R.J., Milliken, G.W., Jenkins, W.M. & Merzenich, M.M. (1996). Use-dependent alterations of movement representations in primary motor cortex of adult squirrel monkeys. *J. Neurosci.*, **16**: 785–807.

Nusser, Z.R., Laube, G., Roberts, J.B.D., Molnr, E. & Somogy, P. (1998). Cell type and pathway dependence of synaptic AMPA receptor number and variability in the hippocampus. *Neuron*, **21**: 545–559.

Pascual-Leone, A., Grafman, J. & Hallet, M. (1994). Modulation of cortical motor output maps during development of implicit and explicit knowledge. *Science*, **263**: 1287–1289.

Plautz, E.J., Milliken, G.W. & Nudo, R.J. (2000). Effects of repetitive motor skill training on movement representations in adult squirrel monkeys: role of use versus learning. *Neurobiol. Learn. Mem.*, **74**: 27–55.

Petralia, R.S., Esteban, J.A., Wang, Y-X. et al. (1999). Selective acquisition of AMPA receptors over postnatal development suggests a molecular basis for silent synapse. *Nat. Neurosci.*, **2**: 31–36.

Power, J.M., Thompson, L.T., Moyer, J.R. & Disterhoft, J.F. (1997). Enhanced synaptic transmission in CA1 hippocampus after eyeblink conditioning. *J. Neurophysiol.*, **78**: 1185–1187.

Rioult-Pedotti, M-S., Friedman, D., Hess, G. & Donoghue, J.P. (1998). Strengthening of horizontal cortical connections following skill learning. *Nat. Neurosci.*, **1**: 230–234.

Rioult-Pedotti, M-S., Friedman, D. & Donoghue, J.P. (2000). Learning-induced LTP in neocortex. *Science*, **290**: 533–536.

Rioult-Pedotti, M-S. & Donoghue, J.P. (2003). Plasticity of the synaptic modification range with extended motor skill training. Submitted.

Rioult-Pedotti, M.S. & Donoghue, J.P. (2002). Learning, retention and persistent strengthening of cortical synapses. *Soc. Neurosci. Abstr.*

Rogan, M.T., Staeubli, U.V. & LeDoux, J.E. (1997). Fear conditioning induces associative long-term potentiation in the amygdala. *Nature*, **390**: 604–607.

Roman, F.S., Truchet, B., Marchetti, E., Chaillan, F.A. & Soumireu-Mourat, B. (1999). Correlations between electrophysiological observations of synaptic plasticity modifications and behavioral performance in mammals. *Prog. Neurobiol.*, **58**: 61–87.

Rousselot, P., Lois, C. & Alvarez-Buylla, A. (1995). Embryonic (PSA) N-CAM reveals chain of migrating neuroblasts between the lateral ventricle and the olfactory bulb of adult mice. *J. Comp. Neurol.*, **351**: 51–61.

Rumpel, S., Hatt, H. & Gottmann, K. (1998). Silent synapses in the developing rat visual cortex: evidence for postsynaptic expression of synaptic plasticity. *J. Neurosci.*, **18**: 8863–8874.

Saar, D., Grossman, Y. & Barkai, E. (1999). Reduced synaptic facilitation between pyramidal neurons in the piriform cortex after odor learning. *J. Neurosci.*, **19**: 8616–8622.

Sakimura, K., Kutsuwada, T., Ito, I. et al. (1995). Reduced hippocampal LTP and spatial learning in mice lacking NMDA receptor epsilon 1 subunit. *Nature*, **373**: 151–155.

Sanes, J.N. & Donoghue, J.P. (1997). Static and dynamic organization of motor cortex. *Adv. Neurol.*, **73**: 277–296.

Sanes, J.N. & Donoghue, J.P. (2000). Plasticity and primary motor cortex. *Ann. Rev. Neurosci.*, **23**: 393–415.

Sanes, J.N., Suner, S., Lando, J.F. & Donoghue, J.P. (1988). Rapid reorganization of adult rat motor cortex somatic representation patterns after motor nerve injury. *PNAS*, **85**: 2003–2007.

Sanes, J.N., Suner, S. & Donoghue, J.P. (1990). Dynamic organization of primary motor cortex output to target muscles in adult rats. I. Long-term patterns of reorganization following motor or mixed peripheral nerve lesions. *Exp. Brain Res.*, **79**: 479–491.

Sanes, J.N., Wang, J. & Donoghue, J.P. (1992). Immediate and delayed changes of rat motor cortical output representation with new forelimb configurations. *Cereb. Cortex*, **2**: 141–152.

Saucier, D. & Cain, D.P. (1995). Spatial learning without NMDA receptor-dependent long-term potentiation. *Nature*, **378**: 186–189.

Shimizu, E., Tang, Y-P., Rampon, C. & Tsien, J.Z. (2000). NMDA receptor-dependent synaptic reinforcement as a crucial process for memory consolidation. *Science*, **290**: 1170–1174.

Shors T.J. & Matzel, L.D. (1997). Long-term potentiation: what's learning got to do with it? *Behav. Brain Sci.*, **20**: 597–655.

Silva, A., Stevens, C.F., Tonegawa, S. & Wang, Y. (1992). Deficient hippocampal long-term potentiation in alpha-calcium-calmodulin kinase II mutant mice. *Science*, **257**: 201–206.

Sorra, K.E. & Harris, K.M. (1998). Stability in synapse number and size at 2 hr after long-term potentiation in hippocampal area CA1. *J. Neurosci.*, **18**: 658–671.

Stevens, C.F. (1998). A million dollar question: does LTP = memory? *Neuron*, **20**: 1–2.

Sutherland, R.J., Dringenberg, H.C. & Hoesing, J.M. (1993). Induction of long-term potentiation at perforant path dentate synapses does not affect place learning or memory. *Hippocampus*, **3**: 141–147.

Tang, Y-P., Shimizu, E., Dube, G.R. et al. (1999). Genetic enhancement of learning and memory in mice. *Nature*, **401**: 63–69.

Teskey, G.C., Monfils, M-H., VandenBerg, P.M. & Kleim, J.A. (2002). Motor map expansion following repeated cortical and limbic seizures is related to synaptic potentiation. *Cereb. Cortex*, **12**: 98–105.

Thiels, E., Barrionuevo, G. & Berger, T.W. (1994). Excitatory stimulation during postsynaptic inhibition induces long-term depression in hippocampus in vivo. *J. Neurophysiol.*, **72**: 3009–3016.

Thompson, L.T., Moyer, J.R. & Disterhoft, J.F. (1996). Transient changes in excitability of rabbit CA3 neurons with a time course appropriate to support memory consolidation. *J. Neurophysiol.*, **76**: 1836–1849.

Toni, N., Buchs, P-A., Nikonenko, I., Bron, C.R. & Mueller, D. (1999). LTP promotes formation of multiple spine synapses between a single axon terminal and a dendrite. *Nature*, **402**: 421–425.

Trepel, C. & Racine, R.I., (1998). LTP in the neocortex of the adult, freely moving rat. *Cereb. Cortex*, **8**: 719–729.

Tsien, J.Z., Huerta, P.T. & Tonegawa, S. (1996). The essential role of hippocampal CA1 NMDA receptor-dependent synaptic plasticity in spatial memory. *Cell*, **87**: 1327–1338.

Turner, A.M. & Greenough, W.T. (1985). Differential rearing effects on rat visual cortex synapses, I. Synaptic and neuronal density and synapses per neuron. *Brain Res.*, **329**: 195–203.

Villareal, D.M., Do, V., Haddad, E. & Derrick, B.E. (2002). NMDA receptor antagonists sustain LTP and spatial memory: active processes mediate LTP decay. *Nat. Neurosci.*, **5**: 48–52.

Woody, C.D. (1986). Understanding the cellular basis of memory and learning. *Annu. Rev. Psychol.*, **37**: 433–493.

Wu, G-Y., Malinow, R. & Cline, H.T., (1996). Maturation of a central glutamatergic synapse. *Science*, **274**: 972–976.

2

Techniques of transcranial magnetic stimulation

John C. Rothwell

Sobell Department, Institute of Neurology, London, UK

In this chapter I discuss the physiology of TMS and describe some of the common techniques that have been applied by those using TMS. I will not describe the details of each method, but outline the general principles and limitations. Most of the work on the basic mechanisms of these techniques has been performed on the motor cortex, where the response to each stimulus is easy to quantify as the amplitude of an MEP response. However, it is thought that the same general principles will apply to stimulation of other areas of cortex, although this may be difficult to prove in practice.

Single pulse transcranial stimulation

Although the majority of studies use TMS to activate the brain, the older method of transcranial electrical stimulation (TES) is still used occasionally. As described below, comparison of the effects of TMS and TES can help distinguish whether an intervention changes cortical excitability at the site of stimulation or at a distant projection target (such as the spinal cord).

Transcranial electrical stimulation of the corticospinal output of the hand area of motor cortex

The corticospinal system forms the largest output of the motor cortex. Experiments in primates have shown that single pulse electrical stimulation of the surface of the exposed cortex activates this output both directly, through depolarization of corticospinal axons in the immediately subcortical white matter, and indirectly via excitatory synaptic input from other cortical neurones (Patton & Amassian, 1954). The latter can evoke repetitive discharge of pyramidal neurones, leading to a sequence of descending volleys in the corticospinal tract at intervals of approximately 1.5 ms. The corticospinal volleys are labelled D (direct axonal stimulation) and I (indirect, or synaptic activation) waves, numbered in order of their appearance.

The polarity of stimulation is important: anodal stimulation tends to activate D waves preferentially, whereas cathodal stimulation recruits I waves more readily. It is thought that a surface anode produces inward current in the dendrites and cell body of vertically oriented pyramidal neurones which exits at the proximal nodes of the corticospinal axon. This current depolarizes the axon, and a D wave volley is initiated. Cathodal stimulation will tend to have the opposite effect, and may depolarize afferents to the pyramidal neurones before discharging pyramidal axons.

The phenomenology of I waves is not well understood. We do not know whether particular classes of excitatory input are necessary to evoke them, nor do we know why they occur with such a rapid periodicity. Amassian and colleagues (Amassian et al., 1987) showed that I waves could be elicited in cats after a large lesion had been made in the ventrolateral thalamus, indicating that thalamocortical inputs were not necessary for I wave generation. They favoured the idea that cortico-cortical inputs from other areas were likely to be responsible. The question of why I waves are periodic has never been addressed in detail. Repetitive firing could be produced by (a) reverberating activity in a neural circuit involving pyramidal neurones, (b) separate chains of synaptic inputs for each I wave, or (c) membrane properties of pyramidal neurones that makes them fire repetitively if they receive a large synchronous synaptic depolarization. In all cases, a mechanism would also need to exist to ensure that the activation was synchronized through the population of pyramidal neurones.

Transcranial electrical stimulation in humans appears to have similar effects to those described in animals. Both EMG studies (Day et al., 1989a) and recordings of descending spinal cord volleys (Di Lazzaro et al., 1998) indicate that anodal stimulation preferentially recruits D waves (see Fig. 2.1). Cathodal stimulation also evokes D waves, but is more likely also to recruit I waves. As the intensity of stimulation is increased, both forms of stimulation evoke I waves. The I3 is usually recruited first, with I1, I2 and later waves at slightly higher intensities. The amplitude of D waves is unaffected by levels of cortical excitability (Di Lazzaro et al., 1999b), supporting the idea that they are initiated at some distance from the cell body of the pyramidal neurone, perhaps several nodes distal to the initial segment.

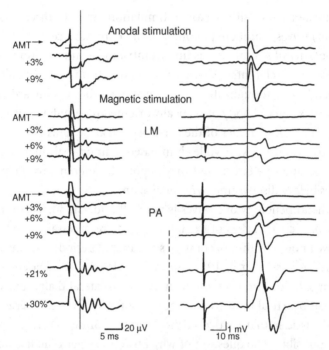

Fig. 2.1   Descending corticospinal volleys (left column) and EMG responses in the first dorsal
interosseous muscle (right column) recorded simultaneously in a conscious subject
with an electrode implanted into the cervical epidural space for control of chronic
pain. The motor cortex was stimulated with anodal TES (top three rows), or TMS
oriented to induce a latero-medial (LM) or posterior–anterior (PA) current in the
brain. The intensity of stimulation was at active motor threshold (AMT) or at different percentages of the maximal stimulator output above threshold. The vertical
lines indicate the peak of the D wave from anodal stimulation, and the onset of the
anodal EMG response. Note that TMS with the LM orientation evokes an I1 wave at
threshold, and that an earlier D wave occurs at AMT + 9%. For TMS with a PA orientation, the D wave is not seen until the intensity of stimulation is AMT + 21%. When
D waves occur, the onset latency of the TMS evoked EMG responses decreases to
equal that seen after anodal TES. (Modified from Di Lazzaro et al., 1998.)

It should be noted that very high intensities of electrical stimulation can
activate corticospinal fibres at deeper levels in the white matter. Recordings
of descending volleys in anaesthetized patients undergoing spinal surgery
show that the latency of the D wave can jump earlier in two discrete steps of
about 0.8 ms each (Burke et al., 1990). It is thought that this corresponds to
spread of the stimulus from the subcortical white matter first to the cerebral

peduncle, and second to the pyramidal decussation. Because the course of the axons changes direction at these points, they may have a particularly low threshold to stimulation (Maccabee et al., 1993).

Stimulation of descending pathways at the level of the brainstem

Transcranial stimulation of the corticospinal pathways is complicated by the fact that, except for near threshold anodal stimulation, a single stimulus pulse usually evokes several descending volleys set up by synaptic activity in the cortex. To avoid this problem, Ugawa and colleagues (Ugawa et al., 1991b) showed that it was possible to stimulate corticospinal fibres directly at the level of the brainstem using a high voltage transmastoidal stimulus. The site of activation may be the pyramidal decussation. It should be noted that, although they used collision techniques to prove that the method activated at least some of the same axons as stimulated by transcranial methods, they could not discount activation of other, perhaps non-corticospinal, pathways as well.

It is also possible to activate these pathways using TMS applied through a large figure-of-eight coil (Ugawa et al., 1994, 1996, 1997). Stimulation occurs best with the coil over the inion, 1–2 cm ipsilateral to the target muscles and with the induced current flowing downwards in the brain. The site of activation is presumably just below the pyramidal decussation (where the pyramidal tract has crossed over from the contralateral side), at the level of the foramen magnum.

Transcranial magnetic stimulation of the corticospinal output of the hand area of motor cortex

The neurones activated depend on the size, shape, orientation, stimulus intensity and stimulus waveform that are produced by the magnetic stimulator.

A monophasic pulse in a figure-of-eight coil

The lowest threshold for activation occurs if monophasic pulses induce current flow from posterior to anterior (AP) in the brain approximately perpendicular to the central sulcus (Mills et al., 1992). Direct recordings of the descending volleys evoked by such stimuli (Di Lazzaro et al., 1998), as well as indirect evidence from the firing pattern of single motor units (Day et al., 1989a), show that such stimulation preferentially evokes an I1 wave (see Fig. 2.1). As the stimulus intensity is increased, this wave increases in size and is followed by later I waves. A D wave appears at the highest intensities. When the D wave is recruited, the latency of the MEP in actively contracting muscles shortens by 1–1.5 ms.

This pattern of recruitment suggests that AP stimulation preferentially activates synaptic inputs to pyramidal neurones. Experiments with a special stimulator that could vary the duration of the stimulus pulse (Barker et al., 1991) showed that the time constant of the structure activated by such stimulation was approximately the same as a large myelinated axon. The implication is that TMS with a monophasic AP current stimulates axons of excitatory inputs to pyramidal neurones.

It is not certain why I waves should be recruited at a lower threshold than D waves. However, it seems likely that the relative threshold of the structures activated depends on their orientation with respect to the current induced by TMS in the brain. For example, if the cortex were unfolded, then pyramidal neurones would all be oriented perpendicular to the skull, whilst many cortico-cortical and local horizontal interneurones would be parallel to the surface. Since the currents induced by TMS flow parallel to the surface of the skull (Tofts, 1990), they would preferentially activate the latter and not the former, resulting in synaptic activation of the corticospinal system rather than direct activation. This argument may hold for the portion of the motor cortex that is exposed on the surface of the precentral gyrus, and it may be this area that is activated at lowest threshold. However, stimulation of the neurones in the anterior bank of the central sulcus would presumably follow a different pattern. These neurones are further from the stimulating coil, and therefore have a higher threshold for activation. At these intensities, perhaps D waves are recruited in preference to I waves.

The tendency of TMS to activate corticospinal output via synaptic mechanisms means that the response to TMS is affected by the level of cortical excitability at the time the stimulus is given. For example, recordings of descending spinal cord volleys in conscious human subjects show that the amplitude and number of I wave volleys is larger when stimuli are given during a voluntary muscle contraction as compared to rest. However, contraction has no effect on the amplitude or threshold of the D wave (Di Lazzaro et al., 1998b). The outcome is that I wave activity can be used as a sensitive indicator of cortical excitability, a fact that is used extensively in the paired pulse studies summarised below. The lack of effect on the D wave component of the volley indicates that it is initiated at some distance from the cell body, probably some nodes distant from the initial segment of the cell. Comparisons of the D wave elicited by latero-medial TMS and transcranial electric stimulation of the hand motor area suggest strongly that both excite the same nodes, perhaps at the point where the axons bend into the white matter before entering the internal capsule (Rothwell et al., 1992).

Changing the orientation of the induced TMS current alters the order in which descending volleys are recruited. A latero-medial (LM) orientation can, in many subjects, preferentially recruit D waves, whereas an anterior–posterior current usually recruits I3 waves before I1 or D waves (Sakai et al., 1997; Di Lazzaro et al., 1998a, 2001b). The latter finding is particularly interesting since it shows that different I waves can be produced by stimulating different populations of inputs to pyramidal neurones (see Fig 2.1).

Circular vs. figure-of-eight coils and monophasic vs. biphasic stimulators

The first magnetic stimulators were supplied with circular coils of about 10 cm diameter. Centred over the vertex of the scalp, the lateral windings lie over the hand area of each hemisphere. An anticlockwise current in the coil as viewed from above induces a PA current across the left motor area and an AP current over the right motor area. Consistent with the pattern of activation with figure-of-eight coils, this preferentially recruits an I1 wave from the left and an I3 from the right hemisphere (Day et al., 1989a). At higher intensities a D wave is recruited. However, this D wave has a slightly longer (0.2 ms) latency than that evoked by a figure-of-eight coil, and its amplitude is affected by the level of cortical excitation at the time the stimulus is given (Di Lazzaro et al., 2002). These differences are thought to indicate that activation is occurring nearer the cell body than with a figure-of-eight coil, at a point where the excitability would be influenced by the membrane potential in the neurone.

Biphasic stimulus pulses are more efficient in stimulating the brain than monophasic pulses even when the initial phase of the stimulus is the same size (Maccabee et al., 1998; Kammer et al., 2001). The reason is that charge transfer is maximal in the swing between the first and second phases of the biphasic pulse. One consequence of this is that the lowest threshold for activating the hand area with a biphasic stimulator occurs when the first phase of the stimulus is in the anterior–posterior direction rather than the posterior–anterior direction. With many commercial stimulators, this means that for optimal stimulation, a biphasic pulse requires a figure-of-eight coil to be held 180 degrees rotated to that when a monophasic pulse is given.

Stimulation of the corticospinal output from the leg area of motor cortex

The data obtained in experiments on the hand area suggest that the effect of TMS is determined by the relative orientation of neurones with respect to the direction of the induced electric field. The leg area provides a test of this hypothesis since the neurones there, buried in the interhemispheric fissure, have a different orientation to the surface of the skull than those in the hand area.

Recordings of MEPs in leg muscles (Priori et al., 1993; Nielsen et al., 1995) and descending volleys in the spinal epidural space (Di Lazzaro et al., 2001a) indicate that, as for the hand area, TMS can evoke a series of volleys at intervals of 1.5 ms. However, there has been some debate over which of these are D waves and which are I waves. The problem is that EMG responses evoked in contracting leg muscle by anodal electrical stimulation can have one of two different latencies. If the anode is at the vertex, the latency can be 1–2 ms later than if the anode is moved 2 cm lateral (Nielsen et al., 1995) (but see conflicting data from Ugawa and colleagues (Terao et al., 1994)). The question is whether the lateral anode is stimulating deep in the white matter and the vertex anode is stimulating the subcortical white matter (a 'true' D wave), or whether the lateral anode is evoking the classic D wave and the vertex anode is recruiting an I wave. Both scenarios would mean a difference in latency of EMG responses of about 1–2 ms. Recent recordings of descending spinal cord volleys (Houlden et al., 1999; Di Lazzaro et al., 2001a) suggest that the latter possibility is more likely. Although not conclusively proven, it seems that lateral anodal stimulation evokes a conventional D wave, and vertex anodal evokes an I1 wave. If this is correct, it illustrates the importance of the orientation of the corticospinal axons with respect to the applied stimulus.

Magnetic stimulation often recruits volleys and EMG responses with the same latency as vertex anodal stimulation. Presumably, as in the hand area, it preferentially activates synaptic inputs to pyramidal neurones.

Mapping the somatotopic organization of the motor cortex

Single cell studies show that the organization of the primate motor cortex is much less discrete than that observed in the primary sensory areas. Individual corticospinal neurones project to several muscles, and the projections to any one muscle may be spread through a wide area of cortex and intermixed with projections to neighbouring muscles (Porter & Lemon, 1993). The result is a mosaic in which a general pattern of hand, arm and shoulder projections can be distinguished, but where true boundaries are imprecise.

Single pulse TMS cannot provide this level of detail, but it is easy to confirm that it can give at least a gross idea of the somatotopy of the human motor cortex and distinguish between the position of the best points to hold the coil in order to activate muscles in shoulder, arm or hand as well as between face, arm and leg (Wassermann et al., 1992). This process of finding the best points to activate various muscles can be standardized by marking a grid of points on the scalp and then plotting the amplitude of EMG responses in various muscles obtained at each point (Wassermann et al., 1993, 1996) (see Fig. 2.2). Such maps provide three pieces of information: the optimal position to obtain the largest responses, the 'centre of gravity' of the area, and the area of the scalp from which responses can be obtained. The optimal position presumably corresponds to the location of the most excitable population of neurones that project to the target. The centre of gravity is effectively the centre of the representation. This often is the same as, or very close to, the best point. The area of the representation is more complex and depends on two factors, (a) the true area on the cortex where neurones are located that project to the target muscle, and (b) the stimulus intensity used to produce the map. If the stimulus intensity is too low, the total extent of map may be underestimated because less excitable elements will not be recruited. If the stimulus intensity is too high, the area will be overestimated because the stimulus current will spread beyond the point of stimulation (Thickbroom et al., 1998). It is simply not possible to reconcile these two opposing factors with TMS, and the area of the map that is recorded is virtually meaningless.

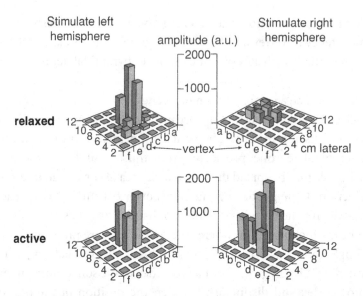

Fig. 2.2   Maps of the representation of the contralateral biceps muscle after TMS of the left
(left column) or right (right column) hemisphere of a subject who had had his right
forearm amputated several years previously. The maps were made either when the
subject was completely relaxed (top row), or when contracting the biceps muscle by
about 5% maximum. In each of the four sections, the grid represents the surface
of the contralateral scalp, marked out into 2 cm squares. The height of the bars
on each square shows the mean amplitude (in arbitrary units) of the EMG evoked
at each point in the biceps muscle. When the subject was relaxed, EMG responses
on the side of the amputation (stimulation of the left hemisphere) were larger and
could be obtained from a wider area of scalp than those on the intact side. However, this difference disappeared when the subject was contracting the muscles.
Stimulus intensity was set to be 15% above threshold for the intact side; a 9 cm
external diameter figure-of-eight coil was used to stimulate the cortex. (Modified
from Ridding & Rothwell, 1995.)

Virtually all mapping studies recognize these inherent limitations in technique, and because of this they focus not on the absolute size of a map, but
on changes in the maps, produced by, for example, anaesthesia, immobilization, or disease. With the exception of a few studies, most interventions
change the size of the map without affecting its optimal point (Cohen et al.,
1991, 1993; Topka et al., 1991; Brasil et al., 1992; Pascual-Leone et al., 1993).
In such cases, changes in the map size are best observed with subjects at

complete rest. If the maps are compared with subjects actively contracting their muscles, the map differences disappear (Ridding & Rothwell, 1995, 1997) (Fig. 2.2). The most likely explanation is that the changes in the maps are the result of changes in the resting excitability of the projection to the target muscle. During voluntary contraction, excitability levels are normalized and therefore the differences disappear.

Changes in optimal map location are much rarer, but have been described for the projections to affected muscle groups in patients with writers' cramp (Byrnes et al., 1998) and in hand muscle projections in patients with facial nerve palsy (Rijntjes et al., 1997). Such changes in location presumably reflect a true reorganization of the anatomical projections to muscles of interest. For example, it may become easier to activate some populations of horizontal connections within the cortex that excite pyramidal projections to the muscles of interest (Sanes & Donoghue, 1997). In terms of a cortical map, this might displace the centre of gravity.

Changes in the direction of movements produced by suprathreshold TMS   Rather than mapping out the EMG activity produced by stimulating over different scalp sites, it is possible to record the movements that are evoked. Woolsey and Penfield used this sort of approach to map the motor homunculus of humans and monkeys. They applied trains of stimuli at 60 Hz for 1 s or so in order to evoke clear motion of the limbs or body. The map that they produced can be regarded as a functional map of cortical output, rather than a physiological or anatomical one.

Single pulse TMS usually only produces clear movement of hand and fingers and therefore is not suitable for mapping the whole motor cortex in this way. However, changes in the movement produced by stimulation at a given point have been used successfully as a measure of cortical excitability before and after behavioural interventions. For example, TMS may tend to produce flexion of the thumb. If the subject then performs several hundred repeated voluntary thumb extension movements, TMS applied afterwards when relaxed will tend to evoke extension, not flexion movements. This persists over the next 15–30 min (Classen et al., 1998). The effects are blocked by giving subjects a single dose of dextromethorphan or lorazepam, drugs that block NMDA receptors and enhance GABA activity, respectively, but unaffected by lamotragine, a drug that affects voltage gated calcium and sodium channels (Butefisch et al., 2000). The authors drew parallels with the role of NMDA and GABA receptors in the form of long-term synaptic potentiation (LTP), and suggested this might be responsible for the effects they observed. However, as with other forms of mapping, such results are as likely to reflect an increase in the resting excitability of the cortical output to muscles involved in thumb extension than changes in synaptic efficacy.

Stimulation of motor cortex: distinguishing cortical from spinal effects

The EMG response to TMS depends on both the excitability of the cortex, which determines the amplitude and number of I waves that are recruited, and the excitability of the spinal motoneurone pool, which determines how many motoneurones are recruited by a given descending input. In many single pulse TMS studies of motor cortex, the size and threshold of MEPs is measured before and after an intervention (e.g. learning, changes in afferent input, drug administration, etc.). Any changes that are seen could therefore be due to changes in excitability at either cortical or spinal level.

Four main techniques are available to distinguish between effects at these two levels, although none of them are sufficient on their own to provide an unequivocal answer.

1. The most direct method is to record the descending volleys evoked by TMS before and after the intervention. This gives a direct measure of changes in the cortical response to stimulation. If the effect being studied is limited to a particular set of muscles, the disadvantage of the technique is that a spinal epidural electrode records all the descending activity set up by the stimulus and not just that destined for the target muscle group. Thus changes in volleys can only be said to correlate with changes in MEPs, and not necessarily to cause them.

2. A second method is to compare the responses to TMS with the responses to TES. If low intensity anodal stimulation is used, then TES evokes a relatively pure D wave that is unaffected by changes in cortical excitability (Di Lazzaro et al., 1999b). If the response to TES is unchanged by the intervention while the response to TMS is, say, facilitated, there may well have been an increase in cortical excitability. The disadvantage is that in most cases, a single D wave is insufficient to evoke an EMG response in relaxed muscle, so that the comparison must be made during voluntary

contraction. However, as noted above, voluntary contraction often conceals changes in excitability that are evident at rest, and this limits the application of the method. One way around this problem is to combine TES with spinal H reflexes. Appropriately timed H reflex input is facilitated by a subthreshold D wave if the two volleys arrive at the spinal motoneurones at the same time. Thus, the amount of H facilitation produced by subthreshold TES in resting subjects is a measure of the amplitude of the D wave input.

3. A third method is to use transmastoid stimulation of the descending tracts, again with the intention to evoke a single descending volley that is unaffected by changes in cortical excitability. As with TES, it may be difficult to evoke a large EMG response in relaxed muscles with this method. In addition it is unknown to what extent activity in other pathways contributes to the size of EMG responses that are evoked. However, this may not be a serious objection if there is no change in the response to transmastoidal stimulation over the time of the study.

4. A fourth method is to use H reflexes or F waves to measure the excitability of spinal reflex pathways and motoneurones. If these remain unchanged by an intervention whilst responses to TMS differ, it is likely that the intervention has caused changes in cortical rather than spinal excitability. The disadvantage of this method is that the motoneurones within a spinal pool may be recruited in a different order by H reflexes or F waves than with TMS (Morita et al., 1999). Since changes in spinal excitability may be distributed differentially to motoneurones of different size or type, this opens the possibility that H and F responses would fail to pick up changes in excitability of the population of spinal motoneurones recruited by TMS.

Paired pulse TMS experiments

Paired pulse experiments involve applying two stimuli, S1 and S2, separated in time by a varying interstimulus interval (ISI). In order to study the motor cortex, S2 is applied over, for example, the hand area, using an intensity sufficient to evoke an MEP in the target muscle; S1 is applied over another (or the same) area of cortex at various times beforehand (Fig. 2.3(a)). If S1 affects the amplitude of the response to S2, there is likely to be a functional connection between the two cortical sites. However, before this can be assumed, it

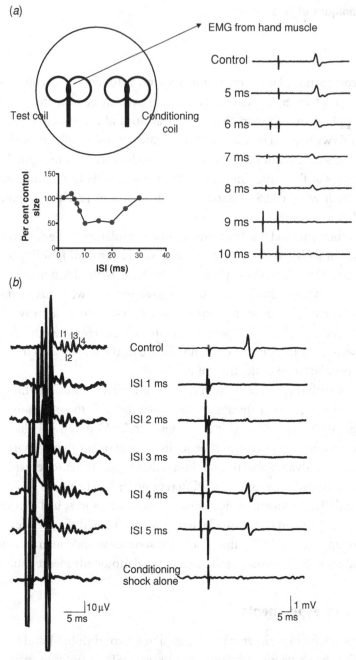

Fig. 2.3   (a) Typical example of a paired pulse design: interhemispheric inhibition. Two mag-
           netic pulses are used to stimulate the brain. One of the stimuli is given to the motor
           cortex contralateral to the muscle being recorded (test coil). The other is placed at
           another point on the scalp, in this case over the opposite hemisphere (conditioning
           coil). The EMG traces on the right show how the size of the EMG response evoked by
           the test stimulus is affected by a prior conditioning stimulus at various interstimulus

is always important to verify that the effect on S2 is at a cortical rather than a spinal level (see above). Connections to the motor cortex have been investigated using this method from the opposite hemisphere (Ferbert et al., 1992), cerebellum (Ugawa et al., 1991a, 1995), premotor cortex (Civardi et al., 2001), and within the motor cortex itself (Kujirai et al., 1993; Tokimura et al., 1996; Ziemann et al., 1998b).

Interhemispheric inhibition between homologous areas of motor cortex results in inhibition of MEPs with a latency of about 7 ms, and a duration that increases with the strength of S1 (Fig. 2.3(a)). There is sometimes a small early period of facilitation at ISI = 3–4 ms (Hanajima et al., 2001). This mixture of early facilitation and predominant later inhibition may reflect the basic neurophysiology of the connection, which is thought to involve a focal point-to-point facilitation with a larger surround inhibition (Asanuma & Okuda, 1962). The amount of inhibition is task dependent, being largest when the hand contralateral to S1 is active and the opposite hand relaxed (Ferbert et al., 1992). The effect of interhemispheric inhibition can be seen in the ongoing voluntary EMG as a silent period with onset latency of about 35 ms and a duration of 30 ms (Meyer et al., 1995). Although the optimal orientation of the coil is the same, the threshold for interhemispheric inhibition is often different from the threshold or evoking a contralateral MEP, suggesting that stimulation of a different set of neurones is required for each effect.

Although interhemispheric inhibition is thought to involve transmission across the corpus callosum, and is absent in patients with lesions that affect the transcallosal motor fibres (Meyer et al., 1995), and present in some

---

Fig. 2.3 (cont.) intervals (ISI) from 5 to 10 ms. Note how the EMG response is suppressed by conditioning stimuli at 6–10 ms. The graph plots the size of the conditioned EMG response as a percentage of its control value at different ISIs. (Modified from Ferbert et al., 1992.) (b) Short latency intracortical inhibition (SICI) illustrated in simultaneous recordings from the epidural space (left column) and EMG (right column) in a patient with a chronically implanted cervical electrode for control of pain. The response to the test (i.e. the second stimulus of the pair) stimulus given alone is shown in the first row. It evokes four I waves in the corticospinal tract, and a clear EMG response. When preceded by the conditioning stimulus, particularly at interstimulus intervals ISIs of 1–3 ms, it is almost abolished, and the number of I waves in the epidural record is reduced. Note that the I1 wave is unaffected by the conditioning stimulus. (Adapted from Di Lazzaro et al., 1998c.)

patients with corticospinal lesions in the internal capsule (Boroojerdi et al., 1996), there is evidence that S1 may produce a small effect on spinal mechanisms (Gerloff et al., 1998), indicating the importance of testing for both cortical and spinal effects.

Cerebello-cortical inhibition provoked by stimulation over the cerebellum inhibits MEPs with a latency of about 5 ms. The effect may be caused by excitation of inhibitory output from the Purkinje cells which secondarily withdraws facilitation from cerebello-thalamo-cortical pathways. The duration of the effect is difficult to define because the initial cerebellar inhibition is followed by a second period of inhibition thought to be due to stimulation of afferent fibres in cervical nerve roots or even in the brainstem (Meyer et al., 1994; Meyer & Roricht, 1995; Rothwell et al., 1995; Werhahn et al., 1996).

Premotor-primary motor cortex inhibition is maximal at an ISI = 6 ms, starting at about 2–3 ms followed by a short period of facilitation with ISI > 8–10 ms (Civardi et al., 2001). In order to study the effect, two small coils must be used so that they can be placed close enough together on the scalp to activate the two areas separately. The best orientation of the conditioning coil is to induce anterior–posterior currents over the premotor area, which indicates that the elements involved are arranged differently with respect to scalp than those needed to evoke MEPs from the primary motor area. The inhibition from premotor cortex is not as powerful as interhemispheric or cerebello-cortical effects.

Cortico-cortical inhibition/facilitation involves giving two stimuli through the same coil (Fig. 2.3(b)). Three types of interaction have been described, each of which tests a different population of intracortical circuits. They are known as: (a) short latency intracortical inhibition and facilitation (SICI and SICF, (b) long latency intracortical inhibition (LICI), and (c) I wave facilitation.

SICI and SICF are seen if the interstimulus interval lies between 1 and 20 ms and the intensity of S1 is below threshold (Kujirai et al., 1993). SICI occurs with ISIs 1–5 ms, and SICF at ISIs > 6–8 ms. Inhibition has a lower threshold than facilitation and is task sensitive, being reduced at the onset and during a voluntary contraction (Ridding et al., 1995; Reynolds & Ashby, 1999). Unlike the usual effect on the MEP, inhibition produced by S1 does not depend on the orientation of the magnetic stimulus current, suggesting that the elements excited are arranged differently in the cortex to those involved in the MEP (Ziemann et al., 1996b). Studies with neuroactive drugs suggest that the inhibition is GABAergic (Ziemann et al., 1996a), and studies with subdural arrays of implanted electrodes in patients with epilepsy suggest that inhibition of a cortical point comes from a relatively focal area of surrounding cortex (Ashby et al., 1999). Examination of much of the published data on SICI shows that SICI at an interstimulus interval of 1 ms often is less responsive to experimental manipulation than at 2–5 ms. This is probably because the mechanism of inhibition at this interval differs from that at later intervals (Fisher et al., 2002).

Long latency intracortical inhibition (LICI) occurs if S1 has an intensity above resting motor threshold (Berardelli et al., 1996). In this case, MEPs evoked by S2 are inhibited at ISI 100–150 ms, depending on the intensity of S1. Inhibition at shorter intervals probably has a spinal contribution due to motoneurone refractoriness after the MEP evoked by S1 (Fuhr et al., 1991).

I wave facilitation can be seen with a more restricted set of parameters than the others forms of interaction. The intensity of S1 must be large enough to generate I wave activity in the cortex. A typical intensity would be at, or just above, resting motor threshold since recordings of descending volleys at this intensity show that at least two or three I waves are recruited (Di Lazzaro et al., 1998b). The intensity of S2 may be similar or larger, and the interval between them between 1 and 5 ms. If this interval is explored in 0.1 or 0.2 ms steps, it is possible to observe peaks of facilitation between the two stimuli at ISIs of approximately 1.3, 2.6 and 4.2 ms (Tokimura et al., 1996; Ziemann et al., 1998b). These are thought to be due to interactions between the I waves evoked by S1 and S2 in the cortex, which have a similar periodicity. Since S1 is above threshold for eliciting a descending volley, some of this interaction could occur in the spinal cord rather than cortex. However, recordings of the epidural volleys generated by such pairs of stimuli show that at least the initial peak at 1.3 ms is likely to be cortical (Di Lazzaro et al., 1999).

Given that the predominant effect of all these interactions (apart from I wave facilitation) is inhibitory, it is reasonable to ask whether they all converge onto the same set of inhibitory interneurones in the motor cortex, or whether there are separate inhibitory circuits private to each pathway. The fact that the time courses of some of the effects are different (e.g. long and short latency ICI) makes it likely that separate pathways can exist. Recent evidence from long and short ICI shows that, even if separate, the pathways may well interact with each other (Sanger et al., 2001). For example, long latency ICI suppresses short latency ICI, possibly through a GABAb system.

In the cases where it has been possible to record descending volleys in the spinal cord, inhibition preferentially suppresses the I3 and later waves, whilst leaving the I1 and (to a lesser extent) the I2 wave unaffected (Di Lazzaro et al., 1998c, 1999a). This suggests that inhibition is not directed directly onto the proximal dendrites or cell body of pyramidal neurones since, if it were, we might expect all I waves to be equally affected. It seems more likely that such inhibition affects the neuronal circuits responsible for I wave generation. In addition, it would be compatible with the idea that some I waves are generated by different circuits than other I waves.

Repetitive TMS

Repetitive TMS (rTMS) refers to stimuli given more frequently than the usual 0.3 Hz that is available from most commercial single pulse stimulators. It is an arbitrary distinction based on the fact that early monophasic TMS machines needed about 3 s to charge up between successive stimuli, whereas TMS machines that delivered a biphasic pulse utilized some of the return current so that they could charge up within 20 ms and deliver pulses at up to 50 Hz. Even today, rapid rates of stimulation can only be achieved with biphasic current pulses.

After-effects of rTMS

rTMS: effects on corticospinal excitability assessed using MEPs

The main interest in using rTMS is that it can produce effects that outlast the application of the stimulus for minutes or hours. As with single pulse TMS, most of our understanding of its actions comes from studies on motor cortex. These show that the after-effects of rTMS depend on the frequency, intensity, and length of time for which the stimulation is given. For stimuli of around resting motor threshold, rTMS for 10 min at low frequency (1 Hz) tends to decrease resting corticospinal excitability (Fig. 2.4) whereas higher frequencies (>5–10 Hz) tend to increase resting excitability (Chen et al., 1997; Maeda et al., 2000b). The same trend appears to hold in the occipital cortex, where a period of 1 Hz rTMS raised the threshold for single pulse TMS to evoke phosphenes by about 3% of stimulator output (Boroojerdi et al., 2000).

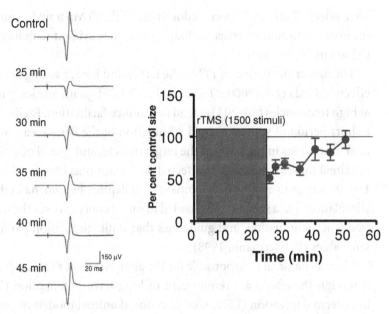

Fig. 2.4   Long-term effects of rTMS on primary motor cortex. The column on the left shows the amplitude of EMG responses in the first dorsal interosseous muscle before (top row) and at different times after 25 min of 1 Hz rTMS using an intensity of 95% resting motor threshold. Note that immediately after the end of rTMS (25 min), the response is dramatically reduced, and that this persists for a further 20 min (45 min from the start of rTMS). The graph on the right plots the mean data from ten subjects. The EMG response recovers gradually over about 20 min. (Adapted from Touge et al., 2001.)

Experiments in the motor cortex show that the interindividual variability of these effects is high, perhaps because of genuine differences in the response of each subject to rTMS. In addition, since the experiments involve comparing MEPs evoked by standard TMS stimuli before and after a period of rTMS, there may be difficulty in maintaining constant MEP amplitudes in resting subjects over long periods (Maeda et al., 2000a).

The interaction between frequency, intensity and duration of rTMS has not been investigated in great detail. For short trains (<20 stimuli) of any frequency, the immediate after-effect on MEP amplitude is more likely to be inhibitory for low intensities of rTMS. Facilitatory after-effects have a higher threshold. However, the number of stimuli in the rTMS train is important, since inhibitory after-effects build up more quickly than facilitatory after-effects. Thus inhibition predominates if the rTMS train has only a small number of stimuli, whereas facilitation becomes evident with longer trains (Modugno et al., 2001).

The longer the period of rTMS the larger and longer lasting are the after-effects (Maeda et al., 2000a; Touge et al., 2001). High intensities, particularly at high frequencies (10–20 Hz) tend to produce facilitation. Facilitation after a short period of suprathreshold stimulation of the hand area can produce after-discharges in the EMG of the target muscle, and spread of activation to proximal muscles normally unaffected by the stimulus (Pascual-Leone et al., 1994b), suggestive of the development of epileptic phenomena in the area of stimulation. Data such as these has led to safety concerns over the use of high frequency stimulation, and guidelines that limit stimulation parameters to safe values (Wassermann, 1998).

The mechanism(s) responsible for the after-effects of rTMS are unknown. Although the effects are reminiscent of long-term potentiation (LTP) and long-term depression (LTD) seen in reduced animal models of cortical circuitry, there is little direct evidence either to support or refute the suggestion. As with experiments on cortical mapping, the effects of rTMS on corticospinal excitability can only be observed in subjects at rest, and disappear when tested during voluntary contraction of the muscle (Touge et al., 2001). An alternative explanation would be that rTMS changes the basal level of excitability when subjects are at rest, and that this is normalized when they contract voluntarily.

rTMS: effects on intracortical circuitry

Repetitive TMS of motor cortex not only has prolonged effects on corticospinal excitability, but also can affect circuits tested by paired pulse designs and the silent period. Subthreshold stimulation at 5 Hz (1250 stimuli) reduces SICI and SICF; rTMS at 1 Hz has no effect in healthy subjects, even though it can increase SICI in patients with focal hand dystonia (Siebner et al., 1999b; Peinemann et al., 2000). Repetitive TMS at 5 Hz can also increase the duration of the silent period in patients with Parkinson's disease, again with no effect on healthy subjects (Siebner et al., 2000a). As with behavioural effects discussed below, these data suggest that a pathological system may be more susceptible to the long-term effects of rTMS than a healthy system.

rTMS: other physiological measures and effects at distant sites

A range of other measures show long-term changes after periods of rTMS. For example, the sensory cortex response to afferent input, as measured by the SEP, may be depressed after 1 Hz stimulation (Enomoto et al., 2001) or increased after paired afferent stimulation and TMS at 0.1 Hz (see section below) (Tsuji & Rothwell, 2002). Bereitschaftspotentials (Rossi et al., 2000), event-related EEG potentials (Jing et al., 2001), and measures of EEG power and coherence between premotor and motor cortex (Jing & Takigawa, 2000; Okamura et al., 2001; Jing et al., 2001) also change after rTMS.

TMS at any one site will activate neurones ortho- and anti-dromically that project to other parts of the CNS. The muscle twitches produced by TMS over motor cortex are an obvious example of effects occurring at a site distant from the point of stimulation. Repetitive TMS will also produce the same effects, leading to the possibility that long-lasting changes can occur in distant structures as well as at the site of stimulation. Electrophysiological studies have shown that rTMS over premotor cortex can affect the excitability of primary motor cortex and change the time course of short latency paired pulse inhibition/facilitation (Gerschlager et al., 2001; Munchau et al., 2002). Functional imaging studies have proved a more valuable technique to explore this question (see below).

Behavioural consequences of rTMS and possible therapeutic uses

In healthy subjects, repetitive TMS of the motor cortex produces no clinically obvious after-effects on movement, nor are there changes in muscle strength or maximal acceleration of isotonic contractions (Muellbacher et al., 2000). Larger behavioural effects have been observed in neurological patients. In Parkinson's disease 5 Hz motor cortex stimulation has been used in attempt to increase motor excitability. Movement speed increased without loss of accuracy for up to 30 min after an rTMS train of 2250 stimuli (Siebner et al., 1999a). In patients with focal dystonia of the arm, 1 Hz stimulation for 30 min improved writing performance for the next hour (Siebner et al., 1999b). It may be that effects on movement are more readily observed in a system already compromised by disease than in healthy subjects.

The question of whether behavioural effects can be seen after rTMS, and for how long, is directly relevant to its possible use as a therapeutic tool. The studies above suggest that at most, after-effects of trains with 1000 or more stimuli may last 1 hour. If this were true in other systems and in other diseases, rTMS would have limited therapeutic use. To try to overcome this limitation, many authors have given repeated sessions of rTMS over days and weeks in order to prolong the duration of the after-effect (George et al., 1995; Pascual-Leone et al., 1996). Strangely enough, no one has ever tested whether repeated application of rTMS has effects that build up from one day to the next, so there is at present no scientific justification for using repeated application. Similarly, there is insufficient data from clinical trials to judge whether one session of rTMS has a greater effect than multiple sessions (George et al., 1999). Even if symptoms improve gradually over the days of rTMS, it is unclear whether this would not have happened even after a single application. The conclusion is that the scientific rationale underpinning the use of rTMS to treat disease is poorly understood, even if some of the results may appear promising (see chapter by Epstein and Rothwell, present volume).

Functional imaging and rTMS

Functional imaging techniques allow direct visualization of the effects of TMS both at the site of stimulation and at distant sites. If they are used in conjunction with an activation paradigm, they can also show whether the pattern of activity associated with a task changes after rTMS (Paus, 1999).

Technically, it is not difficult to use a TMS machine in a PET scanner. The detector coils in the PET are relatively unaffected by the TMS and, with a little magnetic shielding (Mumetal cylinder lining the scanner bore) (Paus et al., 1997), it is possible to obtain data both during and after stimulation. PET studies have shown that rTMS over motor cortex activates the supplementary motor area and the contralateral motor area (Paus et al., 1998) for up to 30 min or so after the end of stimulation (Siebner et al., 2000b). Similar effects have been seen after stimulation of the frontal eye fields (Paus et al., 1997) or medial frontal cortex (Paus et al., 2001). In the latter case, after-effects of rTMS on the excitability of projections from the stimulated site lead to changes in the pattern of activation produced by probing connectivity with pairs of single pulse TMS (Paus et al., 2001).

Repetitive TMS can even be combined with ligand binding studies in PET. Stimulation of frontal cortex can decrease raclopride binding in the head of the caudate nucleus (Strafella et al., 2001). The implication is that

TMS had activated the cortical projection to the caudate and either via an influence on substantia nigra, or through an effect of local glutamate release on nigral terminals in the caudate, increases dopamine release in that region.

Combining TMS and fMRI is more challenging (Bohning et al., 1998). The magnetic fields of the MRI and peak field produced by a TMS coil are of similar size, so that discharging a TMS coil in the MRI bore produces large forces on the coil. With a figure-of-eight coil, reinforcement is needed to stop these forces twisting and bending the coil. They also increase substantially the noise of each discharge pulse. The presence of the coil in the scanner can distort the MRI image, especially in the region under the coil, and finally any image slices obtained when the coil is discharged will be unusable. These factors have meant that only a few studies have been performed to date and these have been mainly to show that the combination of techniques is possible (Bohning et al., 2000a,b; Baudewig et al., 2001).

Interaction of TMS and rTMS with peripheral inputs

Two designs of experiment have investigated the interaction between peripheral sensory input and the response to TMS. In the first type, a single electric shock or a phasic afferent disturbance (such as muscle stretch or a tap to the skin) is used to activate afferent fibres, and the effect on the response to a standard suprathreshold TMS is quantified by measuring the size of the evoked MEP at different times after the sensory input. The design was originally applied to test theories about the possibility of transcortical reflexes. The results showed that afferent input from the upper or lower limb could facilitate MEPs at a latency compatible with transcortical reflexes that involved the motor cortex (Day et al., 1991; Macefield et al., 1996; Christensen et al., 2000). More detailed studies also revealed a short latency inhibitory effect that preceded the later facilitation (Maertens de Noordhout et al., 1992; Tokimura et al., 2000). The cortical mechanism of this unexpected early inhibition is unknown, but since it is abolished by pretreatment with scoplolamine, it may well involve cholinergic transmission (Di Lazzaro et al., 2000).

In an extension of this paradigm, pairs of sensory and TMS stimuli have been given repeatedly at 20 s (Stefan et al., 2000), or every 10 s (Ridding & Taylor, 2001) for 30 min or so. The rationale was based on the fact that, in animal experiments, LTP can be induced at cortical synapses when paired vs. single inputs are applied repeatedly (Hess et al., 1996). In humans, the effect was to increase corticospinal excitability for up to 30 min after the end of stimulation. However, whether these changes are true examples of LTP is unknown. As with other examples of MEP facilitation, the effects are seen only in relaxed muscle, and not if MEPs are tested during voluntary contraction, suggesting that changes in excitability levels at rest may account for the majority of the effect.

In the second design of experiment, sustained changes in sensory input are produced by either anaesthesia or prolonged periods of afferent stimulation. As noted above, anaesthesia increases the excitability of cortical projections to muscles adjacent to the block, whereas prolonged afferent stimulation can increase excitability to muscles around the site of stimulation (Hamdy et al., 1998; Ridding et al., 2000). In many experiments, ischaemic anaesthesia is used. This is rapidly reversible on restoration of the blood supply, so that the time course of recovery of the cortical excitability can be followed. After anaesthesia, excitability recovers almost immediately, whereas after continuous afferent stimulation, the effects may last up to an hour (Brasil et al., 1992; Hamdy et al., 1998). The cause of this asymmetry is unknown. The latter procedure has been used to try to increase muscle strength in patients after stroke (Conforto et al., 2002).

Prolonged changes in afferent input can also affect the responses to rTMS. For example, the usual increase in MEP amplitude of muscles proximal to an anaesthetic block is enhanced by simultaneous application of 0.1 Hz rTMS even though the latter had no effect when applied alone (Ziemann et al., 1998a).

TMS and rTMS as a 'virtual lesion'
Single pulse 'lesions'

The muscle twitch that is produced by single pulse TMS over the primary motor cortex gives the impression that the primary action of TMS is excitatory. However, TMS also has the effect of disrupting any ongoing activity that is occurring at the time the stimulus is applied. There are two reasons for this. First, TMS will tend to synchronize activity in many neurones and, second, after a short period of high frequency discharge, neuronal activity will be reduced by a 50–150 ms period of GABAergic inhibition. The effect has been likened to a reversible or 'virtual' lesion (Walsh & Rushworth, 1999). TMS over non-motor areas of cortex often appears to have no behavioural effects, but that is because the period of disruption is short. If stimuli are given to a part of the cortex at the time that area is engaged in a behavioural task, performance usually changes.

Typical examples of disruption can be seen in both the visual and motor systems (Fig. 2.5). Thus, a single TMS pulse applied over the occiput can suppress perception of a briefly flashed visual stimulus given 80–140 ms earlier (Cracco et al., 1990). It is thought that visual input reaches the primary visual cortex about 80 ms after presentation, and therefore TMS at this time will disrupt processing of the input and cause a transient scotoma in the visual field. In the motor system, a single TMS pulse applied to the motor cortex in the reaction period between a 'go' signal and the expected onset of movement can delay the reaction time by around 50–100 ms (Day et al., 1989b). The explanation may be that the TMS disrupts motor cortex activity so that it cannot respond at the expected time to inputs from other brain areas that trigger release of a movement. In both visual and motor tasks, the duration of the disruption is longer, the higher the intensity of the stimulus.

These two examples also illustrate the two main types of disruption that TMS can produce: the visual task can no longer be performed, whereas in the motor task, performance is delayed, but otherwise unaffected. The final outcome differs in different systems, and may depend, among other things, on whether neural processing relevant to the task continues elsewhere in the brain during the period of disruption. They also show the importance of giving the TMS pulse at the correct time. Neither effect would have been observed if the timing of the pulses had not been within a 100 ms range.

In most cases the disruption of brain activity produced by TMS worsens task performance. However, in some instances, the TMS pulse may remove activity that would otherwise interfere with the task and performance improves. This can be demonstrated by using occipital stimulation to cancel the effect of backward masking in the visual system (Maccabee et al., 1991). Subjects are presented briefly with a dim target, and 100 ms later with a brighter one in the same part of the visual field. The appearance of the bright

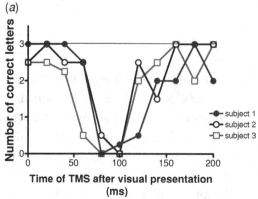

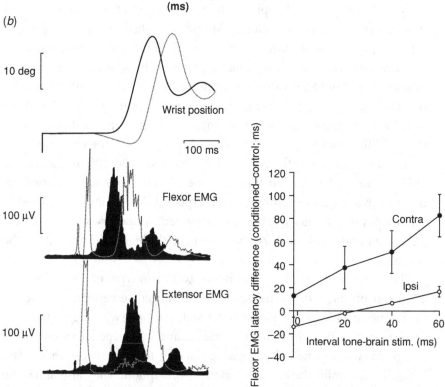

Fig. 2.5   Examples of the 'virtual lesion' effect of TMS. (a) The effect of a single TMS pulse
over the occipital cortex on the ability of three different subjects to identify correctly
three random letter flashed onto a VDU screen at $t = 0$ ms. When the TMS pulse is
given from about 75 to 150 ms after the visual stimulus, subjects cannot identify
all three letters correctly. (Adapted from Maccabee et al., 1991.) (b) Interruption of
a reaction time movement by TMS over the motor cortex. On the left are shown
wrist position (top traces) and rectified EMGs from the flexor (middle) and extensor
(bottom) muscles of the forearm. The filled traces illustrate trials in which no TMS
was given. A clear triphasic EMG pattern can be seen. TMS was applied 100 ms
after the imperative stimulus (at $t = 0$ ms on the traces). It produces a small stimulus

target masks subjects' perception of the dim target (backward masking). However, if a TMS pulse is given to the occiput about 100 ms after the bright target, then subjects can once again perceive the dim target. It is thought that TMS disrupts processing of the bright target and that this prevents it masking prior visual stimuli. Similarly, performance in visual search tasks for stationary objects is improved after TMS over the visual motion sensitive area, V5, whilst visual search of moving objects is disrupted (Walsh et al., 1998). Again, it is thought that the removal of competing input about motion of objects helps subjects perform better when they have to attend only to stationary objects.

The improvement of performance that can occur with removal of competing inputs has been used clinically to improve performance of patients with neglect (Oliveri et al., 1999). TMS of the left frontal region could transiently reduce left-sided neglect in patients with right hemisphere stroke. It was proposed that hemispheric imbalance after stroke leads to an unopposed orienting response towards the side of the lesion. This is corrected by interfering with function in the intact hemisphere.

rTMS induced 'lesions'

Early work on the visual system showed that a pair of pulses can be more effective in disrupting function than either stimulus given alone (Maccabee et al., 1991). Thus, in many studies, short bursts of rTMS have been given in order to increase the time that cortical processing is disrupted (Pascual-Leone et al., 1991; Jahanshahi et al., 1998; Stewart et al., 2001). Although it is easier to show disruption of performance with rTMS compared with single pulse TMS, the disadvantage is that rTMS does not have the temporal specificity of single pulse TMS, so that it cannot be used to address questions about when a region of cortex is active in a task.

Fig. 2.5 (*cont.*) artefact, and an MEP in both sets of muscles 20 ms later. The triphasic burst and the wrist movement are delayed by about 70 ms. Note that the form of the triphasic EMG is the same as when no stimulus was given. The graph on the right shows how the delay in movement onset increases as the TMS pulse is given later and later in the reaction period. Stimuli given over the hemisphere contralateral to the moving hand have the largest effect. Ipsilateral stimulation has only a minor effect. (Adapted from Day et al., 1989b.)

A novel use of rTMS is to interfere with processes involved in consolidation of learning. There is some evidence that the primary motor cortex may be involved in some aspects of motor learning, and that, as learning progresses, these are transferred to other parts of the brain (Pascual-Leone et al., 1994a; Muellbacher et al., 2001). If rTMS at 1 Hz is applied shortly after learning a new task, it may be able to disrupt the learning process, so that, when subjects are tested after stimulation, their performance is the same as it was before practice was given (Muellbacher et al., 2002).

REFERENCES

Amassian, V.E., Stewart, M., Quirk, G.J. & Rosenthal, J.L. (1987). Physiological basis of motor effects of a transient stimulus to cerebral cortex. *Neurosurgery*, **20**: 74–93.

Asanuma, H. & Okuda, O. (1962). Effects of transcallosal volleys on pyramidal tract cell activity of cat. *J. Neurophysiol.*, **25**: 198–208.

Ashby, P., Reynolds, C., Wennberg, R., Lozano, A.M. & Rothwell, J. (1999). On the focal nature of inhibition and facilitation in the human motor cortex. *Clin. Neurophysiol.*, **110**: 550–555.

Barker, A.T., Garnham, C.W. & Freeston, I.L. (1991). Magnetic nerve stimulation: the effect of waveform on efficiency, determination of neural membrane time constants and the measurement of stimulator output. *Electroencephalogr. Clin. Neurophysiol. Suppl.*, **43**: 227–237.

Baudewig, J., Siebner, H.R., Bestmann, S. et al. (2001). Functional MRI of cortical activations induced by transcranial magnetic stimulation (TMS). *Neuroreport*, **12**: 3543–3548.

Berardelli, A., Rona, S., Inghilleri, M. & Manfredi, M. (1996). Cortical inhibition in parkinson's-disease – a study with paired magnetic stimulation. *Brain*, **119**: 71–77.

Bohning, D.E., Shastri, A., Nahas, Z. et al. (1998). Echoplanar BOLD fMRI of brain activation induced by concurrent transcranial magnetic stimulation. *Invest. Radiol.*, **33**: 336–340.

Bohning, D.E., Shastri, A., McGavin, L. et al. (2000a). Motor cortex brain activity induced by 1-Hz transcranial magnetic stimulation is similar in location and level to that for volitional movement. *Invest. Radiol.*, **35**: 676–683.

Bohning, D.E., Shastri, A., Wassermann, E.M. et al. (2000b). BOLD-f MRI response to single-pulse transcranial magnetic stimulation (TMS). *J. Magn. Reson. Imaging*, **11**: 569–574.

Boroojerdi, B., Diefenbach, K. & Ferbert, A. (1996). Transcallosal inhibition in cortical and subcortical cerebral vascular lesions. *J. Neurol. Sci.*, **144**: 160–170.

Boroojerdi, B., Prager, A., Muellbacher, W. & Cohen, L.G. (2000). Reduction of human visual cortex excitability using 1-Hz transcranial magnetic stimulation. *Neurology*, **54**: 1529–1531.

Brasil, N.J., Cohen, L.G., Pascual, L.A., Jabir, F.K., Wall, R.T. & Hallett, M. (1992). Rapid reversible modulation of human motor outputs after transient deafferentation of the forearm: a study with transcranial magnetic stimulation. *Neurology*, **42**: 1302–1306.

Burke, D., Hicks, R.G. & Stephen, J.P. (1990). Corticospinal volleys evoked by anodal and cathodal stimulation of the human motor cortex. *J. Physiol.*, **425**: 283–299.

Butefisch, C.M., Davis, B.C., Wise, S.P. et al. (2000). Mechanisms of use-dependent plasticity in the human motor cortex. *Proc. Natl Acad. Sci., USA*, **97**: 3661–3665.

Byrnes, M.L., Thickbroom, G.W., Wilson, S.A. et al. (1998). The corticomotor representation of upper limb muscles in writer's cramp and changes following botulinum toxin injection. *Brain*, **121**: 977–988.

Chen, R., Classen, J., Gerloff, C. et al. (1997). Depression of motor cortex excitability by low-frequency transcranial magnetic stimulation. *Neurology*, **48**: 1398–1403.

Christensen, L.O., Petersen, N., Andersen, J.B., Sinkjaer, T. & Nielsen, J.B. (2000). Evidence for transcortical reflex pathways in the lower limb of man. *Prog. Neurobiol.*, **62**: 251–272.

Civardi, C., Cantello, R., Asselman, P. & Rothwell, J.C. (2001). Transcranial magnetic stimulation can be used to test connections to primary motor areas from frontal and medial cortex in humans. *Neuroimage*, **14**: 1444–1453.

Classen, J., Liepert, J., Wise, S.P., Hallett, M. & Cohen, L.G. (1998). Rapid plasticity of human cortical movement representation induced by practice. *J. Neurophysiol.*, **79**: 1117–1123.

Cohen, L.G., Bandinelli, S., Findley, T.W. & Hallett, M. (1991). Motor reorganization after upper limb amputation in man. A study with focal magnetic stimulation. *Brain*, **114**: 615–627.

Cohen, L.G., Brasil, N.J., Pascual, L.A. & Hallett, M. (1993). Plasticity of cortical motor output organization following deafferentation, cerebral lesions, and skill acquisition. *Adv. Neurol.*, **63**: 187–200.

Conforto, A.B., Kaelin-Lang, A. & Cohen, L.G. (2002). Increase in hand muscle strength of stroke patients after somatosensory stimulation. *Ann. Neurol.*, **51**: 122–125.

Cracco, R.Q., Amassian, V.E., Maccabee, P.J. & Cracco, J.B. (1990). Excitatory and inhibitory effects of magnetic coil stimulation of human cortex. *Electroencephalogr. Clin. Neurophysiol. Suppl.*, **41**: 134–139.

Day, B.L., Dressler, D., Maertens-de, N.A. et al. (1989a). Electric and magnetic stimulation of human motor cortex: surface EMG and single motor unit responses [published erratum appears in *J. Physiol. Lond.* 1990; **430**:617]. *J. Physiol. Lond.*, **412**: 449–473.

Day, B.L., Rothwell, J.C., Thompson, P.D. et al. (1989b). Delay in the execution of voluntary movement by electrical or magnetic brain stimulation in intact man. Evidence for the storage of motor programs in the brain. *Brain*, **112**: 649–663.

Day, B.L., Riescher, H., Struppler, A., Rothwell, J.C. & Marsden, C.D. (1991). Changes in the response to magnetic and electrical stimulation of the motor cortex following muscle stretch in man. *J. Physiol. Lond.*, **433**: 41–57.

Di Lazzaro, V., Oliviero, A., Profice, P. et al. (1998a). Comparison of descending volleys evoked by transcranial magnetic and electric stimulation in conscious humans. *Electroencephalogr. Clin. Neurophysiol.*, **109**: 397–401.

Di Lazzaro, V., Restuccia, D., Oliviero, A. et al. (1998b). Effects of voluntary contraction on descending volleys evoked by transcranial stimulation in conscious humans. *J. Physiol. Lond.*, **508**: 625–634.

Di Lazzaro, V., Restuccia, D., Oliviero, A. et al. (1998c). Magnetic transcranial stimulation at intensities below active motor threshold activates intracortical inhibitory circuits. *Exp. Brain Res.*, **119**: 265–268.

Di Lazzaro V., Oliviero, A., Profice, P. et al. (1999a). Direct demonstration of interhemispheric inhibition of the human motor cortex produced by transcranial magnetic stimulation. *Exp. Brain Res.*, **124**: 520–524.

Di Lazzaro V., Oliviero, A., Profice, P. et al. (1999b). Effects of voluntary contraction on descending volleys evoked by transcranial electrical stimulation over the motor cortex hand area in conscious humans. *Exp. Brain Res.*, **124**: 525–528.

Di Lazzaro, V., Rothwell, J.C., Oliviero, A. et al. (1999c). Intracortical origin of the short latency facilitation produced by pairs of threshold magnetic stimuli applied to human motor cortex. *Exp. Brain Res.*, **129**: 494–499.

Di Lazzaro, V., Oliviero, A., Profice, P. et al. (2000). Muscarinic receptor blockade has differential effects on the excitability of intracortical circuits in the human motor cortex. *Exp. Brain Res.*, **135**: 455–461.

Di Lazzaro, V., Oliviero, A., Profice, P. et al. (2001a). Descending spinal cord volleys evoked by transcranial magnetic and electrical stimulation of the motor cortex leg area in conscious humans. *J. Physiol.*, **537**: 1047–1058.

Di Lazzaro, V., Oliviero, A., Saturno, E. et al. (2001b). The effect on corticospinal volleys of reversing the direction of current induced in the motor cortex by transcranial magnetic stimulation. *Exp. Brain Res.*, **138**: 268–273.

Di Lazzaro, V., Oliviero, A., Pilato, F. et al. (2002). Descending volleys evoked by transcranial magnetic stimulation of the brain in conscious humans: effects of coil shape. *Clin. Neurophysiol.*, **113**: 114–119.

Enomoto, H., Ugawa, Y., Hanajima, R. et al. (2001). Decreased sensory cortical excitability after 1 Hz rTMS over the ipsilateral primary motor cortex. *Clin. Neurophysiol.*, **112**: 2154–2158.

Ferbert, A., Priori, A., Rothwell, J.C., Day, B.L., Colebatch, J.G. & Marsden, C.D. (1992). Interhemispheric inhibition of the human motor cortex. *J. Physiol. Lond.*, **453**: 525–546.

Fisher, R.J., Nakamura, Y., Bestmann, S., Rothwell, J.C. & Bostock, H. (2002). Two phases of intracortical inhibition revealed by transcranial magnetic threshold tracking. *Exp. Brain Res.*, **143**: 240–248.

Fuhr, P., Agostino, R. & Hallett, M. (1991). Spinal motor neuron excitability during the silent period after cortical stimulation. *Electroencephalogr. Clin. Neurophysiol.*, **81**: 257–262.

George, M.S., Wassermann, E.M., Williams, W.A. et al. (1995). Daily repetitive transcranial magnetic stimulation (rTMS) improves mood in depression. *Neuroreport*, **6**: 1853–1856.

George, M.S., Lisanby, S.H. & Sackeim, H.A. (1999). Transcranial magnetic stimulation: applications in neuropsychiatry. *Arch. Gen. Psychiatry*, **56**: 300–311.

Gerloff, C., Cohen, L.G., Floeter, M.K., Chen, R., Corwell, B. & Hallet, M. (1998). Inhibitory influence of the ipsilateral motor cortex on responses to stimulation of the human cortex and pyramidal tract. *J. Physiol. Lond.*, **510**: 249–259.

Gerschlager, W., Siebner, H.R. & Rothwell, J.C. (2001). Decreased corticospinal excitability after subthreshold 1 Hz rTMS over lateral premotor cortex. *Neurology*, **57**: 449–455.

Hamdy, S., Rothwell, J.C., Aziz, Q., Singh, K.D. & Thompson, D.G. (1998). Long-term reorganization of human motor cortex driven by short-term sensory stimulation. *Nat. Neurosci.*, **1**: 64–68.

Hanajima, R., Ugawa, Y., Machii, K. et al. (2001). Interhemispheric facilitation of the hand motor area in humans. *J. Physiol.*, **531**: 849–859.

Hess, G., Aizenman, C.D. & Donoghue, J.P. (1996). Conditions for the induction of long-term potentiation in layer II/III horizontal connections of the rat motor cortex. *J. Neurophysiol.*, **75**: 1765–1778.

Houlden, D.A., Schwartz, M.L., Tator, C.H., Ashby, P. & MacKay, W.A. (1999). Spinal cord-evoked potentials and muscle responses evoked by transcranial magnetic stimulation in 10 awake human subjects. *J. Neurosci.*, **19**: 1855–1862.

Jahanshahi, M., Profice, P., Brown, R.G., Ridding, M.C., Dirnberger, G. & Rothwell, J.C. (1998). The effects of transcranial magnetic stimulation over the dorsolateral prefrontal cortex on suppression of habitual counting during random number generation. *Brain*, **121**: 1533–1544.

Jing, H. & Takigawa, M. (2000). Observation of EEG coherence after repetitive transcranial magnetic stimulation. *Clin. Neurophysiol.*, **111**: 1620–1631.

Jing, H., Takigawa, M., Hamada, K. et al. (2001). Effects of high frequency repetitive transcranial magnetic stimulation on P(300) event-related potentials. *Clin. Neurophysiol.*, **112**: 304–313.

Kammer, T., Beck, S., Thielscher, A., Laubis-Herrmann, U. & Topka, H. (2001). Motor thresholds in humans: a transcranial magnetic stimulation study comparing different pulse waveforms, current directions and stimulator types. *Clin. Neurophysiol.*, **112**: 250–258.

Kujirai, T., Caramia, M.D., Rothwell, J.C. et al. (1993). Corticocortical inhibition in human motor cortex. *J. Physiol. Lond.*, **471**: 501–519.

Maccabee, P.J., Amassian, V.E., Cracco, R.Q. et al. (1991). Magnetic coil stimulation of human visual cortex: studies of perception. *Electroencephalogr. Clin. Neurophysiol. Suppl.*, **43**: 111–120.

Maccabee, P.J., Amassian, V.E., Eberle, L.P. & Cracco, R.Q. (1993). Magnetic coil stimulation of straight and bent amphibian and mammalian peripheral nerve in vitro: locus of excitation. *J. Physiol. Lond.*, **460**: 201–219.

Maccabee, P.J., Nagarajan, S.S., Amassian, V.E. et al. (1998). Influence of pulse sequence, polarity and amplitude on magnetic stimulation of human and porcine peripheral nerve. *J. Physiol.*, **513**: 571–585.

Macefield, V.G., Rothwell, J.C. & Day, B.L. (1996). The contribution of transcortical pathways to long-latency stretch and tactile reflexes in human hand muscles. *Exp. Brain Res.*, **108**: 147–154.

Maeda, F., Keenan, J.P., Tormos, J.M., Topka, H. & Pascual-Leone, A. (2000a). Interindividual variability of the modulatory effects of repetitive transcranial magnetic stimulation on cortical excitability. *Exp. Brain Res.*, **133**: 425–430.

Maeda, F., Keenan, J.P., Tormos, J.M., Topka, H. & Pascual-Leone, A. (2000b). Modulation of corticospinal excitability by repetitive transcranial magnetic stimulation. *Clin. Neurophysiol.*, **111**: 800–805.

Maertens de Noordhout, A., Rothwell, J.C., Day, B.L. et al. (1992). Effect of digital nerve stimuli on responses to electrical or magnetic stimulation of the human brain. *J. Physiol. Lond.*, **447**: 535–548.

Meyer, B.U. & Roricht, S. (1995). Scalp potentials recorded over the sensorimotor region following magnetic stimulation over the cerebellum in man: considerations about the activated structures and their potential diagnostic use [letter] [see comments]. *J. Neurol.*, **242**: 109–112.

Meyer, B.U., Roricht, S. & Machetanz, J. (1994). Reduction of corticospinal excitability by magnetic stimulation over the cerebellum in patients with large defects of one cerebellar hemisphere. *Electroencephalogr. Clin. Neurophysiol.*, **93**: 372–379.

Meyer, B.U., Roricht, S., Grafin-von, E.H., Kruggel, F. & Weindl, A. (1995). Inhibitory and excitatory interhemispheric transfers between motor cortical areas in normal humans and patients with abnormalities of the corpus callosum. *Brain*, **118**: 429–440.

Mills, K.R., Boniface, S.J. & Schubert, M. (1992). Magnetic brain stimulation with a double coil: the importance of coil orientation. *Electroencephalogr. Clin. Neurophysiol.*, **85**: 17–21.

Modugno, N., Nakamura, Y., MacKinnon, C.D. et al. (2001). Motor cortex excitability following short trains of repetitive magnetic stimuli. *Exp. Brain Res.*, **140**: 453–459.

Morita, H., Baumgarten, J., Petersen, N., Christensen, L.O. & Nielsen, J. (1999). Recruitment of extensor-carpi-radialis motor units by transcranial magnetic stimulation and radial-nerve stimulation in human subjects. *Exp. Brain Res.*, **128**: 557–562.

Muellbacher, W., Ziemann, U., Boroojerdi, B. & Hallett, M. (2000). Effects of low-frequency transcranial magnetic stimulation on motor excitability and basic motor behavior. *Clin. Neurophysiol.*, **111**: 1002–1007.

Muellbacher, W., Ziemann, U., Boroojerdi, B., Cohen, L. & Hallett, M. (2001). Role of the human motor cortex in rapid motor learning. *Exp. Brain Res.*, **136**: 431–438.

Muellbacher, W., Ziemann, U., Wissel, J. et al. (2002). Early consolidation in human primary motor cortex. *Nature*, **415**: 640–644.

Munchau, A., Bloem, B.R., Irlbacher, K., Trimble, M.R. & Rothwell, J.C. (2002). Functional connectivity of human premotor and motor cortex explored with repetitive transcranial magnetic stimulation. *J. Neurosci.*, **22**: 554–561.

Nielsen, J., Petersen, N. & Ballegaard, M. (1995). Latency of effects evoked by electrical and magnetic brain stimulation in lower limb motoneurones in man. *J. Physiol.*, **484**: 791–802.

Okamura, H., Jing, H. & Takigawa, M. (2001). EEG modification induced by repetitive transcranial magnetic stimulation. *J. Clin. Neurophysiol.*, **18**: 318–325.

Oliveri, M., Rossini, P.M., Traversa, R. et al. (1999). Left frontal transcranial magnetic stimulation reduces contralesional extinction in patients with unilateral right brain damage. *Brain*, **122**: 1731–1739.

Pascual-Leone, A., Gates, J.R. & Dhuna, A. (1991). Induction of speech arrest and counting errors with rapid-rate transcranial magnetic stimulation [see comments]. *Neurology*, **41**: 697–702.

Pascual-Leone, A., Cammarota, A., Wassermann, E.M., Brasil, N.J., Cohen, L.G. & Hallett, M. (1993). Modulation of motor cortical outputs to the reading hand of braille readers. *Ann. Neurol.*, **34**: 33–37.

Pascual-Leone, A., Grafman, J. & Hallett, M. (1994a). Modulation of cortical motor output maps during development of implicit and explicit knowledge [see comments]. *Science*, **263**: 1287–1289.

Pascual-Leone, A., Valls, S.J., Wassermann, E.M. & Hallett, M. (1994b). Responses to rapid-rate transcranial magnetic stimulation of the human motor cortex. *Brain*, **117**: 847–858.

Pascual-Leone, A., Rubio, B., Pallardo, F. & Catala, M.D. (1996). Rapid-rate transcranial magnetic stimulation of left dorsolateral prefrontal cortex in drug-resistant depression. *Lancet*, **348**: 233–237.

Patton, H.D. & Amassian, V.E. (1954). Single and multiple unit analysis of the cortical stage of pyramidal tract activation. *J. Neurophysiol.*, **17**: 345–363.

Paus, T. (1999). Imaging the brain before, during, and after transcranial magnetic stimulation. *Neuropsychologia*, **37**: 219–224.

Paus, T., Jech, R., Thompson, C.J., Comeau, R., Peters, T. & Evans, A.C. (1997). Transcranial magnetic stimulation during positron emission tomography: a new method for studying connectivity of the human cerebral cortex. *J. Neurosci.*, **17**: 3178–3184.

Paus, T., Jech, R., Thompson, C.J., Comeau, R., Peters, T. & Evans, A.C. (1998). Dose-dependent reduction of cerebral blood flow during rapid-rate transcranial magnetic stimulation of the human sensorimotor cortex. *J. Neurophysiol.*, **79**: 1102–1107.

Paus, T., Castro-Alamancos, M.A. & Petrides, M. (2001). Cortico-cortical connectivity of the human mid-dorsolateral frontal cortex and its modulation by repetitive transcranial magnetic stimulation. *Eur. J. Neurosci.*, **14**: 1405–1411.

Peinemann, A., Lehner, C., Mentschel, C., Munchau, A., Conrad, B. & Siebner, H.R. (2000). Subthreshold 5-Hz repetitive transcranial magnetic stimulation of the human primary motor cortex reduces intracortical paired-pulse inhibition. *Neurosci. Lett.*, **296**: 21–24.

Porter, R. & Lemon, R.N. (1993). *Corticospinal Function and Voluntary Movement*. Oxford: Oxford University Press.

Priori, A., Bertolasi, L., Dressler, D. et al. (1993). Transcranial electric and magnetic stimulation of the leg area of the human motor cortex: single motor unit and surface EMG responses in the tibialis anterior muscle. *Electroencephalogr. Clin. Neurophysiol.*, **89**: 131–137.

Reynolds, C. & Ashby, P. (1999). Inhibition in the human motor cortex is reduced just before a voluntary contraction. *Neurology*, **53**: 730–735.

Ridding, M.C. & Rothwell, J.C. (1995). Reorganisation in human motor cortex. *Can. J. Physiol. Pharmacol.*, **73**: 218–222.

Ridding, M.C. & Rothwell, J.C. (1997). Stimulus/response curves as a method of measuring motor cortical excitability in man. *Electroencephalogr. Clin. Neurophysiol.*, **105**: 340–344.

Ridding, M.C. & Taylor, J.L. (2001). Mechanisms of motor-evoked potential facilitation following prolonged dual peripheral and central stimulation in humans. *J. Physiol.*, **537**: 623–631.

Ridding, M.C., Taylor, J.L. & Rothwell, J.C. (1995). The effect of voluntary contraction on cortico-cortical inhibition in human motor cortex. *J. Physiol. Lond.*, **487**: 541–548.

Ridding, M.C., Brouwer, B., Miles, T.S., Pitcher, J.B. & Thompson, P.D. (2000). Changes in muscle responses to stimulation of the motor cortex induced by peripheral nerve stimulation in human subjects. *Exp. Brain Res.*, **131**: 135–143.

Rijntjes, M., Tegenthoff, M., Liepert, J. et al. (1997). Cortical reorganization in patients with facial palsy. *Ann. Neurol.*, **41**: 621–630.

Rossi, S., Pasqualetti, P., Rossini, P.M. et al. (2000). Effects of repetitive transcranial magnetic stimulation on movement-related cortical activity in humans. *Cereb. Cortex*, **10**: 802–808.

Rothwell, J.C., Day, B.L. & Amassian, V.E. (1992). Near threshold electrical and magnetic transcranial stimuli activate overlapping sets of cortical-neurons in humans. *J. Physiol. Lond.*, **452**: 109.

Rothwell, J.C., Werhahn, K.J. & Amassian, V.E. (1995). Additional source of potentials recorded from the scalp following magnetic stimulation over the lower occiput and adjoining neck. *J. Neurol.*, **242**: 713–714.

Sakai, K., Ugawa, Y., Terao, Y., Hanajima, R., Furubayashi, T. & Kanazawa, I. (1997). Preferential activation of different I waves by transcranial magnetic stimulation with a figure-of-eight-shaped coil. *Exp. Brain Res.*, **113**: 24–32.

Sanes, J.N. & Donoghue, J.P. (1997). Static and dynamic organization of motor cortex. *Adv. Neurol.*, **73**: 277–296.

Sanger, T.D., Garg, R.R. & Chen, R. (2001). Interactions between two different inhibitory systems in the human motor cortex. *J. Physiol.*, **530**: 307–317.

Siebner, H.R., Mentschel, C., Auer, C. & Conrad, B. (1999a). Repetitive transcranial magnetic stimulation has a beneficial effect on bradykinesia in Parkinson's disease. *Neuroreport*, **10**: 589–594.

Siebner, H.R., Tormos, J.M., Ceballos, B.A. et al. (1999b). Low-frequency repetitive transcranial magnetic stimulation of the motor cortex in writer's cramp. *Neurology*, **52**: 529–537.

Siebner, H.R., Mentschel, C., Auer, C., Lehner, C. & Conrad, B. (2000a). Repetitive transcranial magnetic stimulation causes a short-term increase in the duration of the cortical silent period in patients with Parkinson's disease. *Neurosci. Lett.*, **284**: 147–150.

Siebner, H.R., Peller, M., Willoch, F. et al. (2000b). Lasting cortical activation after repetitive TMS of the motor cortex: a glucose metabolic study. *Neurology*, **54**: 956–963.

Stefan, K., Kunesch, E., Cohen, L.G., Benecke, R. & Classen, J. (2000). Induction of plasticity in the human motor cortex by paired associative stimulation. *Brain*, **123**: 572–584.

Stewart, L., Meyer, B., Frith, U. & Rothwell, J. (2001). Left posterior BA37 is involved in object recognition: a TMS study. *Neuropsychologia*, **39**: 1–6.

Strafella, A.P., Paus, T., Barrett, J. & Dagher, A. (2001). Repetitive transcranial magnetic stimulation of the human prefrontal cortex induces dopamine release in the caudate nucleus. *J. Neurosci.*, **21**: RC157.

Terao, Y., Ugawa, Y., Sakai, K., Uesaka, Y., Kohara, N. & Kanazawa, I. (1994). Transcranial stimulation of the leg area of the motor cortex in humans. *Acta Neurol. Scand.*, **89**: 378–383.

Thickbroom, G.W., Sammut, R. & Mastaglia, F.L. (1998). Magnetic stimulation mapping of motor cortex: factors contributing to map area. *Electroencephalogr. Clin. Neurophysiol.*, **109**: 79–84.

Tofts, P.S. (1990). The distribution of induced currents in magnetic stimulation of the nervous system. *Phys. Med. Biol.*, **35**: 1119–1128.

Tokimura, H., Di, L., V, Tokimura, Y. et al. (2000). Short latency inhibition of human hand motor cortex by somatosensory input from the hand. *J. Physiol.*, **523**: 503–513.

Tokimura, H., Ridding, M.C., Tokimura, Y., Amassian, V.E. & Rothwell, J.C. (1996). Short latency facilitation between pairs of threshold magnetic stimuli applied to human motor cortex. *Electroencephalogr. Clin. Neurophysiol.*, **101**: 263–272.

Topka, H., Cohen, L.G., Cole, R.A. & Hallett, M. (1991). Reorganization of corticospinal pathways following spinal cord injury. *Neurology*, **41**: 1276–1283.

Touge, T., Gerschlager, W., Brown, P. & Rothwell, J.C. (2001). Are the after-effects of low-frequency rTMS on motor cortex excitability due to changes in the efficacy of cortical synapses? *Clin. Neurophysiol.*, **112**: 2138–2145.

Tsuji, T. & Rothwell, J.C. (2002). Long lasting effects of rTMS and associated peripheral sensory input on MEPs, SEPs and transcortical reflex excitability in humans. *J. Physiol.*, **540**: 367–376.

Ugawa, Y., Day, B.L., Rothwell, J.C., Thompson, P.D., Merton, P.A. & Marsden, C.D. (1991a). Modulation of motor cortical excitability by electrical stimulation over the cerebellum in man. *J. Physiol. Lond.*, **441**: 57–72.

Ugawa, Y., Rothwell, J.C., Day, B.L., Thompson, P.D. & Marsden, C.D. (1991b). Percutaneous electrical stimulation of corticospinal pathways at the level of the pyramidal decussation in humans. *Ann. Neurol.*, **29**: 418–427.

Ugawa, Y., Uesaka, Y., Terao, Y., Hanajima, R. & Kanazawa, I. (1994). Magnetic stimulation of corticospinal pathways at the foramen magnum level in humans. *Ann. Neurol.*, **36**: 618–624.

Ugawa, Y., Uesaka, Y., Terao, Y., Hanajima, R. & Kanazawa, I. (1995). Magnetic stimulation over the cerebellum in humans. *Ann. Neurol.*, **37**: 703–713.

Ugawa, Y., Uesaka, Y., Terao, Y. et al. (1996). Clinical utility of magnetic corticospinal tract stimulation at the foramen magnum level. *Electroencephalogr. Clin. Neurophysiol.*, **101**: 247–254.

Ugawa, Y., Uesaka, Y., Terao, Y., Hanajima, R. & Kanazawa, I. (1997). Magnetic stimulation of the descending and ascending tracts at the foramen magnum level. *Electromyogr. Motor Contr. Electroencephalogr. Clin. Neurophysiol.*, **105**: 128–131.

Walsh, V. & Rushworth, M. (1999). A primer of magnetic stimulation as a tool for neuropsychology. *Neuropsychologia*, **37**: 125–135.

Walsh, V., Ellison, A., Battelli, L. & Cowey, A. (1998). Task-specific impairments and enhancements induced by magnetic stimulation of human visual area V5. *Proc. Roy Soc. Lond. B Biol. Sci.*, **265**: 537–543.

Wassermann, E.M. (1998). Risk and safety of repetitive transcranial magnetic stimulation: report and suggested guidelines from the International Workshop on the Safety of Repetitive Transcranial Magnetic Stimulation, June 5–7, 1996. *Electroencephalogr. Clin. Neurophysiol.*, **108**: 1–16.

Wassermann, E.M., McShane, L.M., Hallett, M. & Cohen, L.G. (1992). Noninvasive mapping of muscle representations in human motor cortex. *Electroencephalogr. Clin. Neurophysiol.*, **85**: 1–8.

Wassermann, E.M., Pascual-Leone, A., Valls-Sole, J., Toro, C., Cohen, L.G. & Hallett, M. (1993). Topography of the inhibitory and excitatory responses to transcranial magnetic stimulation in a hand muscle. *Electroencephalogr. Clin. Neurophysiol.*, **89**: 424–433.

Wassermann, E.M., Wang, B., Zeffiro, T.A. et al. (1996). Locating the motor cortex on the MRI with transcranial magnetic stimulation and PET. *Neuroimage*, **3**: 1–9.

Werhahn, K.J., Kunesch, E., Noachtar, S., Benecke, R. & Classen, J. (1999). Differential effects on motorcortical inhibition induced by blockade of GABA uptake in humans. *J. Physiol. Lond.*, **517**: 591–597.

Werhahn, K.J., Taylor, J., Ridding, M., Meyer, B.U. & Rothwell, J.C. (1996). Effect of transcranial magnetic stimulation over the cerebellum on the excitability of human motor cortex. *Electroencephalogr. Clin. Neurophysiol.*, **101**: 58–66.

Ziemann, U., Lonnecker, S., Steinhoff, B.J. & Paulus, W. (1996a). Effects of antiepileptic drugs on motor cortex excitability in humans: a transcranial magnetic stimulation study [see comments]. *Ann. Neurol.*, **40**: 367–378.

Ziemann, U., Rothwell, J.C. & Ridding, M.C. (1996b). Interaction between intracortical inhibition and facilitation in human motor cortex. *J. Physiol. Lond.*, **496**: 873–881.

Ziemann, U., Corwell, B. & Cohen, L.G. (1998a). Modulation of plasticity in human motor cortex after forearm ischemic nerve block. *J. Neurosci.*, **18**: 1115–1123.

Ziemann, U., Tergau, F., Wassermann, E.M., Wischer, S., Hildebrandt, J. & Paulus, W. (1998b). Demonstration of facilitatory I wave interaction in the human motor cortex by paired transcranial magnetic stimulation. *J. Physiol. Lond.*, **511**: 181–190.

3

Developmental plasticity of the corticospinal system

Janet A. Eyre

Department of Child Health, The Royal Victoria Infirmary, Newcastle-upon-Tyne, UK

The young human brain is highly plastic and thus brain lesions during development interfere with the innate development of architecture, connectivity and mapping of functions and trigger modifications in structure, wiring and representations (for review, see Payne & Lomber, 2001). In childhood the motor cortex and/or corticospinal tract is the most common site of brain damage and the pre- or immediately peri-natal period is the most common time for brain damage to occur. It is now increasingly appreciated that the corticospinal system is capable of substantial reorganization after lesions and that such reorganization is likely to underlie spontaneous partial recovery of function (Terashima, 1995; Eyre et al., 2001, 2002; Raineteau & Schwab, 2001). In the mature nervous system synaptic plasticity in pre-existing pathways, and the formation of new circuits through collateral sprouting of lesioned and unlesioned fibres, are the principal components of this recovery process (Raineteau & Schwab, 2001). In the developing nervous system it is clear that there is much greater potential for plasticity, which may involve plasticity not only of the motor areas of the ipsilesional cerebral cortex but also of the contralesional cortex, corticospinal tract formation and the development of spinal cord networks (Benecke et al., 1991; Carr et al., 1993; Cao et al., 1994; Lewine et al., 1994; Maegaki et al., 1995; Terashima, 1995; Muller et al., 1997, 1998; Nirkko et al., 1997; Graveline et al., 1998; O'Sullivan et al., 1998; Hertz-Pannier, 1999; Holloway et al., 1999; Wieser et al., 1999; Balbi et al., 2000; Chu et al., 2000; Eyre et al., 2000a, 2001; Thickbroom et al., 2001). Functional and anatomical evidence demonstrates that spontaneous plasticity can be potentiated by activity, as well as by specific experimental manipulations. Knowledge of the time course and processes of corticospinal system development and plasticity is essential both for a better understanding of current rehabilitation treatments and for the design of new strategies for the treatment of children who sustain damage to the corticospinal system early in life.

Corticospinal tract development and plasticity in subprimate mammals

The development of the corticospinal system has been studied most extensively in the rat. In the neonatal rat the corticospinal projection originates from the whole neocortex including the visual cortex (Stanfield & O'Leary, 1985; Stanfield, 1992). Not all these axons enter the grey matter, those that do initially occupy a larger terminal field and contact more spinal neurones than in the adult (Curfs et al., 1994, 1995, 1996). Corticospinal projections in several mammalian species early in development also have transient ipsilateral projections that are predominantly eliminated when maturity is reached (Stanfield, 1992). Massive axon collateral withdrawal coupled with modest corticospinal cell death leads to complete elimination of the corticospinal projection from inappropriate regions of the cortex, a reduction in the number of corticospinal axons projecting from primary sensorimotor cortex and associated areas such as the premotor cortex (Oudega et al., 1994), and predominant withdrawal of ipsilateral projections (Joosten et al., 1992). Substantial lesions of the sensorimotor cortex or corticospinal tract in subprimate mammals early in postnatal life lead to hypertrophy of the undamaged motor cortex and corticospinal projection (Hicks & D'Amato, 1870, 1877; Huttenlocher & Raichelson, 1989; Huttenlocher & Bonnier, 1991; Rouiller et al., 1991; Jansen & Low, 1996; Uematsu et al., 1996). These changes are associated with maintenance of an increased ipsilateral corticospinal projection from the undamaged hemisphere. The cells of origin of the induced aberrant ipsilateral axons are more widely distributed and are distinct from the cells of origin of the crossed or contralateral corticospinal projection (Huttenlocher & Raichelson, 1989; Reinoso & Castro, 1989; Stanfield, 1992; Jansen & Low, 1996). There is no evidence for double labelling of corticospinal neurones in neonatally hemispherectomized animals that in adulthood had spinal cord injection of fluorescent tracers (Reinoso & Castro, 1989). Thus induced ipsilaterally projecting corticospinal axons from the undamaged cortex do not arise as branches of the contralateral corticospinal projection, but arise from neurones which extend axons into the ipsilateral spinal cord during development, and whose axons would normally be withdrawn. The distribution of aberrant ipsilateral axons within the spinal grey matter resembles that of the contralateral corticospinal projection (McClung & Castro, 1975; Barth & Stanfield 1990) and synaptic contacts have been demonstrated (McClung & Castro, 1975; Leong, 1976). Ipsilateral forelimb movements are observed following stimulation of the intact cortex at abnormally low current thresholds, which are abolished by medullary pyramidotomy (Kartje-Tillotson et al., 1985, 1987).

Corticospinal development and plasticity in monkeys

It has been proposed that corticospinal innervation in primates may not be governed by the same processes nor have the degree of plasticity described in subprimate mammals (Stanfield, 1992; Armand et al., 1997). However, in the Macaque monkey a halving of the area of the cerebral cortex, from which corticospinal axons originate, has been demonstrated during the first 8 postnatal months, when brain volume overall increases by more than 30%. These changes are associated with a threefold reduction in the number of retrogradely labelled cortical neurones providing convincing evidence for an initially exuberant corticospinal projection and significant corticospinal axonal withdrawal (Galea & Darian-Smith, 1995). Although Kuypers (1962) and Armand et al. (1997) found no evidence for postnatal reduction in corticospinal synapses in the cervical spinal cord during the same period in Macaque monkeys, this may reflect the methodology employed. Both studies used anterograde labelling of axons projecting from the hand area of the primary motor cortex. Such focal anterograde labelling would not detect projection and withdrawal of corticospinal axons and synapses from other areas of the cortex, including other areas of the motor cortex. It is from these other areas that the majority of supernumerary axons arise both in subprimate mammals (Stanfield et al., 1982) and also in the Macaque monkey (Galea & Darian-Smith, 1995). Furthermore, elimination of supernumerary synapses occurs in conjunction with the proliferation of synapses from the subset of axons that are maintained. It is the subset of axons that are maintained which would be labelled by anterograde tracers. Net increases in synaptic density have been observed during significant axonal withdrawal in other primate systems (LaMantia & Rakic, 1990, 1994).

Studies in monkeys have failed to reveal plasticity of corticospinal tract development following lesions. However, no study has yet replicated the circumstances in which plasticity has been demonstrated in subprimate mammals and in human (see below). Passingham et al. (1983) performed lesions too late with all but one being between postnatal days 23 and 89. Rouiller et al. (1991) made very focal lesions in the motor cortex and demonstrated substantial reorganization of the surrounding motor cortex on the same side as the lesion. Reorganization of the ipsilateral projection from the undamaged hemisphere in subprimate mammals has only been observed following large lesions such as ablation or extensive infarction of the motor cortex, or following pyramidotomy. Finally, Galea and Darian Smith (1997) performed hemisection of the cervical spinal cord in the monkey. Thus the lesion was below the pyramidal decussation and involved the projections from both hemispheres. Galea and Darian Smith's detailed study did, however, exclude significant branching of corticospinal axons at spinal levels in response to early lesions of the corticospinal tract.

Corticospinal development and plasticity in human

Studies within our laboratory of embryonic human brain development between 6 and 7 weeks postconceptional age (PCA) reveal that the cortical plate is barely formed at that time and no outgrowth of GAP43 positive axons can be detected (Hagan et al., 1999). It is surprising therefore that the most widely quoted studies of human corticospinal tract development (Humphrey, 1960; O'Rahily & Müller, 1994) claim that corticospinal axons reach the medulla by 8 weeks PCA. Decussation is thought to occur before 15 weeks PCA and corticospinal axons to have reached as far as the lumbar enlargement by 18 weeks PCA. Remarkably little neuroanatomical work on the developing human corticospinal tract has been done since these original observations. We have recently confirmed that human corticospinal axons reach the lower cervical spinal cord by 24 weeks PCA at the latest (Fig. 3.1). Following a waiting period of up to a few weeks they progressively innervate the grey matter such that there is extensive innervation of spinal neurones, including motoneurones, prior to birth (Eyre et al., 2000b, 2002). By 40 weeks PCA corticospinal axons have begun to express neurofilaments and to undergo myelination (Fig. 3.2). These anatomical findings of early corticospinal

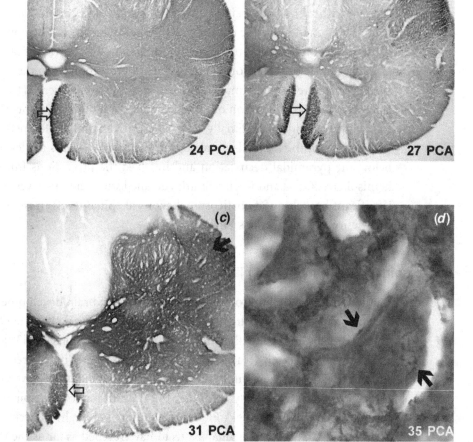

Fig. 3.1   Anatomical studies of human spinal cord $C_{5,6}$ (*a*) 24 weeks PCA. GAP43 immunore-activity is widespread in white and grey matter (*b*) 27 weeks PCA. Corticospinal tracts are the only major axon tracts expressing GAP43 from which weaker immunoreactivity extends into the intermediate grey matter. (*c*) 31 weeks PCA. Immunoreactivity is also now intense in the intermediate grey matter and present in motoneuronal pools and dorsal horn. (*d*) 35 weeks PCA. Section counterstained with cresyl violet. M, Nissl stained motoneuronal cell body; solid arrows, GAP43 expressing varicose axons. Motoneurone cell bodies are closely apposed by GAP43 immunoreactive varicose axons. (*a*), (*b*) and (*c*), Scale bar, 500 μm. Solid arrows mark the lateral, and open arrows the anterior corticospinal tracts. (*d*) Scale bar, 20 μm. (From Eyre et al., 2000.)

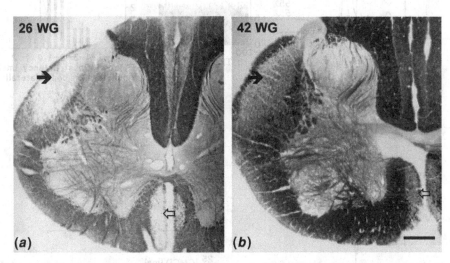

Fig. 3.2   Onset of myelination of the human corticospinal tract in the lower cervical spinal cord. Sections of human spinal cord, level $C_{5,6}$ (*a*) 24 weeks PCA and (*b*) 40 weeks PCA stained for myelin. The filled arrows mark the lateral corticospinal tract and the open arrows the anterior corticospinal tract, both of which stand out because of their lack of myelination relative to most other white matter tracts. From our studies of GAP43 immunoreactivity (Fig. 3.1) we know that corticospinal axons are present at 24 weeks PCA and it appears at this age that only occasional fibres within the tract may be myelinated. By birth, myelination is under way, although far from complete. Myelination appears to be proceeding in a ventromedial to dorsolateral direction in the lateral tract. Note also the marked asymmetry of the two anterior corticospinal tracts, a common feature of the human spinal cord. (From Eyre et al., 2002.)

innervation are confirmed by neurophysiological studies demonstrating that functional synaptic corticospinal projections to motoneurones and spinal interneurones are established prenatally during the final trimester of pregnancy (Eyre et al., 2000). These combined morphological and neurophysiological observations provide strong evidence for the prenatal establishment of functional corticospinal innervation in human even though it is not associated with a significant developmental milestone of motor behaviour. It is likely that this early innervation, rather than furthering motor control *per se*, occurs to allow activity in the corticospinal system as a whole to shape development of the motor cortex and spinal motor centres (Eyre et al., 2000, 2001).

In the newborn we have demonstrated significant bilateral innervation of spinal motoneuronal pools from each motor cortex. Thus, focal TMS of

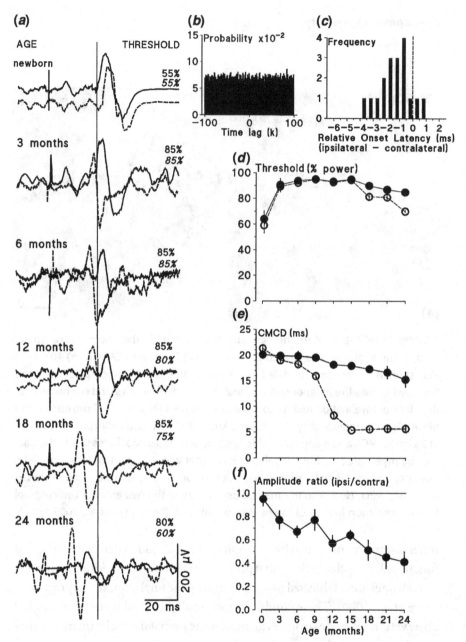

Fig. 3.3   (a) Serial ipsilateral and contralateral responses recorded in the EMG of biceps following TMS of the left cortex in the same normal subject at increasing ages. The continuous line traces are from ipsilateral (left) biceps and dashed line traces are from contralateral (right) biceps. The stimulus artefact marks the application of TMS. The vertical line indicates the onset of the ipsilateral response when the subject was newborn. Thresholds for the responses are recorded on the right above the traces. Those in italics are for contralateral responses. (Adapted from Eyre et al., 2001.)

the motor cortex evokes responses in ipsilateral and contralateral muscles that have similar thresholds and amplitudes but shorter onset latencies ipsilaterally, consistent with the shorter ipsilateral pathway length (Eyre et al., 2001) (Fig. 3.3). In longitudinal and cross-sectional studies of normal babies and children, neurophysiological findings are consistent with the significant withdrawal of corticospinal axons over the first 24 postnatal months (Eyre et al., 2001), as has been observed in subhuman primates (Galea & Darian-Smith, 1995) (Figs. 3.3 and 3.4(j)–(l)). Furthermore, rapid differential development of the ipsilateral and contralateral projections occurs over this time, so that responses at 2 years postnatal age in ipsilateral muscles are less frequent, significantly smaller, and have longer onset latencies and had higher thresholds than responses in contralateral muscles (Figs. 3.3 and 3.4 (j)–(l)). This differential development of the ipsilateral responses is consistent with a greater withdrawal of ipsilateral corticomotoneuronal projections than contralateral, as has been observed during development of the corticospinal tract in animals (Joosten et al., 1992; Stanfield, 1992). In addition, it is consistent with faster growth of axonal diameters in the

---

Fig. 3.3 (*cont.*) (*b*) Cross-correlogram of multi-unit EMGs from contracting right and left biceps in the same newborn subject illustrated in (*a*) demonstrating no evidence for common drive to the motoneuronal pools. (*c*) The relative onset latencies for the ipsilateral and contralateral responses in the 18 neonates studied, calculated by subtracting the onset of the ipsilateral response from that of the contralateral. These data demonstrate the significantly shorter onset latency of ipsilateral responses in the newborn period. (*d*)–(*f*) Longitudinal data from nine subjects, including the subject illustrated in (*a*), studied at 3-monthly intervals. Filled symbols and continuous lines represent data from ipsilateral and open symbols and dashed lines from contralateral responses. The symbols represent the mean and the vertical lines the 95% confidence limits for mean. Threshold was measured as the % of maximum stimulator output. CMCD is the central conduction delay within the corticospinal tract. The amplitude ratio was calculated by dividing the peak to peak amplitude of the ipsilateral responses by that of the contralateral. The horizontal dashed line in (*d*) indicates a ratio of one where responses are of equal size. These data demonstrate differential development of ipsilateral and contralateral responses evoked by TMS so that by 15 months ipsilateral responses have significantly higher thresholds, longer CMCDs and smaller amplitudes compared to contralateral responses.

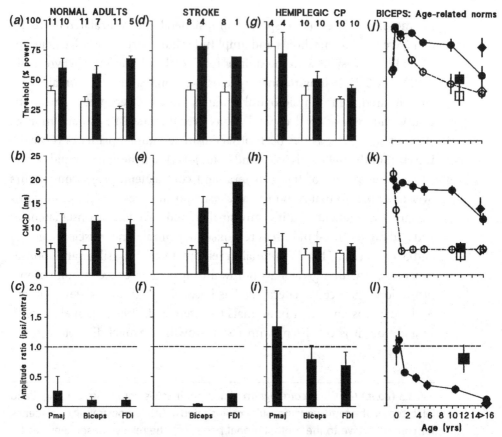

Fig. 3.4   (a)–(i) Means ± 95% confidence limits for threshold (a), (d), (g), central motor
conduction delay (CMCD) (b), (e), (h) and amplitude ratio (c), (f), (i) for ipsilateral
responses (solid bars) and contralateral responses (open bars) evoked by TMS of
the left hemisphere in normal adults (a)–(c), and the intact hemisphere in subjects
with hemiplegia following stroke (d)–(f) and those with spastic hemiplegic cerebral palsy (CP) (g)–(i). (j)–(l) Ontogeny of ipsilateral and contralateral responses
in biceps muscle. Data from the cross-sectional study of 84 subjects, TMS of the left
cortex in normal subjects •; TMS of the intact cortex in subjects with spastic hemiplegic cerebral palsy ■; and subjects with stroke ♦. Filled symbols and continuous
lines represent data from ipsilateral responses and open symbols and dashed lines
from contralateral. The symbols represent the mean and the vertical lines the 95%
confidence limits. Threshold (a), (d), (g), (j) is measured as the % of maximum
stimulator output. The CMCD (b), (e), (h), (k) is the central motor conduction delay
within the corticospinal tract. The amplitude ratio (c), (f), (i), (l) was calculated by
dividing the amplitude of the ipsilateral responses by that of the contralateral. The
dashed horizontal line indicates a ratio of one where responses are of equal size.
(From Eyre et al., 2001.)

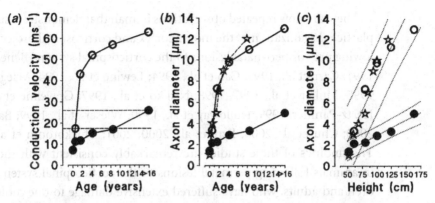

Fig. 3.5   (a) Development of corticospinal axon conduction velocities in (o) contralateral and
(•) ipsilateral corticospinal projections in man. The conduction velocities are estimated from central motor conduction delays (Eyre et al., 1991, 2000) and estimates
of the conduction distance within the corticospinal tract (see Eyre et al., 1991, 2000).
(b) and (c) The diameter of the largest corticospinal axons in human subjects in
relation to age and mean body height. Open stars represent data obtained by direct
measurement at the level of the pyramid in a newborn baby and in subjects aged 4,
8 and 18 months and 2, 3, 4 and 7 years, reported by Verhaart (1950) and in a subject aged 13 years reported by Häggpvist (1937). Open and closed circles represent
the mean axonal diameters in the contralateral and ipsilateral corticospinal tract, respectively. The axonal diameters were estimated from the conduction velocities of
the subjects in (a) using the ratio of 5.2 m s^{-1}/μm between the conduction velocity
of corticospinal axons and their diameters in the medullary pyramid (Olivier et al.,
1997).

contralateral corticospinal projection than in the ipsilateral projection
(Fig. 3.5). The small and late ipsilateral responses observed in older children and adults are consistent with the persistence of a small ipsilateral
corticomotoneuronal projection, with slower conducting axons than contralateral projections. This conclusion is supported by anatomical studies in
human and monkeys that demonstrate in maturity the corticospinal tract
has approximately 8–15% of uncrossed axons (Nathan et al., 1990; Galea &
Darian-Smith, 1994; Armand et al., 1997). These ipsilaterally projecting axons have been shown in human to arise from similar areas of the cortex and
to have a similar pattern of spinal innervation to the contralateral projection (Liu & Chambers, 1964; Nathan et al., 1990; Galea & Darian-Smith,
1994).

There are now repeated observations in man that demonstrate substantial plastic reorganization of the motor cortex and corticospinal projections following pre- or peri-natal lesions to the corticospinal system (Benecke et al., 1991; Carr et al., 1993; Cao et al., 1994; Lewine et al., 1994; Maegaki et al., 1995; Muller et al., 1997, 1998; Nirkko et al., 1997; Graveline et al., 1998; Hertz-Pannier, 1999; Holloway et al., 1999; Wieser et al., 1999; Balbi et al., 2000; Chu et al., 2000; Eyre et al., 2000, 2001; Thickbroom et al., 2001). The findings of these studies are remarkably consistent with those made in animals following perinatal lesions to the corticospinal system. In children and adults, who have suffered extensive damage to one motor cortex early in development, significant bilateral corticospinal innervation of spinal motoneuronal pools persists from the undamaged hemisphere. Thus focal TMS of the intact motor cortex evokes large responses in ipsilateral and contralateral muscles, which have similar latencies and thresholds (Figs. 3.4 and 3.6). These observations have been made following perinatal unilateral brain damage arising from a variety of pathologies including infarction, dysplasia, and arteriovenous malformations (Benecke et al., 1991; Carr et al., 1993; Maegaki et al., 1995; Balbi et al., 2000; Eyre et al., 2000, 2001; Thickbroom et al., 2001). Short latency ipsilateral responses do not occur in normal subjects outside the perinatal period. Nor do they occur in subjects who acquired unilateral cortical lesions in adulthood, establishing that fast ipsilateral responses are not simply unmasked by unilateral lesions (Netz et al., 1997; Eyre et al., 2001) (Figs. 3.4 and 3.6). Furthermore, the responses in contralateral muscles evoked by stimulation of the intact motor cortex, although within the normal range for age, are abnormally clustered towards short onset latencies and low thresholds (Fig. 3.4) (Eyre et al., 2001). Together, these findings imply not only bilateral innervation of motoneuronal pools but also an increase in the number of both fast conducting ipsilateral and contralateral corticospinal axons from the intact hemisphere following perinatal unilateral lesions of the corticospinal system. This conclusion is supported by direct measurement of corticospinal axonal number in the bulbar pyramid obtained at postmortem. These measurements demonstrate significant increases in the numbers of corticospinal axons, particularly larger diameter axons, projecting from the intact hemisphere in adult subjects with spastic hemiplegic cerebral palsy, in comparison to normal subjects and those with lesions acquired in adulthood (Verhaart, 1950; Scales & Collins, 1972) (Fig. 3.7). Similarly, MRI studies of

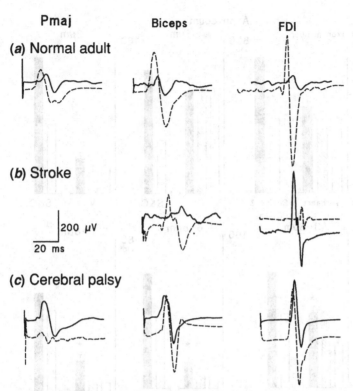

Fig. 3.6   Ipsilateral and contralateral responses recorded in the EMG of pectoralis major (Pmaj), biceps brachii (biceps) and the first dorsal interosseous muscle (FDI) following TMS of (*a*) the left hemisphere in a normal adult and (*b*) the intact hemisphere in a subject with stroke which occurred in adulthood and (*c*) a subject with spastic hemiplegic cerebral palsy. The continuous traces in (*a*), (*b*) and (*c*) are from ipsilateral muscles and dashed traces are from contralateral muscles. TMS was delivered at the onset of each trace. (Adapted from Eyre et al., 2001).

subjects with early unilateral brain damage demonstrate an increased size of the corticospinal projection from (Sener, 1995) and a shift of cortical sensorimotor functions to the intact hemisphere (Cao et al., 1994; Lewine et al., 1994; Maegaki et al., 1995; Muller et al., 1997, 1998; Nirkko et al., 1997; Graveline et al., 1998; Hertz-Pannier, 1999; Holloway et al., 1999; Wieser et al., 1999; Chu et al., 2000). Finally, short onset ipsilateral responses observed bilaterally in subjects with Kallman's syndrome are associated with significant bilateral hyperplasia of the corticospinal tract (Mayston et al., 1997). Taken together these observations support persistence of ipsilateral

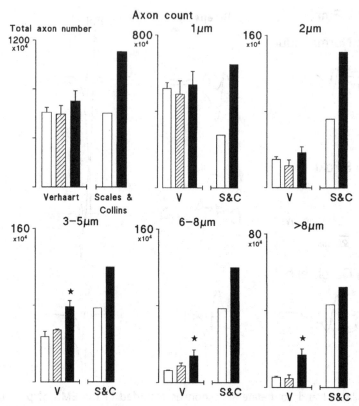

Fig. 3.7   Total axonal count and counts for axons of the specified diameters in the medullary
pyramids in normal subjects and the medullary pyramid ipsilateral to the undamaged hemisphere in subjects with unilateral brain damage involving the motor cortex. Data from Verhaart (1950) (V) who studied postmortem material from three
normal adults (open bars), four adults with hemiplegia following stroke in adulthood (hashed bars) and two adults who suffered unilateral brain damage in the
perinatal period (solid bars); Scales and Collins (S&C) who studied postmortem
material from one normal adult (open bars) and an adult who suffered unilateral
brain damage in the perinatal period (solid bars). Stars indicate statistically significant increases in axonal numbers from values in the normal adults.

and contralateral corticospinal projections from the intact hemisphere following unilateral brain damage early in development, which would normally have been withdrawn during subsequent development. Whilst some
studies indicate the increased ipsilateral corticospinal projections arise from
the primary motor cortex of the intact hemisphere (Sabatini et al., 1994;
Nirkko et al., 1997) a more common finding is of the projection arising

from non-primary motor and multimodal association areas of the non-affected hemisphere (Pascual-Leone et al., 1992; Cao et al., 1994; Lewine et al., 1994; Muller et al., 1997; Graveline et al., 1998; Bernasconi et al., 2000; Brittar et al., 2000; Chu et al., 2000). These observations imply the maintenance of corticospinal projections from areas of the cortex where axons projecting to the spinal cord would normally have been withdrawn during development.

In our laboratory, we observed different patterns of corticospinal system development after unilateral and bilateral lesions to the corticospinal tract when we compared the contralateral corticospinal projections in subjects with severe spastic hemiplegic and severe spastic quadriplegic cerebral palsy, who had similarly severe pathology of hand and upper limb movement control (Eyre et al., 1989, 2000, 2001). In subjects with spastic hemiplegic cerebral palsy, TMS of the damaged cortex either failed to evoke responses or evoked responses with abnormally high thresholds and prolonged onset latencies. In contrast, responses with relatively short onset latencies and low thresholds were evoked from the intact hemisphere. In subjects with spastic quadriparesis, responses from both hemispheres lay predominantly within the normal range (Fig. 3.8). These observations are consistent with a significant reduction in the corticospinal projection from damaged hemisphere and an increased projection from the intact hemisphere in subjects with unilateral lesions, whilst those with bilateral lesions maintain qualitatively normal projections from both hemispheres. An explanation for these apparently contradictory findings may be found in the studies of Martin and his colleagues (Martin et al., 1999; Martin & Lee, 1999). In the kitten, unilateral inhibition of the motor cortex causes exuberant ipsilateral and contralateral corticospinal projections from the uninhibited cortex to be maintained, at the expense of those from the inhibited cortex, which becomes much reduced (Martin et al., 1999). Martin and his coworkers established that the reduction in the inhibited contralateral projection was due to competition between the two projections and not due to reduced activity *per se*, since in a subsequent experiment bilateral inhibition of the motor cortices led to qualitatively normal projections from both cortices (Martin & Lee, 1999) (Fig. 3.9). Competitive activity-dependent refinement of bilateral corticospinal projections demonstrates parallels between the mechanisms governing early postnatal development of the corticospinal system and that of the visual system. Monocular retinal activity blockade,

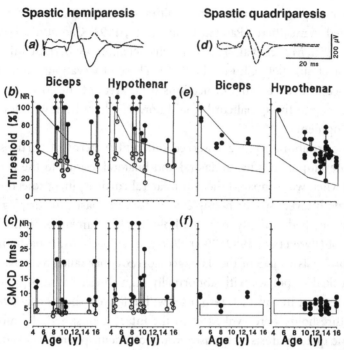

Fig. 3.8   (a) and (d) Contralateral responses evoked in biceps following TMS of the intact (continuous line) and lesioned (dashed line) motor cortices in (a) a subject with spastic hemiplegic cerebral palsy and (d) the left and right motor cortices in a subject with spastic quadriplegic cerebral palsy. TMS was applied at the start of each trace. In the graphs (b), (c), (e) and (f) the vertical lines join data from stimulation of each motor cortex in the same subject. Filled circles represent stimulation of lesioned cortices and open of the intact cortex. The boxed areas represent the ±2 standard deviation ranges for age obtained in 372 normal subjects (Eyre et al., 1991). (b) and (e) Thresholds in subjects with spastic hemiplegic and quadriplegic cerebral palsy respectively. Threshold is expressed as % of maximum power delivered by the stimulator. (c) and (f) Central motor conduction delay (CMCD) in the corticospinal tract (in subjects with spastic hemiplegic and quadriplegic cerebral palsy, respectively. NR = no response. (Adapted from Eyre et al., 1989.)

for example, reduces the thalamic territory occupied by silenced retinogeniculate terminals and expands the active terminal's territory. By contrast, binocular activity blockade, which similarly eliminates interocular competition, does not (Penn & Shatz, 1999).

Activity-dependent competition between the two cerebral hemispheres for spinal synaptic space implies that the degree of abnormality of the

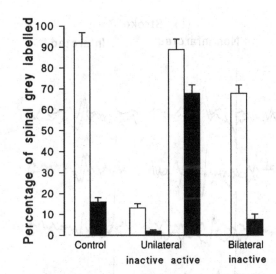

Fig. 3.9   The percentage of spinal grey matter labelled in the cervical spinal cord by anterograde transport of label placed on the forelimb area of the sensorimotor cortex in
three groups of animals: four normal control cats; four cats who had unilateral infu-
sion of muscimol and four cats who had bilateral muscimol infusions. All infusions
were made 3 mm below the pial surface at the centre of the forelimb area of the
motor cortex. The infusions were continuous between postnatal weeks 3 and 7,
which is the period of postnatal refinements of corticospinal terminations in cats.
The open bars represent cervical spinal cord contralateral to the cortex labelled
and the solid bars the ipsilateral cervical spinal cord. Inactive: data obtained from
labelling projections from motor cortices infused with muscimol. Active: data obtained from labelling projections from normal motor cortices. (Data derived from
Martin et al., 1999; Martin & Lee, 1999.)

corticospinal projection following unilateral lesions may not reflect simply the extent of the initial lesion, but also the consequential competitive
disadvantage of surviving corticospinal projections. Such competitive disadvantage would lead to corticospinal projections from the intact hemisphere progressively replacing the surviving corticospinal projections from
the damaged hemisphere and thus to progressively worsening hemiplegia
with development. Recent observations in longitudinal study of babies who
have suffered a stroke at birth involving the motor cortex unilaterally,
supports these conclusions. In these babies we have observed responses
to TMS of the damaged cortex soon after birth, which become progressively more difficult to elicit over the subsequent 3 to 6 months and which
then disappear. This pattern of development is associated with the rapid

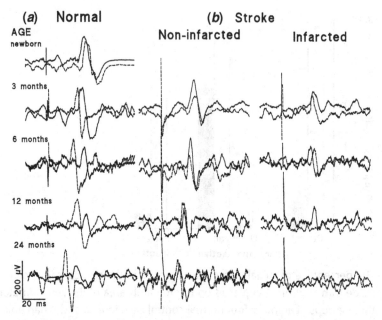

Fig. 3.10   Serial ipsilateral and contralateral responses recorded in the EMG of biceps at increasing ages following TMS of: (*a*) the left cortex in a normal subject and (*b*) the
non-infarcted and the infarcted hemisphere in a subject who suffered a unilateral
stroke at birth. The continuous line traces are from biceps ipsilateral to the cortex
stimulated and the dashed line traces are from the contralateral biceps. The stimulus
artefact marks the application of TMS.

development in parallel of the contralateral and ipsilateral corticospinal projections from the undamaged hemisphere such that both have abnormally
short onset latencies by 24 months of age (Smith, Villagra & Eyre, unpublished data) (Fig. 3.10). This pattern of development is also consistent with
the clinical observation that signs of hemiplegia may not become established
in children until the second year of life (Bouza et al., 1994).

Our longitudinal studies of the development of the corticospinal system
following perinatal infarction (Smith, Villagra and Eyre, unpublished data)
also confirm the observations of Rouiller et al. (1998) that reorganization
of the ipsilesional cortex can also occur with functional resiting of the area
of the motor cortex within the damaged hemisphere (Alkadhi et al., 2000).
This can either be in immediately adjacent areas of the primary motor cortex
(Maegaki et al., 1995), within non-primary motor areas (Alkadhi et al., 2000;

Brittar et al., 2000) and in other cases reorganization of function may occur to more remote sites in the same hemisphere (Chollet et al., 1991). The exact factors that govern intrahemispheric vs. interhemispheric reorganization after sensorimotor lesions during development are not understood. It is likely that reorganization is influenced by overall cortical development and specification at the time of the lesion, the fractional size of the lesion, the availability of sufficient and appropriate juxta-lesional cortex, the absence or presence of transient corticospinal projections (Martin et al., 1999; Martin & Lee, 1999; Eyre et al., 2001) and the maturational status of the system as a whole at the time of the lesion (Eyre et al., 2000).

The temporal limit of plasticity of both the ipsi- and contra-lesional motor cortices and their corticospinal projections is at present unknown. The existence of critical periods for substantial experience-dependent plasticity has been clearly demonstrated for the visual, auditory and somatosensory systems and for language development in humans. By starting periods of monocular deprivation at progressively older ages, Hubel and Wiese (1970) first documented that ocular dominance plasticity is confined to a critical period which in the cat extends from 3 weeks to about 3 months of age. Deprivation-induced plasticity occurs rapidly at the height of the critical period. In their original studies Wiesel and Hubel monocularly deprived animals for months. In later work, they found that robust effects were observed with as little as a week of deprivation. Subsequent studies by many other investigators showed that as little as 8 hours of deprivation could produce synaptic depression in the visual cortex (Bear & Rittenhouse, 1999). The neurophysiological consequences are maximal after 48 hours of monocular deprivation in animals at the height of the critical period. It is possible therefore, that during critical periods, relatively short periods of relative inactivity of motor cortex, induced by ischemia, or over-activity induced by seizures, may lead to permanent plastic changes in the development of the motor cortex and corticospinal projections.

Finally, many diverse studies in animals and in human establish that spinal cord development during a critical period early in development is also shaped by activity in descending motor pathways including the corticospinal tract (Wolpaw & Tennissen, 2001). Spinally mediated muscle stretch reflexes and flexion withdrawal reflexes, which are poorly focused in the newborn, become precisely and appropriately focused during early life

(O'Sullivan, 1991; Levinsson et al., 1999). When lesions occur in the perinatal period to the corticospinal system, the development of α-motoneurones and their afferent segmental reflex control is secondarily disrupted (O'Sullivan et al., 1991, 1998; Levinsson et al., 1999; Gibson et al., 2000; Wolpaw & Tennissen, 2001). This implies a role for the corticomotoneuronal system in the activity-dependent regulation of the development of spinal motor centres. Existing literature in animals including monkeys establishes a critical period in early development, in which synaptic inputs from descending motor pathways and from segmental afferents shape spinal motor centre development. Motoneuronal cell soma size, dendritic morphology and the pattern of synaptic input have been shown to be altered by activity deprivation during critical periods in early development (McCouch et al., 1968; Kalb & Hockfield, 1992; Commissiong & Sauve, 1993; O'Hanlon & Lowrie, 1993, 1995; Kalb, 1994; Kalb & Fox, 1997; Dekkers & Navarrete, 1998; Gibson et al., 2000). The neurotransmitters of the corticospinal tract are glutamate and aspartate (Giuffrida & Rustioni, 1989; Valtschanoff et al., 1993). Activity-dependent development of corticospinal synapse formation and spinal motor centres is likely to be contingent upon NMDA receptor activation in a similar manner to activity-dependent development of the vertebrate visual system (Constantine-Paton et al., 1990; Constantine-Paton & Cline, 1998; Bear & Rittenhouse, 1999). Molecular markers for neural differentiation indicate that motoneurones in developing kittens and rats undergo activity-dependent development during a circumscribed critical period, and this requires activation of NMDA receptors (Kalb & Hockfield, 1992; Kalb, 1994; Maier et al., 1995). Significant levels of high affinity NMDA receptors are transiently expressed in humans in the ventral horn from 24 weeks PCA to 2 months postnatally (Kalb & Fox, 1997), indicating that a critical period for plasticity in α-motoneurone development is also likely to occur in humans in the perinatal period. Corticospinal axons are actively growing, innervating spinal cord and expressing GAP43 during this period and are thus also likely to have a high degree of plasticity (Benowitz & Routtenberg, 1997). Such observations throw new light on 'cerebral palsy', a term originally used by William Osler (1889) to highlight the significant consequences on motor development of lesions to the brain which occur in the perinatal period. It is likely that William Osler's seminal observations identify the perinatal period, not only because of the special vulnerability of the motor system to damage at this time (Johnston, 1998), but also because abnormal or decreased activity in the corticospinal system during this critical perinatal period will secondarily disrupt development of the motor cortex, corticospinal projections and spinal motor centres.

Functional and anatomical evidence exists that spontaneous plasticity can be potentiated and shaped by activity. The clinical importance and urgency of understanding further the potential for, and different patterns of, plasticity in the corticospinal system with age is best illustrated by the recent development of constraint-induced movement therapy to promote cortical plasticity for adults after stroke. Postlesional plasticity of representational maps in the motor cortex in the adult depends strongly on use of the affected hand (Nudo & Milliken, 1996; Nudo et al., 1996). Constraint-induced movement therapy has therefore been developed for adults recovering from stroke. It consists of two components: (i) constraining movement of the non-paretic upper limb for prolonged periods and (ii) intensive training of the paretic upper limb. Motor performance in the impaired arm has been demonstrated to improve and this is associated with increases in the size of the cortical area where TMS evokes responses in paretic muscles, suggesting improved functional reorganization of the damaged cortex (Taub et al., 1999). The application of this therapy to improve functional outcome following unilateral infarction in the neonate or young infant is being discussed and may even be being applied in some centres. Restraint of a limb in animal experiments during development, however, significantly increases the ipsilateral and contralateral corticospinal projections to spinal segments innervating that limb (Huttenlocher & Bonnier, 1991) possibly because corticospinal axons are in competition with segmental afferents for synaptic space and limb restraint reduces segmental afferent activity. Thus in very young children it may be more appropriate to restrain the affected limb to reinforce its corticospinal projection. In this context note that early inhibitive casting of affected limbs is currently used in rehabilitation of infants with spastic cerebral palsy. The rationale for its use is to prevent the development of contractures. Although inhibitive casting has not been systematically evaluated, there are several descriptive reports of a 'permanent reduction in spasticity and enhanced hand function' (Yasukawa, 1990; Law et al., 1991) following a period of serial casting.

Restraining the non-paretic limb in very young children has the potential to exacerbate the disability by increasing the competitive advantage of the corticospinal axons of the intact hemisphere compared to those of the damaged hemisphere. Understanding the potential for plastic reorganization of the corticospinal system during development in humans is therefore essential, not only to prevent inappropriate and potentially harmful application of therapies developed for adults, but also to allow development of appropriate interventions that would maximize functional reorganization.

The use of enriched environments and appropriately targeted training strategies are likely to potentiate the capacity of the brain to compensate for lesion-induced deficits and allow relatively normal organized behaviour. Pharmacological interventions and transplants of embryonic and fetal material are also likely to have important roles in repair and regeneration of the corticospinal system during development. Understanding of the developmental plasticity of the corticospinal system is likely therefore to lead to treatments and interventions that maximize the functional outcome for children with cerebral palsy.

REFERENCES

Alkadhi, H., SS K, Crelier, G. et al. (2000). Plasticity of the human motor cortes in patients with arteriovenous malformations: a functional MR imaging study. *Am. J. Neuroradiol.*, **21**: 1423–1433.

Armand, J., Olivier, E., Edgley, S.A. & Lemon, R.N. (1997). Postnatal development of corticospinal projections from motor cortex to the cervical enlargement in the Macaque monkey. *J. Neurosci.*, **17**: 261–266.

Balbi, P., Trojano, L., Ragno, M., Perretti, A. & Santoro, L. (2000). Patterns of motor control reorganization in a patient with mirror movements. *Clin. Neurophysiol.*, **111**: 318–325.

Barth, T.M. & Stanfield, B.B. (1990). The recovery of forelimb placing behaviour in rats with neonatal unilateral cortical damage involves the remaining hemisphere. *J. Neurosci.*, **10**: 3449–3459.

Bear, M. & Rittenhouse, C. (1999). Molecular basis for induction of ocular dominance plasticity. *J. Neurobiol.*, **41**: 83–91.

Benecke, R., Meyer, B.U. & Freund, H.J. (1991). Reorganisation of descending motor pathways in patients after hemispherectomy and severe hemispheric lesions demonstrated by magnetic brain stimulation. *Exp. Brain Res.*, **32**: 419–426.

Benowitz, L.I. & Routtenberg, A. (1997). GAP-43 an intrinsic determinant of neuronal development and plasticity. *Trends Neurosci.*, **20**: 84–91.

Bernasconi, A., Bernasconi, N., Lassonde, M. et al. (2000). Sensorimotor organization in patients who have undergone hemispherectomy: a study with 15 O-water PET and somatosensory evoked potentials. *Neuroreport*, **11**: 3085–3090.

Bouza, H., Dubowitz, L., Rutherford, M. & Pennock J. (1994). Prediction of outcome in children with congenital hemiplegia: a magnetic resonance imaging study. *Neuropediatrics*, **25**: 60–66.

Brittar, R., Pitto, A. & Reutens, D. (2000). Somatosensory representation in patients who have undergone hemispherectomy: a functional magnetic resonance imaging study. *J. Neurosurg.*, **92**: 45–51.

Cao, Y., Vikingstad, E.M., Huttenlocher, P.R., Towle, V.L. & Levin, D.N. (1994). Functional magnetic resonance studies of the reorganisation of human sensorimotor area after unilateral brain injury in the perinatal period. *Proc. Natl Acad. Sci., USA*, **91**: 9612–9616.

Carr, L.J., Harrison, L.M., Evans, A.L. & Stephens, J.A. (1993). Patterns of central motor reorganisation in hemiplegic cerebral palsy. *Brain*, **166**: 1223–1247.

Chollet, F., Di Piero, V., Wise, R. et al. (1991). The functional anatomy of motor recovery after stroke in humans: a study with positron emission tomography. *Ann. Neurol.*, **29**: 63–71.

Chu, D., Huttenlocher, P., Levin, D. & Towle, V. (2000). Reorganization of the hand somatosensory cortex following perinatal unilateral brain injury. *Neuropediatrics*, **2000**: 63–69.

Commissiong, J.W. & Sauve, Y. (1993). Neurophysiological basis of functional recovery in the neonatal spinalised rat. *Exp. Brain Res.*, **96**: 473–479.

Constantine-Paton, M., Cline, H. & Debski, E. (1990). Patterned activity, synaptic convergence and the NMDA receptor in developing visual pathways. *Annu. Rev. Neurosci.*, **13**: 129–154.

Constantine-Paton, M. & Cline, H.T. (1998). LTP and activity-dependent synaptogenesis: the more alike they are the more different they become. *Curr. Opin. Neurobiol.*, **8**: 139–148.

Curfs, M.H.J.M., Gribnan, A.A.M. & Dederen, P.J.W.C. (1994). Selective elimination of transient corticospinal projections in the rat cervical spinal grey matter. *Brain Res. Dev. Brain Res.*, **78**: 182–190.

Curfs, M.H.J.M., Gribnan, A.A.M., Dedren, P.J.W.C. & Bergervoet-Vernooij, H.W.M. (1995). Transient functional connections between the developing corticospinal tract and cervical spinal interneurone as demonstrated by c-fos immunohistochemistry. *Dev. Brain Res.*, **87**: 214–219.

Curfs, M.H.J.M., Gribnan, A.A.M. & Dederen, P.J.W.C. (1996). Direct cortico-motoneuronal synaptic contacts are present in the adult rat cervical spinal cord and are first established at postnatal day 7. *Neurosci. Lett.*, **205**: 123–126.

Dekkers, J. & Navarrete, R. (1998). Persistence of somatic and dendritic growth associated processes and induction of dendritic sprouting in motoneurones with neonatal axonal injury in rats. *Neuroreport*, **9**: 1523–1527.

Eyre, J., Gibson, M., Koh, T. & Miller, S. (1989). Corticospinal transmission excited by electromagnetic stimulation of the brain is impaired in children with spastic hemiparesis but not those with quadriparesis. *J. Physiol. (Lond.)*, **414**: 9P.

Eyre, J.A., Miller, S. & Ramesh, V. (1991). Constancy of central conduction delays during development in man: investigation of motor and somatosensory pathways. *J. Physiol. (Lond.)*, **434**: 441–452.

Eyre, J.A., Miller, S., Clowry, G.J., Conway, E.A. & Watts, C. (2000a). Functional corticospinal projections are established prenatally in the human foetus permitting involvement in the development of spinal motor centres. *Brain*, **123**: 51–64.

Eyre, J., Taylor, J., Villagra, F. & Miller, S. (2000b). Exuberant ipsilateral corticospinal projections are present in the human newborn and withdrawn during development probably involving an activity-dependent process. *Dev. Med. Child Neurol.*, **82**: 12.

Eyre, J., Taylor, J., Villagra, F., Smith, M. & Miller, S. (2001). Evidence of activity dependent withdrawal of corticospinal projections during development in man. *Neurology*, **57**: 1543–1554.

Eyre, J.A., Miller, S. & Clowry, G.J. (2002). Development of the corticospinal tract in man. In *Handbook of Transcranial Magnetic Stimulation*, ed. A. Pascual-Leone, A. Davey, G. Wasserman, E.M. & J. Rothwell, pp. 235–249. London: Arnold.

Galea, M. & Darian-Smith, I. (1994). Multiple corticospinal neuron populations in the macaque monkey are specified by their unique cortical origins, spinal terminations, and connections. *Cereb. Cortex*, **4**: 166–194.

Galea, M.P. & Darian-Smith, I. (1995). Postnatal maturation of the direct corticospinal projections in the macaque monkey. *Cereb. Cortex*, **5**: 518–540.

Galea, M.P. & Darian-Smith, I. (1997). Corticospinal projection patterns following unilateral section of the cervical spinal cord in the newborn and juvenile macaque monkey. *J. Comp. Neurol.*, **381**: 282–306.

Gibson, C.L., Arnott, G.A. & Clowry, G.C. (2000). Plasticity in the rat spinal cord seen in response to lesions to the motor cortex during development but not to lesions in maturity. *Exp. Neurol.*, **166**: 422–434.

Giuffrida, R. & Rustioni, A. (1989). Glutamate and aspartate immunoreactivity in corticospinal neurones of rats. *J. Comp. Neurol.*, **288**: 154–164.

Graveline, C.J., Mikulis, D.J., Crawley, A.P. & Hwang, P.A. (1998). Regionalised sensorimotor plasticity after hemispherectomy fMRI evaluation. *Ped. Neurol.*, **19**: 337–342.

Hagan, D.M., Lisgo, S., Strachan, T. et al. (1999). Mapping gene expression domains and neuronal cell differentiation during human embryonic forebrain development. *Am. J. Hum. Gen.*, **65**: 403.

Haggqvist, G. (1937). Faseranalytische studien uber die pyramidenbahn. *Acta Psychiat. Neurol.*, **12**: 457–466.

Hertz-Pannier, L. (1999). Plasticite au cours de la maturation cerebrale:bases physogiques et etude par IRM fontionelle. *J. Neuroradiol.*, **26**: IS66–IS74.

Hicks, S. & D'Amato, C. (1870). Motor-sensory and visual behaviour after hemispherectomy in newborn and mature rats. *Exp. Neurol.*, **29**: 416–438.

Hicks, S. & D'Amato, C. (1877). Locating corticospinal neurons by retrograde axonal transport of horseradish peroxidase. *Exp. Neurol.*, **56**: 410–420.

Holloway, V., Chong, W., Connelly, A., Harkness, W. & Gadian, D. (1999). Somatomotor fMRI and the presurgical evaluation of a case of focal epilepsy. *Clin. Radiol.*, **54**: 301–303.

Hubel, D. & Wiesel, T. (1970). Laminar and columnar distribution of geniculocortical fibres in the Macaque monkey. *J. Comp. Neurol.*, **146**: 421–450.

Hittenlocher, P. & Bonnier, C. (1994). Effects of changes in the periphery on development of the corticospinal system in the rat. *Brain Res. Dev. Brain Res.*, **60**: 253–260.

Huttenlocher, P.R. & Raichelson, R.M. (1989). Effects of neonatal hemispherectomy on location and number of corticospinal neurons in the rat. *Dev. Brain Res.*, **47**: 59–69.

Humphrey, T. (1960). The development of the pyramidal tracts in human fetuses, correlated with cortical differentiation. In *Structure and Function of the Cortex*, ed. D.B. Tower & J.B. Schade. Proceedings of the Second International Meeting of Neurobiologists, pp. 93–103. Amsterdam: Elsevier.

Jansen, E.M. & Low, W.C. (1996). Quantitative analysis of contralateral hemisphere hypertrophy and sensorimotor performance in adult rats following unilateral neonatal ischemic–hypoxic brain injury. *Brain Res.*, **708**: 93–99.

Johnston, M-L. (1998). Selective vulnerability in the neonatal brain. *Am. J. Neurol. Assoc.*, **44**: 155–156.

Joosten, E.A., Schuitman, R.L., Vermelis, M.E. & Dederen, P.J. (1992). Postnatal development of the ipsilateral corticospinal component in rat spinal cord: a light and electron microscopic anterograde HRP study. *J. Comp. Neurol.*, **326**: 133–146.

Kalb, R.G. (1994). Regulation of motor neuron dendrite growth by NMDA receptor activation. *Development*, **120**: 3063–3071.

Kalb, R.G. & Fox, A.J. (1997). Synchronized over production of AMPA kainate and NMDA glutamate receptors during human spinal chord developent. *J. Comp. Neurol.*, **384**: 200–210.

Kalb, R.G. & Hockfield, S. (1992). Activity-dependent development of spinal cord motor neurons. *Brain Res. Rev.*, **17**: 283–289.

Kartje-Tillotson, G., Neafsey, E.J. & Castro, A.J. (1985). Electrophysiological analysis of motor cortical plasticity after cortical lesions in newborn rats. *Brain Res.*, **332**: 103–111.

Kartje-Tillotson, G., O' Donoghue, D.L., Dauzvardis, M.F. & Castro, A.J. (1987). Pyramidotomy abolishes the abnormal movements evoked by intracortical microstimulation in adult rats that sustained neonatal cortical lesions. *Brain Res.*, **415**: 172–177.

Kuypers, H.G.J.M. (1962). Corticospinal connections: postnatal development in the rhesus monkey. *Science*, **138**: 678–680.

LaMantia, A.S. & Rakic, P. (1990). Axonal over production and elimination in the corpus callosum of the developing rhesus monkey. *J. Neurosci.*, **10**: 2156–2175.

LaMantia, A.S. & Rakic, P. (1994). Axon over production and elimination in the anterior commissure of the developing rhesus monkey. *J. Comp. Neurol.*, **340**: 328–336.

Law, M., Cadman, D., Rosenbaum, P. et al. (1991). Neurodevelopmental therapy and upper limb extremity inhibitive casting for children with cerebral palsy. *Dev. Med. Child Neurol.*, **33**: 377–378.

Leong, S.K. (1976). A qualitative electron microscopic investigation of the anomalous corticofugal projections following neonatal lesions in the albino rat. *Brain Res.*, **107**: 1–8.

Levinsson, A., Luo, X-L., Holmberg, H. & Schouenborg, J. (1999). Developmental tuning in a spinal nociceptive system: effects of neonatal spinalisation. *J. Neurosci.*, **19**: 10397–10403.

Lewine, J.D., Astur, R.S., Davis, L.E. et al. (1994). Cortical organization in adulthood is modified by neonatal infarct: a case study. *Radiology*, **190**: 93–96.

Liu, C. & Chambers, W. (1964). An experimental study of the cortico-spinal system in the monkey. The spinal pathways and preterminal distribution of degenerating fibres following discrete lesions of the pre- and postcentral gyri and bulbar pyramid. *J. Comp. Neurol.*, **123**: 257–284.

McClung, J.R. & Castro, A.J. (1975). An ultrastructional study of ipsilateral corticospinal projections after frontal cortical lesions in newborn rats. *Anat. Rec.*, **181**: 417–418.

McCouch, G.P., Austin, G.M. & Liu, C.Y. (1968). Sprouting as a cause of spasticity. *J. Neurophysiol.*, **21**: 205–216.

Maegaki, Y., Yamamoto, T. & Takeshita, K. (1995). Plasticity of central motor and sensory pathways in a case of unilateral extensive cortical dysplasia. Investigation of magnetic resonance imaging, transcranial magnetic stimulation and short latency somatosensory evoked potentials. *Neurology*, **45**: 2255–2261.

Maier, L., Kalb, R. & Stelzner, D. (1995). NMDA antagonism during development extends sparing of hindlimb function to older spinally transected rats. *Dev. Brain Res.*, **87**: 135–144.

Martin, J.H. & Lee, S.J. (1999). Activity-dependent competition between developing corticospinal terminations. *Neuroreport*, **10**: 2277–2282.

Martin, J.H., Kably, B. & Hacking, A. (1999). Activity-dependent development of cortical axon terminations in the spinal cord and brain stem. *Exp. Brain Res.*, **125**: 184–199.

Mayston, M., Harrison, L., Quinton, R. et al. (1997). Mirror movements in X-linked Kallmann's syndrome. I. A neurophysiological study. *Brain*, **120**: 1199–1216.

Muller, R.A., Rothermel, R.D., Behen, M.E. et al. (1997). Plasticity of motor organization in children and adults. *Neuroreport*, **8**: 3103–3108.

Muller, R.A., Watson, C.E., Muzik, O., Chakraborty, P.K. & Chugani, H.T. (1998). Motor organization after early middle cerebral artery stroke: a PET study. *Pediatr. Neurol.*, **19**: 294–298.

Nathan, P., Smith, M. & Deacon, P.V. (1990). The corticospinal tracts in man. Course and location of fibres at different segmental levels. *Brain*, **113**: 303–324.

Netz, J., Lammers, T. & Hömberg, V. (1997). Reorganization of motor output in the non-affected hemisphere after stroke. *Brain*, **120**: 1579–1586.

Nirkko, A.C., Rosler, K.M., Ozdoba, C. et al. (1997). Human cortical plasticity. Functional recovery with mirror movements. *Neurology*, **48**: 1090–1093.

Nudo, R. & Milliken, G. (1996). Reorganisation of movement representations in primary motor cortex following focal ischaemic infarcts in adult squirrel monkeys. *J. Neurophysiol.*, **75**: 2144–2149.

Nudo, R., Wise, B., SiFuentes, F. & Milliken, G. (1996). Neural substrates for the effects of rehabilitative training on motor recovery after ischaemic infarct. *Science*, **271**: 1791–1794.

O'Hanlon, G.M. & Lowrie, M.B. (1993). Neonatal nerve injury causes long-term changes in growth and distribution of motoneuron dendrites in the rat. *Neuroscience*, **56**: 453–464.

O'Hanlon, G. & Lowrie, M. (1995). Nerve injury in rats causes abnormalities in motoneurone dendritic fields that differ from those that follow neonatal nerve injury. *Exp. Brain Res.*, **103**: 243–250.

Olivier, E., Edgley, S., Armand, J. & Lemon, R. (1997). An electrophysiological study of the postnatal development of the corticospinal system in the Macaque monkey. *J. Neurosci.*, **17**: 267–276.

O'Rahily, R. & Müller, F. (1994). *The Human Embryonic Brain: an Atlas of Developmental Stages.* New York: Wiley-Liss.

Osler, W. (1889). The cerebral palsies of children. In *A Clinical Study from the Infirmary for Nervous Diseases.* Philadelphia: Blakiston.

O'Sullivan, M. (1991). The development of the phasic stretch reflex in man and its pathophysiology in central motor disorders. PhD Thesis, University of Newcastle upon Tyne.

O'Sullivan, M.C., Eyre, J.A. & Miller, S. (1991). Radiation of the phasic stretch reflex in biceps brachii to muscles of the arm in man and its restriction during development. *J. Physiol. (Lond.)*, **439**: 529–543.

O'Sullivan, M.C., Miller, S. & Ramesh, V. et al. (1998). Abnormal development of biceps brachii phasic stretch reflex and persistence of short latency heteronymous excitatory responses to triceps brachii in spastic cerebral palsy. *Brain*, **121**: 2381–2395.

Oudega, M., Varon, S. & Hagg, T. (1994). Distribution of corticospinal motor neurons in the postnatal rat: quantitative evidence for massive collateral elimination and modest cell death. *J. Comp. Neurol.*, **347**: 115–126.

Pascual-Leone, A., Chugani, H. & Cohen, L. (1992). Reorganisation of human motor pathways following hemispherectomy. *Ann. Neurol.*, **32**: 261.

Passingham, R.E., Perry, R.E. & Wilkinson, F. (1983). The long term effects of removal of sensorimotor cortex in infant and adult rhesus monkeys. *Brain*, **106**: 675–705.

Payne, B. & Lomber, S. (2001). Reconstructing functional systems after lesions of the cerebral cortex. *Nat. Rev. Neurosci.*, **2**: 911–919.

Penn, A. & Shatz, C. (1999). Brain waves and brain wiring: the role of endogenous and sensory-driven neural activity in development. *Pediatr. Res.*, **45**: 447–458.

Raineteau, O. & Schwab, M. (2001). Plasticity of motor systems after incomplete spinal cord injury. *Nat. Rev. Neurosci.*, **2**: 263–273.

Reinoso, B.S. & Castro, A.J. (1989). A study of corticospinal remodelling using retrograde fluorescent tracers in rats. *Exp. Brain Res.*, **74**: 387–394.

Rouiller, E.M., Liang, P., Moret, V. & Wiesendanger, M. (1991). Trajectory of redirected corticospinal axons after unilateral lesion of the sensorimotor cortex in neonatal rat; a phaseolus vulgaris-leucoagglutinin (PHA-L) tracing study. *Exp. Neurol.* **114**: 53–65.

Rouiller, E.M., Yu, X.H., Moret, V. et al. (1998). Dexterity in adult monkeys following early lesion of the motor cortical hand area: the role of cortex adjacent to lesion. *Eur. J. Neurosci.*, **10**: 729–740.

Sabatini, U., Toni, D., Pantone, P. et al. (1994). Motor recovery after early brain damage. A case of brain plasticity. *Stroke*, **25**: 514–517.

Scales, D.A. & Collins, G.H. (1972). Cerebral degeneration with hypertrophy of the contralateral pyramid. *Arch. Neurol.*, **26**: 186–190.

Sener, R.N. (1995). Unilateral cortical dysplasia associated with contralateral hyperplasia of the brainstem. *Ped. Radiol.*, **25**: 440–441.

Stanfield, B.B. (1992). The development of the corticospinal projection. *Prog. Neurobiol.*, **38**: 169–202.

Stanfield, B.B. & O'Leary, D.D. (1985). The transient corticospinal projection from the occipital cortex during postnatal development of the rat. *J. Comp. Neurol.*, **238**: 236–248.

Stanfield, B.B., O'Leary, D.D.M. & Fricks, C. (1982). Selective collateral elimination in early postnatal development restricts cortical distribution of rat pyramidal tract neurones. *Nature*, **298**: 371–373.

Taub, E., Uswatte, G. & Pidikiti, R. (1999). Constraint-induced movement therapy: a new family of techniques with broad application to physical rehabilitation – a clinical review. *J. Rehabil. Res. Dev.*, **36**: 237–251.

Terashima, T. (1995). Anatomy, development and lesion induced plasticity of rodent corticospinal tract. *Neurosci. Res.*, **22**: 139–161.

Thickbroom, G., Byrnes, M., Archer, S., Nagarajan, L. & Mastaglia, F. (2001). Differences in sensory and motor cortical organization following brain injury early in life. *Ann. Neurol.*, **49**: 320–327.

Uematsu, J., Ono, K., Yamano, T. & Shimanda, M. (1996). Development of corticospinal tract fibres and their plasticity II Neonatal unilateral cortical damage and subsequent development of the corticospinal tract in mice. *Brain Dev.*, **18**: 173–178.

Valtschanoff, J., Weinberg, R. & Rustioni, A. (1993). Amino acid immunoreactivity in corticospinal terminals. *Exp. Brain Res.*, **93**: 95–103.

Verhaart, J.W.C. (1950). Hypertrophy of the pes pedunculi and pyramid as a result of degeneration of the contralateral corticofugal fibre tracts. *J. Comp. Neurol.*, **92**: 1–15.

Wieser, H., Henke, K., Zumsteg, D. et al. (1999). Activation of the left motor cortex during left leg movements after right central resection. *J. Neurol. Neurosurg. Psychiatry*, **67**: 487–491.

Wolpaw, J. & Tennissen, A. (2001). Activity-dependent spinal cord plasticity in health and disease. *Annu. Rev. Neurosci.*, **24**: 807–843.

Yasukawa, A. (1990). Upper extremity casting: adjunct treatment for a child with cerebral palsy hemiplegia. *Am. J. Occup. Ther.*, **44**: 840–846.

4

Practice-induced plasticity in the human motor cortex

Joseph Classen[1] and Leonardo G. Cohen[2]

[1]Human Cortical Physiology Laboratory, Department of Neurology, Bayerische Julius-Maximilians Universität, Würzburg, Germany
[2]Human Cortical Physiology Section, NINDS, National Institutes of Health, Bethesda, MD, USA

Introduction

It is common knowledge that 'practice makes perfect'. Many types of human motor behaviour seem to rely heavily on the fact that the performance of subsequent movements is facilitated by prior performance of similar movements. Therefore, the capacity to build a memory trace of previously practised movements appears to be a fundamental property of the human motor system. Recent studies have focused on this theme in an attempt to gain insight into the physiology of motor memory. Such understanding may contribute to the development of techniques to promote recovery of function following brain damage in humans.

Use-dependent plasticity

Since the 1990s, numerous reports, by employing TMS, demonstrated plasticity induced by motor learning, motor practice or use. One of the earliest reports showed that the excitability of the muscle representation of the 'reading' finger is increased in Braille readers (Pascual-Leone et al., 1993). Pearce and coworkers found that, in highly trained Olympic badminton players, the excitability of the first dorsal interosseus muscle of the skilled hand is increased and its topographical representation is altered when compared to the unskilled hand or to the representations in untrained players (Pearce et al., 2000). These studies provided evidence that the organization of motor activity is modifiable. They also raised questions about the particular factors involved in long-term practice that were instrumental in triggering these profound changes. Was repetition of movements alone, attention paid to the task, or the explicit or implicit intention of establishing a novel movement scheme, or the novel movement scheme itself the crucial element in triggering and sustaining the plastic changes? In addition, what might be the underlying physiological mechanisms? Recent TMS studies have shed light on some of these questions while raising new ones.

If representational plasticity in the motor cortex were to be related to a specific skill acquired, one would expect the plastic changes to depend on the presence of behavioural improvement and, more specifically, to correlate with the magnitude of the improvement. This has not generally been found to be the case. Pascual-Leone and coworkers studied changes associated with the acquisition of a fine motor skill over a period of several weeks (Pascual-Leone et al., 1995). Subjects trained over a period of 2 hours each on 5 successive days to perform a particular sequence of key strokes on a piano. Motor maps were generated by stimulating the representation of forearm muscles at various points on the scalp and displaying the MEP amplitudes as a function of the topographical location of the stimulation site. Training the sequence of key presses was followed by an improvement of motor behaviour (as evidenced by a reduced number of errors in key strokes), as well as an expansion of the region from which MEPs in the practising muscle could be evoked (Pascual-Leone et al., 1995). This result indicates that performing repetitive movements, over a relatively short time period, with the explicit goal of establishing a novel movement scheme is capable of triggering specific excitability changes in the corticomotoneuronal system. A control group that performed key presses for the same amount of time as the subjects who learned a new sequence, but with no particular instruction to optimize performance, also showed a change in motor maps, although the magnitude of that change was substantially smaller than in the first group. This result indicated that enlargement in motor maps (interpreted as an increase in corticomotor excitability targeting the practicing muscles) relied on the greater attentional demand or difficulty involved in learning a complex motor sequence.

In a different set of experiments, Cohen and coworkers (1996) asked subjects to perform synchronous movements of the thumb and shoulder. The subjects were instructed to minimize the time difference between the onset of the thenar and of the deltoid muscle activity fed back to them on an EMG monitor. After training for 60 min, the centre of gravity (CoG) of the thenar muscle representation on the scalp shifted medially towards the shoulder representation. Liepert and coworkers (1999) confirmed this finding by showing that the training of synchronous movements of the thumb and the leg produced a similar shift of the CoG of the thumb motor map. The CoG of the thumb motor map moved medially in the direction of the foot representation area and returned to its original location within 1 h. These experiments showed that a short training was sufficient to elicit changes in the organization of the corticomotor system controlling the training muscles. No change of the CoG was noted when asynchronous thumb and foot muscles were performed (Liepert et al., 1999), indicating a critical dependence on the conjoint activation of two different muscle representations. When thenar muscles were activated synchronously with facial muscles, the CoG of the thumb moved laterally (Cohen et al., 1996) demonstrating spatial specificity and pointing to the cortex as the site of the plastic reorganization. Thus, the representational changes reflected specific timing aspects of the training task. Importantly, however, neither in the study by Cohen et al. (1996) nor by Liepert et al. (1999) in the motor cortex, nor by Schwenkreis et al. (2001) who studied plasticity in the somatosensory cortex induced by the same paradigm, did the magnitude of the shift correlate with the improvement in synchronising the EMG onset of muscle activity.

Muellbacher and colleagues (2001) studied changes in motor cortical excitability following a training period consisting of ballistic or ramp pinch contractions for 60 min at a pace of 0.5 Hz. After the first of two successive periods practising ballistic contractions, but not after practising ramp contractions, peak pinch acceleration and force increased. The increase in force and acceleration correlated with an increase in MEP amplitude in a muscle involved in the training (flexor pollicis brevis) but not in a muscle unrelated to the task (abductor digiti minimi). The practice-induced changes in MEP amplitude were observable only with TMS of M1 but not with direct stimulation of the corticospinal tract, pointing to the cortex as the likely site of the changes. Thirty days after the completion of the first training session, which had been sufficient for the subjects to acquire a new skill, MEPs were found to have returned to their baseline amplitude. No changes in MEP amplitude were induced by subsequent periods of practice, which were also ineffective in inducing a further improvement of motor performance, as measured by peak force or peak acceleration, after the initial improvement following the first training session. This study demonstrated a training-related behavioural gain that was also associated with increases in corticomotor excitability targeting the training muscles. The skill was retained even when corticomotor excitability returned to baseline levels. The failure of subsequent training to induce changes in cortical excitability could indicate that there was no further capacity for the brain to improve behaviour. An alternative explanation is provided by the documented role of attention in modulation of motor performance gains (McNevin et al., 2000). It is conceivable that, during early training, more attention is required to reach a target behavioural goal. With repetition, the task becomes simpler and consequently corticomotor excitability is not modified. Such rationale could have contributed to the results reported by Pascual-Leone et al. (1994). These authors found an excitability change in the representation of finger flexors, while the subjects implicitly learned a particular sequence of key presses. The changes of cortical excitability were reversible after the subject reached explicit knowledge of the task and became fully aware of the sequence to be learned. Possibly, in this task the attentional load decreased at the moment when explicit knowledge was achieved. It is conceivable that the return to baseline cortical excitability was a reflection of task difficulty and attentional load, similar to the return to baseline of excitability in the task of Muellbacher et al. (2001).

Classen and coworkers (1998) showed that performing a brief training of simple thumb movements specifically and temporarily generated an elementary motor memory. In this paradigm, the authors studied the effects of training consisting of voluntary thumb movements in a specific direction on the direction of TMS-evoked thumb movements. After establishing the optimal scalp position for activation of the abductor pollicis brevis muscle, the investigators determined TMS-evoked thumb movement directions ('baseline'). Brisk voluntary 'training' movements of the thumb were then made for 30 min in a direction approximately opposite that of the baseline movements. Post-training, the direction of TMS-evoked movements changed, towards the direction of training (Fig. 4.1). The directions of movement evoked by transcranial electric stimulation were not significantly changed post-training indicating a cortical site of changes. This directional change elicited by training was interpreted as the generation of an elementary motor memory that was present on average for about 20 min, but outlasted this duration in individual subjects up to an additional 20–30 min. These results suggest that the motor cortex builds up, and loses, in a short time,

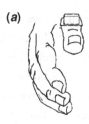

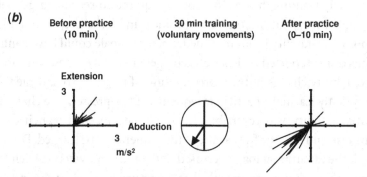

Fig. 4.1   Direct evidence for practice-induced plasticity in the human motor cortex. (a) Acceleration along two orthogonal axes was assessed simultaneously using miniature
accelerometers fixed to the proximal phalanx of the thumb. Movement direction
was assessed as the direction of the vector constructed from the first peaks of the
orthogonal accelerations in the principal movement plane. (b) Directional change of
first peak acceleration vector of TMS-evoked movements. Before practice (baseline),
TMS-evoked extension and abduction thumb movements. Training consisted of
voluntary thumb movements in the direction opposite to that of TMS-evoked
movements (adduction and flexion, middle panel). Following practice, TMS-evoked
movement direction changed from baseline to the practiced direction. (Modified
from Classen et al., 1998.)

memory traces of movements retaining the subject's recent history of performance. Plasticity of movement representations in this paradigm could be
repeatedly induced across sessions, seemingly at variance with the observations made by Muellbacher and colleagues (2001) that subsequent training
could not induce cortical excitability changes after a performance plateau was
reached.

From the experiments described above, it is hard to separate the role of
skill acquisition from that of attentional load in eliciting practice-induced
plasticity. It is possible, however, that both factors contribute to this effect.

To investigate the training time required to build this elementary motor memory, the 30-min period of training was broken up into six 5-min epochs (Classen et al., 1998). It was found that the direction of TMS-evoked movements began to change in most subjects after just 15 minutes' training. The rapid conformation of this memory trace is consistent with the idea that the motor cortex is constantly adapting to new environmental requirements. If so, it is likely that maintenance of such memory traces in the motor cortex may require a minimum amount of attended movements performed regularly at relatively short time intervals.

This proposal would predict that cortical organization of movements should change as a consequence of non-use. Three studies have addressed this issue. Liepert and coworkers (1995) showed that, following unilateral immobilization of the ankle joint, the representation of the inactivated anterior tibial muscle in the motor cortex shrank compared to the unaffected leg. Because H-reflex amplitudes remained constant, these changes were probably generated at a supraspinal level. The area reduction correlated with the duration of immobilization. It could be quickly reversed by voluntary muscle contraction indicating a functional (as opposed to structural) origin of the phenomenon. At variance from the results of Liepert and colleagues (1995), Zanette and coworkers (1997) showed that motor maps representing wrist muscles increased as a consequence of immobilization. Recently, Facchini and others (2002) demonstrated that excitability of the human motor system decreased specifically upon immobilization of two hand fingers. MEPs elicited in the immobilized left abductor digiti minimi (ADM) decreased while those elicited in the non-immobilized first dorsal interosseous muscles remained constant. The decrease of MEP amplitudes of the ADM went along with an increase of resting motor thresholds. No time-related changes of peripheral (M-wave) and spinal (F-wave) excitability were noted, suggesting a likely cortical origin of ADM changes. The findings of Liepert and coworkers, and of Facchini and coworkers, are consistent with the hypothesis that levels of corticomotor excitability depend heavily on use.

Mechanisms underlying use-dependent plasticity

Modulation of intracortical inhibition

The cerebral cortex is richly equipped with mechanisms capable of supporting reorganization. Modulation of intracortical inhibition is one powerful mechanism of reshaping function in the motor cortex. Focal application of the GABA$_A$ receptor antagonist bicuculline (Jacobs & Donoghue, 1991) modified intracortical inhibition and led to representational changes in the motor cortex.

Paired-pulse inhibition, a technique developed by Kujirai et al., and thought to convey information on function of postsynaptic GABA$_A$ receptors (Kujirai et al., 1993), is modulated in training paradigms. For example, in a motor task involving repetitive activation of the APB muscle in the presence of relaxation of the fourth dorsal interosseous muscle (Liepert et al., 1998) paired-pulse inhibition was profoundly reduced in APB, but increased in the fourth dorsal interosseus muscle. Following repetitive unidirectional thumb movements, intracortical inhibition was greater in the training antagonist than in the agonist, during the first 10 min following the training (Classen et al., 1999). However, it is increasingly recognized that the magnitude of paired-pulse inhibition depends on the magnitude of the unconditioned response. Because neither the study of Liepert et al. (1998) nor that of Classen et al. (1999) controlled explicitly for this factor, the role of intracortical inhibition in practice-induced plasticity remains uncertain. A proper assessment of paired-pulse inhibition in intrinsic hand muscles acting as agonists or antagonists in performing finger movements is difficult because of volume conduction between the muscles. To overcome this problem, Wolters and coworkers (2001) studied excitability changes associated with repetitive wrist movements which allow to dissociate more reliably the muscle activity related to the training agonist from that of the training antagonist. Subjects performed repetitive wrist flexions or extensions at a rate of 0.5 Hz over a period of 30 min. MEPs were recorded from the extensor carpi radialis and flexor carpi ulnaris muscles. Excitability of the agonist and antagonist representations was assessed by single-pulse TMS as well as by paired-pulse TMS. Following training, single-pulse excitability of the training agonist increased, while that of the training antagonist increased to a lesser extent (not shown). Therefore, the difference between agonist and antagonist normalized MEP size (agonist–antagonist) increased after training (Fig. 4.2(a)) suggesting that the training had changed the pattern of single-pulse TMS cortical excitability in a way specifically reflecting the recently practised movements. Resting motor thresholds remained constant both in the agonist and in the antagonist muscles. Following training, paired-pulse inhibition was decreased both

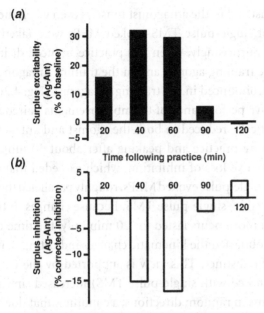

Fig. 4.2   No evidence for specific role of GABAergic inhibition in generating practice-induced plasticity as evidenced in paired-pulse studies. (*a*) Corticomotor excitability changes associated with training unidirectional wrist movements. Results from ten subjects. Recordings from wrist flexors (mainly flexor carpi ulnaris (FCU)) and wrist extensors (mainly extensor carpi radialis (ECR)) acting as training agonist or antagonist in repetitive (0.5 Hz, 30 min) wrist flexions or extensions. MEP amplitudes evoked by single-pulse TMS at suprathreshold (1.2 times resting motor threshold) intensity were normalized to baseline. Practice-induced changes of excitability were assessed as difference between training agonist and antagonist ('surplus excitability'). Positive values indicate changes in favour of agonist excitability. Excitability was more increased in training agonists and antagonists reaching a peak at about 25–30 min. (*b*) Changes of corrected intracortical inhibition as assessed by the paired-pulse stimulation paradigm (Kujirai et al., 1993) associated with training unidirectional wrist movements. The amplitude of the MEP in FCU and ECR evoked by paired-pulse TMS (ISI = 1ms) was assessed, expressed as per cent of the unconditioned baseline amplitude and corrected for the magnitude of the unconditioned response. Practice-induced changes of paired-pulse inhibition were then assessed as difference between paired-pulse inhibition of training agonist and that of the training antagonist ('surplus inhibition'). Paired-pulse inhibition was more reduced in training antagonist as compared to the training agonist indicating greater disinhibition. (Modified from Wolters et al., 2001.)

in the training agonist and in the antagonist muscles even when the changes in the magnitude of single-pulse TMS-evoked MEPs were taken into account (not shown). Surprisingly, when this practice-induced disinhibition was compared in the training agonist and in the training antagonist, disinhibition was more pronounced in the training antagonist (Fig. 4.2(b)).

Following repetitive performance of thumb movements paired pulse inhibition was dramatically reduced in both the agonist and antagonist during ~50 min following practice and peaking after about 30 min (Classen et al., 1999). This relative loss of inhibition, which exceeded that expected from the increase of single-pulse evoked MEPs, roughly paralleled the increase of excitability as tested by single-pulse TMS. Because changes in the direction of TMS-evoked movements lasted for 20 min only, the time course of excitability changes outlasted the kinematic changes indicating that the two phenomena might be distinct. This view is supported by the observation that excitability (as tested with single-pulse TMS) increased similarly after practice of movements in random directions, a condition that does not lead to a directional change of TMS-evoked movements. Thus, although the results of Classen et al. (1999) and Wolters et al. (2001) suggest that practice triggers dramatic changes of intracortical inhibition, its time course and pattern of modulation do not support a role for modulation of intracortical inhibition to represent the single-most important mechanism in establishing a high degree of specificity of practice-related alterations in cortical organization.

Disinhibition of the arm representation in the motor cortex can be induced experimentally by ischemic nerve block at the forearm. Ziemann and colleagues (2001) asked subjects to practise repeated ballistic contractions of the biceps muscle in the presence of ischemic nerve block. This intervention elicited an increase in the size of the MEP recorded from the biceps muscle. No substantial excitability increases were noted when subjects performed biceps contractions in the absence of ischemic nerve block, or when ischemic nerve block was applied in the absence of practising biceps contractions. This finding suggests that decreases in intracortical inhibition could facilitate practice-dependent plasticity in the human motor cortex. If cortical disinhibition facilitates plasticity, enhancing cortical inhibition may depress it. In a recent study, it was shown that drugs that enhance intracortical inhibition by its interaction with $GABA_A$ receptors like lorazepam substantially

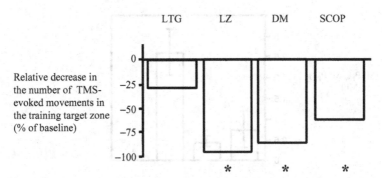

Fig. 4.3   Blockade of practice-induced plasticity by pharmacological intervention. Proportional increase in the number of TMS-evoked movements that fell in the trained
direction after training (mean ± SE). In the control condition, training resulted in
a significant increase in the proportion of TMS-evoked movements in the training direction of between 40 and 65%. Premedication with lorazepam (LZ), dextromethorphan (DM), or scopolamine (SCOP) led to a reduction of this increase.
Lamotrigine (LTG) did not induce significant changes in reference to control.
*$P < 0.025$. (Modified from Buetefisch et al., 2001 and Sawaki et al., 2002a.)

attenuated practice-dependent plasticity (Bütefisch et al., 2000). Administration of lamotrigine, a Na^+/Ca^{2+} channel blocker with similar sedating
properties, did not modify significantly practice-induced plasticity (Fig. 4.3).
Similar results were obtained by Ziemann and colleagues (2001), who showed
that plasticity induced by motor training in the presence of ischemic nerve
block was blocked in the presence of lorazepam (Fig. 4.4). Of additional
interest is the observation that the performance of voluntary movements is
associated with reduction of intracortical inhibition (Ridding et al., 1995;
Reynolds & Ashby, 1999). Together, these results suggest a role for cortical
inhibition as a mechanism gating the capacity for repetitive movements to
induce motor memories in the motor cortex.

In addition to gating practice-induced plasticity, the finding of lasting
changes in intracortical inhibition after motor practice suggests a role for
disinhibition in motor memory consolidation (Classen et al., 1999). This
hypothesis is consistent with recent results by Muellbacher and colleagues
(2002) showing that excitability changes as well as consolidation of skill
following training of a pinch-grip task can be suppressed by slow-rate (1 Hz)
rTMS applied immediately after practice.

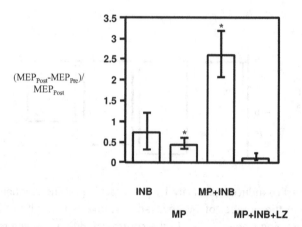

$$(MEP_{Post}\text{-}MEP_{Pre})/MEP_{Post}$$

INB   MP+INB

MP   MP+INB+LZ

Fig. 4.4   Facilitation of practice-induced plasticity by disinhibition through ischemic nerve block. MEP amplitudes at the end of intervention are displayed as increments of the baseline measurements (mean±standard error). Asterisks indicate significant differences from zero ($P < 0.05$). INB=ischemic nerve block at the forearm; MP= motor practice; MP+INB motor practice during ischemic nerve block; MP+INB+ LZ motor practice during INB with subject being premedicated with lorazepam. (Modified from Ziemann et al., 2001.)

Modulation of synaptic efficacy

Changes in synaptic efficay are thought to represent mechanisms subserving information storage in the brain, and, therefore, are natural candidates underlying practice-induced plasticity. Long-term potentiation (LTP) is regarded as the prototype of mechanisms altering the efficacy of synapses. Although, for obvious reasons, the operation of LTP cannot directly be proven in humans, the fact that it has distinct properties allows testing for its presence in vivo. As most types of LTP are dependent on the activation on NMDA receptors, practice-induced plasticity was investigated while volunteers were exposed to dextromethorphan, a NMDA receptor blocker. When taken prior to the practice of unidirectional thumb movements, dextromethorphan prevented practice-induced plasticity (Fig. 4.3) (Bütefisch et al., 2000). Acetylcholine and cholinergic agents enhance the relative amplitude of long-term potentiation in neocortical structures (Hasselmo & Barkai, 1995), most likely by enhancing NMDA currents (Maalouf et al., 1998). In a double-blind placebo-controlled study, practice-induced plasticity of thumb-movement representation was substantially attenuated by scopolamine, a blocker of muscarinic acetylcholine receptors (Fig. 4.3)

(Sawaki et al., 2002). Thus, the pharmacological profile of plasticity induced by repetitive performance of thumb movements carries a remarkable similarity with properties of LTP induction in vitro. In addition to pharmacological manipulation, the induction of LTP may be influenced by physiological interventions. For example, stimulation methods leading to depression of synaptic efficacy (LTD) or saturating the local capacity of the neuronal population to express LTP should interfere with the induction of LTP-like mechanisms elicited by practice (Rioult-Pedotti et al., 2000). An example of this phenomenon may be the blocking effect of transcranial direct current stimulation (tDCS) (Nitsche & Paulus, 2000) on the formation of the motor memory trace (Rosenkranz et al., 2000). The results reported by Muellbacher and colleagues (2002) (see above) are also consistent with a role of LTP-like mechanisms in the consolidation of a motor skill. Subjects optimized pinch-grip force and acceleration by performing repetitive movements over a period of 60 min (Muellbacher et al., 2001). Repetitive TMS at 1 Hz, known to depress cortical excitability possibly through mechanisms related to LTD (Chen et al., 1997), was applied to the motor cortex immediately after a practice period. This intervention resulted in failure to maintain enhanced performance at later retesting. However, when rTMS was applied 6 hours after the first practice period, retention of performance gain remained unaffected.

An interesting addition supporting the role of GABA in LTP-related mechanisms of recovery of function after cortical lesions comes from the work of Hagemann et al. (1998). Brain regions surrounding focal cortical ischemic lesions experience a down-regulation of GABA receptor activity that modifies cortical excitability (Schiene et al., 1996) and facilitates the induction of LTP (Hagemann et al., 1998). Therefore, it is an intriguing question whether changes of cortical inhibition either as a result of pathology, or through pharmacological or physiological intervention could promote practice-dependent plasticity in health and disease. Because removal of GABAergic inhibition and activation of NMDA receptors are two conditions synergistically involved in the induction of LTP in cortical synapses (Hess et al., 1996), the results reviewed above suggest that practice-induced cortical plasticity heavily relies on changes of synaptic efficacy.

Pharmacological enhancement of practice-induced plasticity

That practice-induced plasticity may be enhanced pharmacologically has been shown by two recent studies testing the effect of amphetamine on

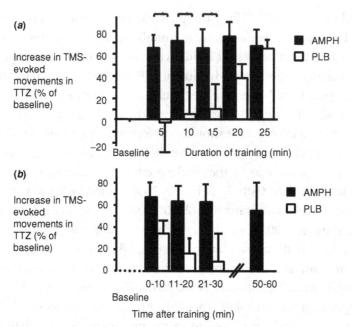

Fig. 4.5   Enhancement of practice-induced plasticity by amphetamine. (*a*) Training time required to elicit directional changes. Results from six subjects. Five to 10 minutes of
training sufficed to induce a proportional increase of more than 60% in the transcranial magnetic stimulation (TMS)-evoked movements falling in the training target
zone in the d-amphetamine (AMPH) condition (dark bars). In the placebo condition,
changes of similar magnitude required 25 minutes of training (white bars). By
25 minutes of training, similar directional changes were seen in both conditions.
TTZ training target zone: (*b*) Duration of directional changes after completion of
training. Results from six subjects. Transcranial magnetic stimulation (TMS)-evoked
movements falling in the training target zone disappeared within 10 to 20 minutes
in the placebo condition (white bars) but lasted for more than 1 hour in the
D-amphetamine (AMPH) condition (dark bars). (Modified from Bütefisch et al.,
2002.)

plasticity of movement representation following repetitive unidirectional
thumb movements. In one study, amphetamine accelerated the development
and prolonged the duration of practice-induced plasticity (Bütefisch et al.,
2002) (Fig. 4.5). Additionally, it increased the magnitude of plastic changes
elicited by short periods of motor training (Bütefisch et al., 2002). In another
study (Sawaki et al., 2002) the effect of amphetamine on practice-induced
plasticity was studied in six subjects in whom training had previously failed to

elicit plasticity. A single oral dose of 10 mg D-amphetamine preceding training succeeded in generating an elementary motor memory in two of these
subjects. The mechanism(s) by which amphetamine exerts its facilitatory
effect is unknown. However, it is likely that alpha adrenergic neurotransmission, previously proposed to explain the facilitatory effects of amphetamine
on motor recovery after stroke (Feeney, 1997) plays a role, possibly through
modulation of LTP-like mechanisms.

Conclusions

Repetitive performance of voluntary movements is associated with plasticity
of the corticomotoneuronal system. Motor training is a useful strategy geared
to the acquisition of motor skills of different complexities. TMS has been
used in a variety of settings to evaluate changes in corticomotoneuronal excitability and representational plasticity. Performance of thumb movements
in a specific direction results in the establishment of an elementary motor memory. This event is associated with a practice-dependent differential
modulation of excitability of muscles acting as training agonists or antagonists. These forms of short-term plasticity are influenced by the status of
intracortical $GABA_A$ receptor mediated inhibition. (a) Following, training a
lasting cortical disinhibition was identified in muscles acting as training agonist and training antagonist. (b) Pharmacological experiments showed that
practice-induced plasticity was blocked when training was performed under
the influence of a $GABA_A$ receptor agonist. (c) Practice-induced plasticity was
enhanced following forearm ischemic nerve block, an intervention that elicits
cortical disinhibition. (d) Performance of voluntary movements is associated with reduction of intracortical inhibition. Pharmacological experiments
demonstrated that blockade of NMDA receptors and of muscarinic receptors
abolished the effect of practice. The improvement in motor behaviour that
follows in some experimental paradigms after practising simple repetitive
movements can be blocked by applying low-frequency repetitive magnetic
stimulation immediately after practice over the primary motor cortex. These
findings suggest the involvement of LTP-like processes, a form of synaptic
plasticity, as a substrate mechanism. It is possible to enhance the training effects by premedication of amphetamine, a drug thought to operate through
its effects on alpha adrenergic function. These findings may be relevant

for therapeutic strategies employed in rehabilitation of patients with brain injury.

Acknowledgements

This work was supported by Cl 95/3-1. The authors thank C. Bütefisch, L. Sawaki, and A.Wolters for helpful discussions.

REFERENCES

Baker, J.T., Donoghue, J.P. & Sanes, J.N. (1999). Gaze direction modulates finger movement activation patterns in human cerebral cortex. *J. Neurosci.*, **19**: 10044–10052.

Bütefisch, C.M., Davis, B.C. & Wise, S.P. (2000). Mechanisms of use-dependent plasticity in the human motor cortex. *Proc. Natl Acad. Sci., USA*, **97**: 3661–3665.

Bütefisch, C.M., Sawaki, L., Davis, B.C. et al. (2002). Modulation of use-dependent plasticity by D-amphetamine. *Ann. Neurol.*, **51**: 59–68.

Chen, R., Classen, J., Gerloff, C. et al. (1997). Depression of motor cortex excitability by low-frequency transcranial magnetic stimulation. *Neurology*, **48**: 1398–1403.

Classen, J., Liepert, A., Wise, S.P., Hallett, M. & Cohen, L.G. (1998). Rapid plasticity of human cortical movement representation induced by practice. *J. Neurophysiol.*, **79**: 1117–1123.

Classen, J., Liepert, J., Hallett, M. & Cohen, L.G. (1999). Plasticity of movement representation in the human motor cortex. In *Transcranial Magnetic Stimulation*, ed. W. Paulus, J.C. Rothwell, M. Hallett & P.M. Rossini, vol. 51, pp. 162–173. Amsterdam: Elsevier Press.

Cohen, L.G., Gerloff, C., Faiz, L. et al. (1996). Directional modulation of motor cortex plasticity induced by synchronicity of motor outputs in humans. *Soc. Neurosci. Abstr.*, **22**: 576.11.

Facchini, S., Romani, M., Tinazzi, M. & Aglioti, S.M. (2002). Time-related changes of excitability of the human motor system contingent upon immobilisation of the ring and little fingers. *Clin. Neurophysiol.*, **113**: 367–375.

Feeney, D.M. (1997). From laboratory to clinic: noradrenergic enhancement of physical therapy for stroke or trauma patients. *Adv. Neurol.*, **73**: 383–394.

Hagemann, G., Redecker, C., Neumann-Haefelin, T., Freund, H.J. & Witte, O.W. (1998). Increased long-term potentiation in the surround of experimentally induced focal cortical infarction. *Ann. Neurol.*, **44**: 255–258.

Hasselmo, M.E. & Barkai, E. (1995). Cholinergic modulation of activity-dependent synaptic plasticity in the piriform cortex and associative memory function in a network biophysical simulation. *J. Neurosci.*, **15**: 6592–6604.

Hess, G., Aizenman, C.D. & Donoghue, J.P. (1996). Conditions for the induction of long-term potentiation in layer II/III horizontal connections of the rat motor cortex. *J. Neurophysiol.*, **75**: 1765–1778.

Jacobs, K.M. & Donoghue, J.P. (1991). Reshaping the cortical motor map by unmasking latent intracortical connections. *Science*, **251**: 944–947.

Kujirai, T., Caramia, M.D., Rothwell, J.C. et al. (1993). Corticocortical inhibition in human motor cortex. *J. Physiol.*, **471**: 501–519.

Liepert, J., Tegenthoff, M. & Malin, J.P. (1995). Changes of cortical motor area size during immobilization. *Electroencephalogr. Clin. Neurophysiol.*, **97**: 382–386.

Liepert, J., Classen, J., Cohen, L.G. & Hallett, M. (1998). Task-dependent changes of intracortical inhibition. *Exp. Brain Res.*, **118**: 421–426.

Liepert, J., Terborg, C. & Weiller, C. (1999). Motor plasticity induced by synchronized thumb and foot movements. *Exp. Brain Res.*, **125**: 435–439.

McNevin, N.H., Wulf, G. & Carlson, C. (2000). Effects of attentional focus, self-control, and dyad training on motor learning: implications for physical rehabilitation. *Phys. Ther.*, **80**: 373–385.

Maalouf, M., Dykes, R.W. & Miasnikov, A.A. (1998). Effects of D-AP5 and NMDA microiontophoresis on associative learning in the barrel cortex of awake rats. *Brain Res.*, **793**: 149–168.

Muellbacher, W., Ziemann, U., Boroojerdi, B., Cohen, L. & Hallett, M. (2001). Role of the human motor cortex in rapid motor learning. *Exp. Brain Res.*, **136**: 431–438.

Muellbacher, W., Ziemann, U., Wissel, J. et al. (2002). Early consolidation in human primary motor cortex. *Nature*, **415**: 640–644.

Nitsche, M.A. & Paulus, W. (2000). Excitability changes induced in the human motor cortex by weak transcranial direct current stimulation. *J. Physiol.*, **527**: 633–639.

Pascual-Leone, A., Cammarota, A., Wassermann, E.M., Brasil-Neto, J.P., Cohen, L.G. & Hallett, M. (1993). Modulation of motor cortical outputs to the reading hand of braille readers. *Ann. Neurol.*, **34**: 33–37.

Pascual-Leone, A., Valls-Sole, J., Wassermann, E.M. & Hallett, M. (1994). Responses to rapid rate transcranial magnetic stimulation of the human motor cortex. *Brain*, **117**: 847–858.

Pascual-Leone, A., Nguyet, D., Cohen, L.G. Brasil-Neto, J.P., Cammarota, A. & Hallett, M. (1995). Modulation of muscle responses evoked by transcranial magnetic stimulation during the acquisition of new fine motor skills. *J. Neurophysiol.*, **74**: 1037–1045.

Pearce, A.J., Thickbroom, G.W., Byrnes, M.L. & Mastaglia, F.L. (2000). Functional reorganisation of the corticomotor projection to the hand in skilled racquet players. *Exp. Brain Res.*, **130**: 238–243.

Reynolds, C. & Ashby, P. (1999). Inhibition in the human motor cortex is reduced just before a voluntary contraction. *Neurology*, **53**: 730–735.

Ridding, M.C., Taylor, J.L. & Rothwell, J.C. (1995). The effect of voluntary contraction on cortico-cortical inhibition in human motor cortex. *J. Physiol. (Lond.)*, **487**: 541–548.

Rioult-Pedotti, M.S., Friedman, D. & Donoghue, J. P. (2000). Learning-induced LTP in neocortex. *Science*, **290**: 533–536.

Rosen Kranz, K., Nitsche, M.A., Tergau, F. & Paulus, W. (2000). Diminution of training-induced transient motor cortex plasticity by weak transcranial direct current stimulation in the human. *Neurosc. Lett.*, **296**: 61–63.

Sawaki, L., Boroojerdi, B., Kaelin-Lang, A. (2002a). Cholinergic influences on use-dependent plasticity. *J. Neurophysiol.*, **87**: 166–171.

Sawaki, L., Cohen, L.G., Classen, J., Davis, B. & Butefisch, C.M. (2002b). Enhancement of use-dependent plasticity by D-amphetamine. *Neurology*, **59**: 1262–1264.

Schiene, K., Bruehl, C., Zilles, K. et al. (1996). Neuronal hyperexcitability and reduction of GABAA-receptor expression in the surround of cerebral photothrombosis. *J. Cereb. Blood Flow Metab.*, **16**: 906–914.

Schwenkreis, P., Pleger, B., Hoffken, O., Malin, J.P. & Tegenthoff, M. (2001). Repetitive training of a synchronised movement induces short-term plastic changes in the human primary somatosensory cortex. *Neurosci. Lett.*, **312**: 99–102.

Wolters, A., Kunesch, E., Benecke, R. & Classen, J. (2001). Zeitgang verschiedener Parameter kortikaler Exzitabilitätsveränderungen nach repetitiven Handgelenksbewegungen. *Akt. Neurol.*, **Suppl. 28**: 68.

Zanette, G., Tinazzi, M., Bonato, C. et al. (1997). Reversible changes of motor cortical outputs following immobilization of the upper limb. *Electroencephalogr. Clin. Neurophysiol.*, **105**: 269–279.

Ziemann, U., Muellbacher, W., Hallett, M. & Cohen, L.G. (2001). Modulation of practice-dependent plasticity in human motor cortex. *Brain*, **124**: 1171–1181.

5

Skill learning

Edwin M. Robertson, Hugo Theoret and Alvaro Pascual-Leone

Behavioral Neurology Unit, Beth Israel Medical Center Boston, MA, USA

Plasticity as an intrinsic property of the brain

In the course of brain development, very complex processes take place to establish an intricate and highly specific network of millions of cells interconnected by billions of dendritic arborizations and synapses. It is reasonable to think that the brain might be resistant to change once development is completed, given the daunting complexity of these processes and of the resulting 'end-product'. This notion of a rather static and unchanging brain was the pervasive belief for many years. However, in the meantime, it has become clear that this notion is wrong. The brain does not only undergo reorganization, but it is constantly reorganizing (Fuster, 1995; Kaas, 1997) and this entire volume provides ample support for the emerging concept of a dynamically changing brain.

The brain's capacity to change is referred to as plasticity and we might think of it as an intrinsic property of the human nervous system that persists throughout the human lifespan. An obvious example to lend support to this claim is the acquisition of new skills, to which the present chapter is devoted. The brain is designed to be able to change in response to changes in the environment. This is the mechanism for growth and development, but also for learning. In the process of learning, the brain has to change to be able to code for, and appropriately implement, the new knowledge. Neuroimaging studies have found decreases, increases, and shifts in activations as effects of practice depending on the amount of repetition and relating to priming, proficient learning, and overlearning with automatization (Poldrack, 2000; Schachter & Buckner, 1998; van Mier, 2000). Plastic changes are also induced by a large number of pathological conditions, including injury to central and peripheral nervous system (Chollet, 2000; Kaas, 2000). In this setting, plasticity is likely to represent the mechanisms by which recovery of function after the injury is possible (Chollet & Weiller, 2000).

However, it is important to recognize that plasticity at the neural level does not speak to the question of behavioural change and certainly does not imply necessarily functional recovery or even functional change. It is reasonable to assume that plasticity is a characteristic of the nervous system that evolved for coping with changes in the environment associated with learning and development and that are co-opted as a response to brain injury. Yet, as these mechanisms did not specifically evolve to cope with injury, they are not altogether successful in this regard. It is also safe to say, at this stage of our knowledge, that structural plasticity does not predict for behavioural plasticity. However, a fuller understanding of the mechanisms underlying plasticity will probably eventually allow such predictions.

An intuitive concept of plasticity is of a definable starting point, which can be established and a process followed that leads to an observable and measurable change of function or structure in the nervous system. This, however, is incorrect and the situation is far more complicated. The brain is never at rest and never switches off at the start of an experiment or a period of observation. Any given event is the consequence of all other events, past and present, and will in its turn combine with all others to give rise to new events. We should therefore not conceive of the brain as a stationary object capable of activating a cascade of changes that we shall call plasticity, nor as an orderly stream of events, driven by plasticity. We might be better served thinking of the nervous system as a moving target, a continuous changing system in which plasticity is an integral property and the obligatory consequence of each sensory input, each visuomotor transformation, motor command, reward signal, action plan, or awareness. In this framework, notions such as psychological processes as distinct from organic-based functions or dysfunctions cease to be meaningful. Behaviour will lead to changes in brain circuitry, hence establishing organic underpinnings of learned attitudes, dispositions, or thinking styles, as much as faulty brain circuits will lead to specific behavioural patterns.

Rapid plastic changes and potential risks

As an intrinsic property of brain function, plasticity does not necessarily have to be beneficial for the subjects. Plastic changes might result in a behavioural gain or loss for a given subject and may underlie the development of symptoms in a given disease. The concept of 'maladaptive plasticity' was introduced to capture the idea of potentially functionally undesirable consequences of plasticity. However, the concept of an obligatory link between plasticity and adaptation may be all together incorrect. Instead it may be more appropriate to think of plasticity as the obligatory consequence of each activation of a given neural pathway. In this framework the potential separation between brain changes and behavioural desirability becomes obvious.

The role played by plasticity in task-specific dystonia, for example in 'pianist's cramp', is a useful example for this issue and relates to rapid plastic changes during skill acquisition. Playing a musical instrument, requires more than factual knowledge about the musical instrument and about the mechanics of how it is played. The central nervous system has to acquire and implement a 'translation mechanism' to convert knowledge into action. These translation capabilities constitute the skill that enable the pianist to act on memory systems, select the relevant facts, choose the proper response goals, activate the necessary sensory–motor structures, and execute the sonata successfully. In general, we think of such a skill as being acquired with practice. The pianist confronted with a new composition, after understanding the task and its demands, develops a cognitive representation of it, and initiates a first, centrally guided response that results in sensory–motor feedback and movement correction. It seems certain that both sensory and motor aspects have to be exquisitely coordinated. At the beginning, the limbs move slowly, with fluctuating accuracy and speed, and success requires visual, proprioceptive, and auditory feedback. Eventually, each single movement is refined, the different movements chained into the proper sequence with the desired timing, a high probability of stability in the ordered sequence attained, and a fluency of all movement developed. Only then can the pianist shift his or her attentional focus away from the mechanical details of the performance towards the emotional content of the task. We can think of the acquisition of such a skill as the conversion of declarative knowledge (facts) into procedural knowledge (actions, skills).

Normal subjects taught to perform, with one hand, a five-finger exercise on a piano keyboard require several days of practice to acquire proficiency (Pascual-Leone et al., 1995a). Eventually, over the course of 5 days with 2 hours of practice per day, the number of sequence errors and variability of the intervals between key pushes (as marked by the metronome beats)

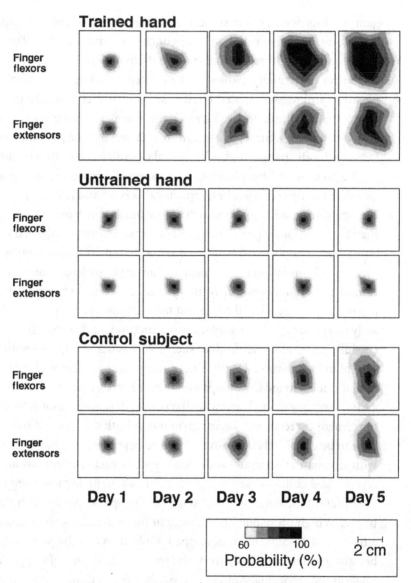

Fig. 5.1   Representative examples of the cortical motor output maps for the long finger flexor and extensor muscles on days 1–5 in a test subject (trained and untrained hand) and a control subject. The maps express the probability of evoking a motor potential with a peak-to-peak amplitude of at least 50 μV in the contralateral muscles with a stimulus intensity of 10% above motor threshold at the optimal scalp position. Eight stimuli were given at each scalp position. Each contour map represents 25 scalp positions (1 cm apart) arranged in a 5 × 5 grid around the optimal position. (Modified from Pascual-Leone et al., 1995a.)

decrease significantly and the accuracy improves. These behavioural gains are associated with changes in the motor output maps to the muscles involved in the task that can be demonstrated using TMS mapping. As the subjects' performance improves, the threshold for TMS activation of the finger flexor and extensor muscles decreases steadily and, even taking this change in threshold into account, the size of the cortical representation for both muscle groups increases significantly (Fig. 5.1).

Rather than showing the activation during the task as would be the case with neuroimaging studies, this TMS mapping technique demonstrates a trace or memory of the activation of the motor cortical outputs that took place while the task was performed. During learning, the cortical output maps obtained following task performance show a progressive increase in size. This implies that skill acquisition is associated with a change in the pattern of cortical activation. These changes cannot be demonstrated before task performance, hence it seems that developing an appropriate pattern of cortical output recruitment is an important neurophysiological component of learning. Eventually, as performance improves further and skill becomes overlearned, other neural structures (including subcortical structures) may take an increasingly prominent role in the behaviour. Consequently, following the initial flexible and short-term modulation across the motor cortex, there are probably longer-term structural changes in the intracortical and subcortical networks, as skill becomes increasingly automatic.

Such plastic reorganization is driven by efferent demand and afferent input. However, a system capable of such flexible reorganization harbours the risk of unwanted change. Increased demand of sensory–motor integration poses such a risk. We can postulate that faulty practice may result in unwanted cortical rearrangement and set the stage for motor control problems such as overuse syndrome and focal, task-specific dystonias. For example, the style of piano playing, Russian vs. German school, seems to play a critical role in the risk of development of motor control problem. The forceful playing with the fingers held bent and executing hammer-like movements is more frequently associated with overuse syndrome and dystonia than the softer playing with extended fingers 'caressing' the keys. This stresses the importance of proper, well-guided practice.

Musicians with dystonia during guitar playing, show significantly larger activation of the contralateral primary sensorimotor cortex and bilateral underactivation of premotor areas, when compared to the activation pattern obtained in the same subjects during other hand movements or in matched guitar players without dystonia while executing the same guitar playing ex-cercises (Pujol et al., 2000). Furthermore, the somatosensory homunculus of patients with focal, task-specific dystonia has been shown to be abnormal (Bara-Jimenez et al., 1998; Pascual-Leone, 2001). For example, patients with hand dystonia have distortions in the representation of adjacent fingers and excessive overlap between them. This might be due to extensive practice of coordinated hand postures in which various digits function as a unit, e.g. in arpeggios. In this case, digits repeatedly receive concurrent sensory inputs that can eventually lead to a blurring of the segregation of different digits in the somato sensory homonculus. Such might be particularly the case when small repeated traumas are added, for example in forceful, 'hammer-finger' piano playing. Disorganization and consequent confusion of sensory inputs could potentially lead to poorly differentiated control of motor representa-tions and be the mechanisms underlying the risk of faulty motor control in some instrumentalists.

Long-term plastic reorganization

The demonstration of short-term plastic changes following skill acquisition in normal subjects raises interesting questions relating to possible long-term plastic reorganization in populations with highly developed motor skills. In violin players, the cortical representation of the digits of the left hand is larger than that in controls (Elbert et al., 1995). Thus, long-lasting plastic changes seem to occur following repetitive performance of a complex and skilled motor task. Another example of skill-dependent plastic reorganization in professional musicians is that of the corpus callosum (CC). Schlaug et al. (1995) reported hypertrophy of the anterior half of the CC in subjects whose musical training began before the age of seven.

By using the paired-pulse TMS (Ferbert et al., 1992; Kujirai et al., 1993), Ridding and collaborators (2000) set out to explore whether the increased volume of the CC in musicians was associated with changes in the interhemi-spheric process of inhibition. A single TMS pulse applied to the motor cortex of one hemisphere can reduce MEP amplitudes elicited by a second TMS pulse applied 10–20 ms later to the contralateral hemisphere (Ferbert et al., 1992). In professional musicians, the interhemispheric inhibitory effects of the conditioning stimulus are markedly reduced compared to a control group (Ridding et al., 2000). Since interhemispheric facilitation or inhibition of the motor cortex is probably involved in bilateral movements of the hands (Schnitzler et al., 1996) it may be argued that extensive practice in musicians results in plastic changes, which have a behavioural correlate. Whether or not this is the case awaits further studies but none the less raises very interesting questions regarding practice-dependent long-term plastic changes of cortical organization.

Another study recently demonstrated the plastic reorganization of motor cortex following long-term skill acquisition. Like musicians, athletes require fine motor skills for the effective performance of their sport, which might result in alterations in motor cortex organization. Pearce et al. (2000) investigated motor cortical topography and excitability of the first dorsal interosseous (FDI) muscle in five highly trained badminton players. The results were contrasted with those obtained from five social-level players and ten normal subjects. Cortical motor maps of the FDI were obtained, in addition to MEP amplitudes, latencies and silence period durations. Results showed increases in MEP amplitudes and/or decreases in MEP thresholds of the playing hand of elite athletes indicating a change in corticomotor excitability, which is not present in control populations. Motor cortical representation maps of the FDI muscle were also modified in elite athletes. Comparing the playing and non-playing hands, the centre of the map was displaced medially in three subjects and laterally in two others. Conversely, no map modifications were observed in casual players or normal subjects. These data, in addition to those obtained in musicians, demonstrate the potential for practised skilled motor tasks to result in long-term plasticity of the motor cortex.

Competition for substrates

Another population in which questions of skill learning-induced plasticity can be addressed is Braille readers. Braille reading requires the processing of tactile stimuli information into meaningful shapes. Consequently, motor and sensory representations of the reading finger could be changed in response to the novel use it subserves in proficient Braille readers. Pascual-Leone et al. (1993) used TMS to map motor cortical representation of the FDI muscle

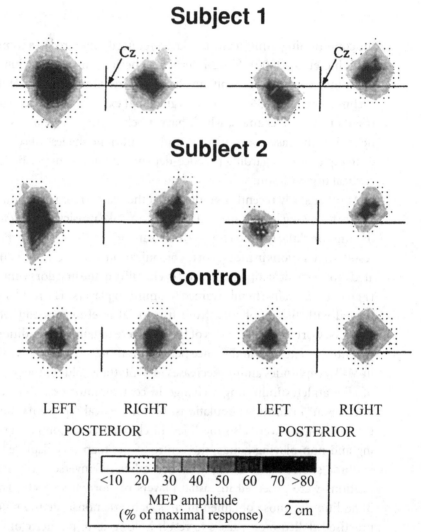

Fig. 5.2   Representative example of contour maps of two early blind, proficient Braille readers (subjects 1 and 2) and in a non-proficient Braille reading blind control (control). All three subjects were right-handers and both proficient Braille readers used
their right index finger as preferred reading digit. Motor output maps for the first
dorsal interosseous (FDI) and the abductor pollicis brevis (ADM) muscles are presented. The FDI is the primary agonist of the side-to-side index finger movement
required for Braille reading. Note the larger representation of the FDI and the relatively smaller representation of the ADM in the Braille reader as compared with the
blind, non-proficient Braille reading control. (Modified from Pascual-Leone et al.,
1993.)

in a population of blind Braille readers divided into two groups on the basis of Braille proficiency. In proficient Braille readers, the representation of the FDI muscle in the reading hand was significantly larger than that in the non-reading hand. This increase in the cortical representation of the reading finger was absent in the non-proficient Braille readers. The increase in FDI area was accompanied with a decrease in the cortical representation of the abductor digiti minimi (ADM) muscle (Fig. 5.2). Thus, these results suggest that the motor cortical representation of the reading finger in proficient Braille readers is enlarged at the expense of the representation of other fingers (Pascual-Leone et al., 1993).

These long-term plastic changes may be due to the increased sensory stimulation resulting in an increased representation in sensory cortex. The modifications observed in motor cortex would then be secondary to those changes. On the other hand, motor strategies and movements used by the Braille readers might also play a role in the modulation of motor cortical outputs. In much the same way as when amputation results in the reorganization of motor outputs, increased use and enhanced sensory feedback associated with learning a highly specialized motor skill may shift the balance of intracortical networks toward the overused body part (Pascual-Leone et al., 1993).

It appears then that plastic changes associated with acquisition of a skill take place in competition for resources for established behavioural capabilities: the enlargement of the motor output maps to the FDI was associated with the reduction of the maps to the ADM. Therefore, the gain in one domain might lead to the loss in another. If so, even long-term, established, plastic changes ought to show a significant amount of flexibility to adapt to changing behavioural demands.

Stability of long-term plastic reorganization

In a subsequent study, Pascual-Leone and collaborators (1995b) set out to determine how stable modifications in sensory–motor cortex are in blind proficient Braille readers. Remarkably, preceding activity does play a critical role in the size of the motor output maps in Braille readers. We determined cortical motor output maps of the FDI in six blind proficient Braille readers with the use of TMS. Maps obtained on a day in which proficient Braille

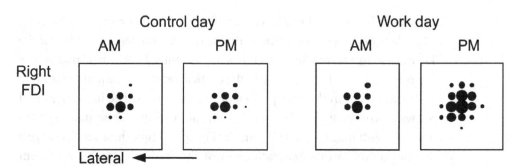

Fig. 5.3   Representative example of the modulation of cortical output maps in an early
blind, proficient Braille reader depending on the amount of Braille reading during the study day. On a regular work day (Braille reading for about 6 hours) there
is notable increase in the motor output map to the primary mover of the reading finger. On a control day, when the subject did not read Braille there is no
significant modification of the output maps. The diameter of the bubbles represents the peak-to-peak amplitude of the motor evoked potentials at each location of a 5×5 cm grid centred around the optimal position for activation of the
right first dorsal interosseous muscle (FDI). (Modified from Pascual-Leone et al.,
1995b.)

readers worked as Braille proofreaders were compared with those obtained
on a day they took off from work. At the end of the work-day, FDI motor thresholds were lower than those collected before work. In addition, on
days when the subjects worked, the cortical output maps of the reading finger were significantly larger than maps of the contralateral finger (Fig. 5.3).
When subjects did not go to work, no such differences were observed. In
other words, comparison of the motor output maps following a day of intensive work or after having been off from work for 2 days demonstrates
significant differences in the cortical representation of the reading finger of
proficient Braille proofreaders. Disuse, in this case by virtue of the 2 days
off from work, results in a decrease in the cortical output maps. Vacation,
with a week of minimal Braille reading leads to even more dramatic reduction in motor output maps. Such disuse related changes might underlie the
common experience of 'rustiness' upon returning to work following some
time off, and may be viewed as functionally undesirable consequences of
plasticity.

Rat MI representation patterns

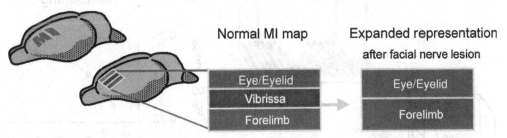

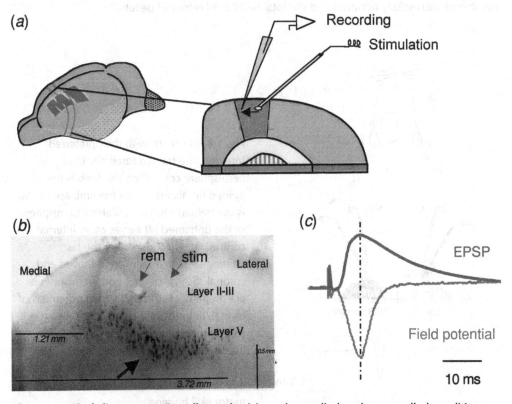

Fig. 1.1 Plasticity of adult motor cortex. The three main output representations of the rat motor cortex under normal condition (left). With a lesion of the peripheral vibrissa motor nerve, the adjacent cortical territories expand into the cortical zone that previously represented output to the vibrissa (right). Within 1 hour of lesion, forelimb movements can be evoked from the former MI whisker representation.

Fig. 1.2 Cortical slice preparation allows plasticity to be studied under controlled condition. (*a*) Configuration of stimulating and recording electrodes in coronal slices containing the forelimb area (FL) of the primary motor cortex (MI). (*b*) The location of stimulation and recording electrodes in the MI–FL area has been verified by layer V labelling with Fast Blue injections in the cervical spinal cord. (*c*) Evoked layer II/III intrinsic extracellular field potentials (blue) and excitatory postsynaptic responses (EPSPs, red).

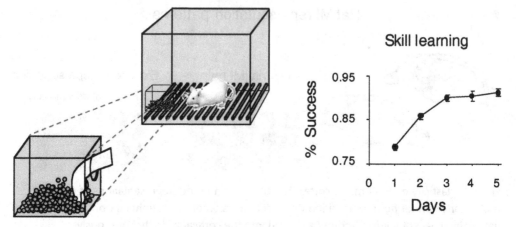

Fig. 1.3 Training apparatus and learning curve. Rats were shaped to reach inside a Plexiglas box to obtain small food pellets. The progression of learning is indicated by the increase in success rate over 3–5 days of motor skill training. Success was defined as the ratio of the number of successfully retrieved and the total number of retrieved pellets.

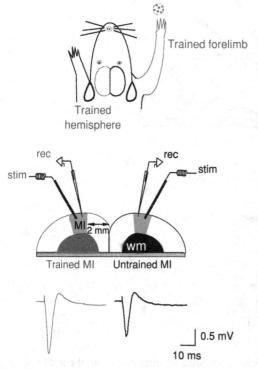

Fig. 1.4 Rats learn with their preferred forelimb, the trained forelimb. The hemisphere controlling this limb is the trained hemisphere. The forelimb area in MI is the trained MI. The ipsilateral hemisphere or the untrained MI serves as an internal control. One or 2 days after the last training session, brains are removed and coronal slices including both hemispheres are prepared. Extracellular field potentials of layer II/III horizontal connections are recorded simultaneously in both hemispheres. Field potentials evoked in the trained MI are consistently larger than that in the untrained MI after at least 3–5 days of motor skill training.

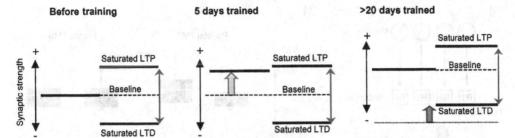

Fig. 1.5 Modification of synaptic strength and synaptic modification range with motor skill learning and continued practice. Synaptic strengthening following 5 days of skill training occludes LTP and increases LTD (middle) by an upward shift of baseline synaptic strength (orange arrow) within a fixed synaptic modification range. Extended training maintains enhanced synaptic strength but restores the synaptic modification range. The upward shift of the range (blue arrow) returns synaptic efficacy to the middle of its operating range allowing pre-learning levels of LTP and LTD. The extent of the synaptic modification range remained unchanged.

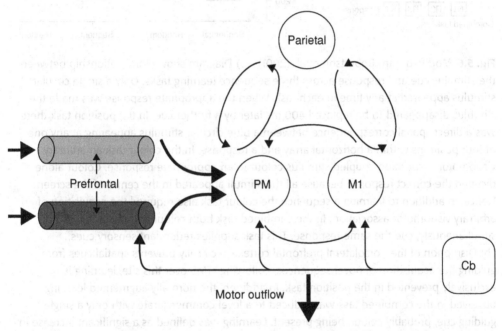

Fig. 5.5 Schematic diagram showing the neural principles underlying a model of sequence learning. We envisage sequence learning to result from an interaction between upstream cue-dependent with downstream cue-independent circuits. Upstream, is a parallel array of circuits each dedicated to a single guiding cue. Hence, spatial and non-spatial information is segregated resembling the functional organization of the dorsolateral and ventrolateral prefrontal cortex, respectively. This segregated organization breaks down at the dorsal premotor cortex, where an integration and transformation of multiple cues occurs allowing them all to be expressed within a common framework. Downstream from this confluence site is a circuit dedicated to the general aspects of sequence learning, consisting of both cortical areas such as the primary motor cortex and the basal ganglia and cerebellum.

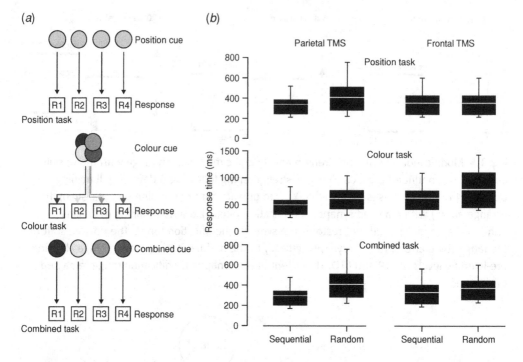

Fig. 5.6 Modified from Robertson et al. (2001). (*a*) Diagram shows the relationship between the stimulus cue and response across three sequence learning tasks. Only a single circular stimulus appeared at any time in each task. When the appropriate response was made the stimulus disappeared to be replaced 400 ms later by a further cue. In the position task there was a direct spatial correspondence between a blue circular stimulus appearing at any one of four positions within a horizontal array and a response. In the colour task an arbitrary visuomotor association coupled stimulus colour to an appropriate response. Colour alone dictated the correct response because all the stimuli appeared in the centre of the screen. Hence, in addition to learning a sequence the colour task also required the acquisition of an arbitrary visuomotor association. In the combined task both colour and position, simultaneously, cue the same response. This task supplies redundant sensory cues.
(*b*) Disruption of the dorsolateral prefrontal cortex specifically prevents spatial cues from guiding the acquisition of novel sequences. Following rTMS over this site, learning is exclusively prevented in the position task. In addition, the normally augmented learning observed in the combined task was reduced to a level commensurate with only a single guiding cue, probably colour, being present. Learning was defined as a significant increase in response times during performance in the random trials following earlier performance of a repeating ten-item sequence (after-effect).

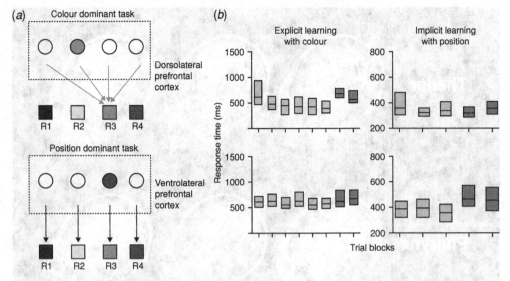

Fig. 5.7 (*a*) Diagram shows the relationship between the stimulus cue and response in the dual task. Two sequences are presented simultaneously, one using colour, the other using position cue. Subjects' responses can be driven by colour or position (colour dominant versus position dominant versions). (*b*) A two-by-two truth table, with one axis devoted to the site of rTMS stimulation (dorsolateral or ventrolateral prefrontal cortex) and the other to the effect of sensory cue and awareness. Each cell shows a box graph of the response times for blocks of 50 sequential (light coloured) and random trials (dark coloured), a significant rise in response time during the random trials is evidence of having acquired skill in performing a sequence. A significant difference between the sequential and random trials was observed during explicit learning guided by a colour cue, despite earlier disruption of the dorsolateral prefrontal cortex. This was in contrast to the absence of learning when an implicit sequence was guided by position. Conversely, following disruption of the ventrolateral prefrontal cortex skill was not acquired in the colour guided and explicit sequence, but there was a significant difference between the response times of the random and sequential trials when position guided the acquisition of the implicit sequence. Therefore, the findings support the notion of parallel, modality specific processing streams in the prefrontal cortex that are engaged during learning regardless of awareness.

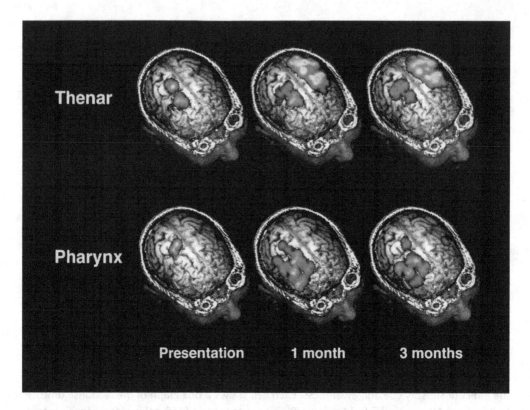

Fig. 11.1 Surface-rendered MRI brain images from a patient following left-sided hemispheric stroke. TMS topographic data of the pharyngeal and contralateral thenar muscles has been coregistered. The patient was dysphagic at presentation but had recovered swallowing at 1 month. It is evident that, after stroke, the representation of the pharynx in the anterior aspect of the motor cortex and premotor areas expands anterolaterally in the right unaffected hemisphere at both 1 and 3 months, with little change in the affected left hemisphere. In contrast, the representation of the thenar muscles in superior motor cortex increases anteriorly and posteriorly in the affected left hemisphere over time, but remains unchanged in the unaffected right hemisphere. (Reproduced with kind permission, Hamdy et al., 1998a.)

NO STIMULATION

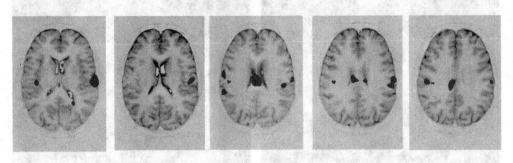

STIMULATION

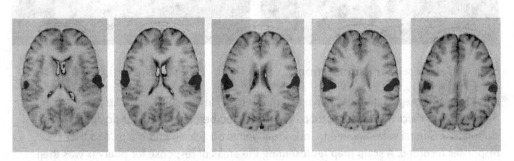

Fig. 11.3 Effect of pharyngeal stimulation on cortical BOLD (blood oxygenation level dependent) fMRI signal in healthy subjects during normal swallowing. Activated pixels in red. Greater bilateral functional activation occurs within sensorimotor cortex (BA 3,4) in those subjects receiving pharyngeal stimulation compared to sham stimulation. (From Fraser et al., 2001a.)

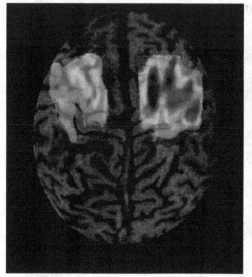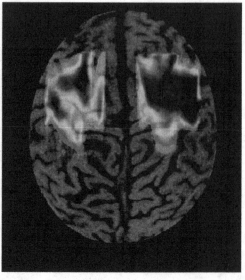

Before sensory stimulation   After sensory stimulation

Fig. 11.4 MRI coregistration of pharyngeal motor maps in a dysphagic stroke patient after left basal ganglia infarct. Topographic maps were acquired before and 1 hour postpharyngeal stimulation. Stimuli were applied to individual points on a scalp grid matrix and the responses recorded. A scalp map representing the areas of response for pharynx was then generated and coregistered anatomically with the patient's motor cortices using MRI. After stroke, most of the pharyngeal representation is on the undamaged (right) hemisphere. The greatest changes are also seen in the intact hemisphere after pharyngeal stimulation (From Fraser et al., 2001b.)

Recruitment of distant brain areas and functional significance

The acquisition of Braille-reading skill poses an interesting problem of neural logistics, because it imposes a marked increase in afferent input and efferent demands onto a restricted body space (the pads of Braille-reading fingers). Blind Braille readers must discriminate, with exquisite sensitivity and accuracy, between subtle patterns of raised and depressed dots with the pads of their fingers and translate this spatial code into meaningful information. Faced with the complex cognitive demands of Braille reading, striking adaptive changes occur in the sensorimotor representation of the reading finger in the human brain as discussed in previous sections of this chapter. Longitudinal studies of the cortical outputs of blind subjects learning Braille reveal that this enlargement seems to have two phases (Fig. 5.4): (a) a rapid, dramatic, and transient enlargement that is likely due to the unmasking of connections or upregulation of synaptic efficacy, and (b) a slower, less prominent, but more stable enlargement of the cortical representation of the

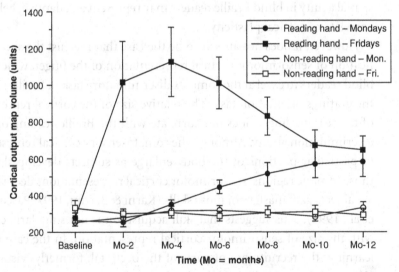

Fig. 5.4   Line graph of the cortical motor output map volumes to the right and left FDI and the Braille reading speed over the course of 10 months of Braille learning. Result display mean ± standard deviation values for ten subjects. Monday and Friday maps refer to the time of testing in relation to the week of daily Braille classes.

reading finger that may represent structural plasticity (Pascual-Leone et al., 1998a). If these findings regarding the acquisition of Braille reading skills can be extrapolated to other forms of skill learning, we might infer that learning involves transient rapid changes in efficacy of existing connections that lead the way for enduring structural changes in the face of continued practice.

The expanded cortical representation of fingers used in Braille reading appears to be associated with an enhanced fidelity in the neural transmission of spatial details of a stimulus and result in a heightened tactile spatial acuity. Using the grating orientation discrimination task, in which threshold performance is accounted for by the spatial resolution limits of the neural image evoked by a stimulus, van Boven et al. (2000) quantified the psychophysical limits of spatial resolution at the middle and index fingers of blind Braille readers and sighted control subjects. The mean grating orientation threshold was significantly lower in the blind group compared with the sighted group. The self-reported dominant reading finger in blind subjects had the lowest grating orientation threshold in all subjects and was significantly better than other fingers tested. Therefore, these findings suggest that superior tactile spatial acuity in blind Braille readers may represent an adaptive, behavioural correlate of cortical plasticity.

However, it does not appear to be the case that it is just the sheer magnification of sensorimotor cortical representation of the finger, which enables blind readers to excel at the complex discriminatory task of Braille reading or the gratings orientation task. The relative size of the cortical representation of the reading finger does not correlate with the Braille reading or sensory discrimination ability. Although the somatosensory cortical representations of particular portions of the body enlarge as subjects develop skills using those somatic regions, sensorimotor cortical representations decrease in size as subjects gain mastery of those skills (Karni & Bertini, 1997; Pascual-Leone et al., 1994). This suggests that skill acquisition is not singularly correlated with the size of sensorimotor cortical representation. In the case of Braille learning, the recruitment of parts of the occipital, formerly 'visual', cortex (V1 and V2) for tactile information processing appears to be a critical contributor to the improved tactile acuity. There appears to be a significant correlation between the amount of activation in striate and peristriate cortex to tactile stimulation of the finger pads as measured by functional magnetic resonance imaging (fMRI) and the gratings-orientation thresholds for the different fingers of proficient Braille readers (Kiriakopoulos et al., 1999; van Boven et al., 2000). The blood-oxygen level dependent (BOLD) activation in occipital cortex is significantly greater during stimulation of the preferred reading finger than during stimulation of adjacent fingers in the same hand or of the homologous finger in the other hand.

Plasticity in the context of normal behaviour: sequence learning

We have discussed thus far how acquisition of new motor skills is associated with a change in brain circuitry and function that can be revealed with TMS. However, we have also pointed out that plasticity is not a special state of the nervous system; plasticity is the normal state of the nervous system. A full, coherent account of any sensory or cognitive function has to build into its framework the ongoing changes that occur as the brain is moulded and modified by experience. The evidence for this view is overwhelming: adaptation in the short- and long-term, priming, order effects in experiments, the effects of feedback in experiments. As we try to address such plastic brain changes experimentally, we need to consider that the brain also acts on the world and it will not turn off at the start of an experiment simply to allow the experimenter to begin with a clean slate. The solution can be twofold. First, one can design experiments that as far as possible negate the small changes that may occur in brain circuits over the course of experiments, a hugely successful strategy as the current state of cognitive neuroscience testifies. The experiments we have discussed thus far take this strategy and, while addressing plasticity during skill acquisition, they assume an initial, 'stable' starting point for the finding. Alternatively, one can try to understand plasticity in the context of normal behaviour. Studies of sequence learning provide a useful example of this approach.

An ability to order thoughts, events and actions in time, so-called sequencing, is fundamental to many aspects of human behaviour. Some sequences are acquired explicitly as rules, for example a prerequisite to obtaining a driving licence is to know the order and meaning of changes in traffic light colours. Acquiring an ability to play a musical instrument such as the piano would be a further example of this form of learning, where initially there is conscious awareness of a pattern but with practice and time this gives way to highly skilled actions associated with relatively little awareness. However, in other situations, humans are initially oblivious even to the presence of a repeating and orderly pattern of events. This extends from perhaps the common-place preparation and cooking of food that allows the entire meal to be ready simultaneously, to the slow and intuitive realization of previously hidden order amongst a series of events.

The serial response time task

Over the past 20 years, the serial response time task (SRTT) has become increasingly popular as a means to investigate this later type of sequence acquisition (Nissen & Bullemer, 1987). In the basic form of this task, a stimulus appears at one of four positions with each position corresponding to a button on a response pad. The subject sits in front of a monitor holding a response pad and is instructed to push, as quickly and accurately as possible, the appropriate response button upon presentation of a visual stimulus on the monitor. The interval between the appearance of the stimulus and selection of the correct button on the response pad is termed the response time (RT). When selected, the correct response triggers the presentation of a further stimulus. This is an iterative process with the relationship amongst the stimuli being, unbeknown to the subject, either random or following an ordered pattern, i.e. a repeating sequence.

During the random trials RT is related exclusively to movement performance and may be affected by non-specific factors such as familiarity with the task and equipment. However, RTs over the sequential trials are related to both movement performance and knowledge of the sequence. Hence a significant rise in RT during a series of random trials following earlier exposure to a sequence, is related exclusively to learning. This so-called after-effect has been used widely both for sequence learning and visuomotor adaptation because it is related exclusively to the acquisition of a skill rather than any non-specific improvement in task performance (Martin et al., 1996; Robertson & Miall, 1999).

Although this paradigm has afforded a considerable improvement in our understanding of sequence learning, there are still important neural principles, which remain undiscovered. While vital to guiding the attainment of new skills, relatively little work has examined the importance of sensory information. Recent observations from a behavioural paradigm, designed to systematically explore the influence of sensory information upon learning, have helped to develop a conceptual model of sequence learning (Robertson & Pascual-Leone, 2001). In this, we envisage sequence learning arising from an interaction and co-operation between cue-dependent and -independent circuits. TMS can be used to experimentally test this proposal. In doing so, TMS is used to reveal functional roles of a dynamically changing system in the context of an ongoing, learning-related, plastic adaptation.

A model of sequence learning

Generally, two almost mutually exclusive approaches have been taken to deepen our understanding of sequence learning. Some models have explored the computations underlying the acquisition of sequences, for instance, simple recurrent networks can establish the temporal context of an item based upon previous items (Elman, 1990; Jordan, 1996). These approaches offer potential insights into the neuronal mechanisms of sequence learning and help to demonstrate how the solution to inherent problems of sequencing emerges from relatively simple mechanisms. Other models have developed an integrated framework in which observations from functional imaging studies and the sequence learning deficits in patient populations can be understood. These models have established a network of areas, over which there is reasonable consensus, thought to play at least some role in sequence learning (Doyon, 1997; Doyon et al., 1997; Hazeltine, 2001; Hazeltine et al., 1997; Willingham et al., 1989). However, the nature of this role and how the role changes in time remains relatively unexplored. A notable exception has been an attempt to distinguish between those brain areas making a contribution early or late in the learning process (Hikosaka et al., 1999). This has been applied to animals, in particular to non-human primates, where the issue of awareness is less of a confounding factor, and using a paradigm that greatly expands the time over which learning takes place. In humans, a similar approach informed by a model that attempts to discern a network of areas supporting sequence learning and gives some insight into the computational contribution made by each of these areas has been lacking.

Regions of the premotor and parietal cortices have been implicated in sequence learning, along with the striatum, cerebellum, supplementary motor area, cingulate cortex, and bilateral primary motor and somatosensory strips

(Doyon et al., 1996; Grafton et al., 1992, 1994, 1995, 1998; Hazeltine et al., 1997; Honda et al., 1998; Rauch et al., 1995). Only awareness of the underlying sequence was thought to alter this pattern, with the recruitment of the prefrontal cortex perhaps responsible for the augmented learning observed in explicit learning. Consequently, many contemporary studies have concentrated upon drawing an anatomical distinction between those areas involved in implicit and explicit sequence learning. Whether this transition is accomplished by chance (Grafton et al., 1995, 1998; Hazeltine et al., 1997) or design (Honda et al., 1998; Rauch et al., 1995) the pattern of brain activation always shows some overlap between the circuits associated with these two modes of sequence learning. A circuit of primary motor cortex, supplementary and premotor areas is implicated in supporting implicit sequence learning (Grafton et al., 1995; Honda et al., 1998). During the development of explicit learning the prefrontal (Doyon et al., 1996; Grafton et al., 1995; Honda et al., 1998) and possibly the parietal cortex (Grafton et al., 1995) are recruited to this circuit.

Without a doubt, the identification of partly separate circuits in implicit and explicit sequential learning has been a major advance of cognitive neuroscience in the past 20 years. However, concentrating on the role of explicit vs. implicit strategies on sequence learning has occurred with the relative disregard of other potentially important influences upon the neural substrate of sequence learning. For example, while sensory information is critical to guiding sequence acquisition, relatively little work has examined the effects which differences in the sensory environment have upon sequence learning.

We have proposed a model that integrates neuroanatomical, neurophysiologic and neuroimaging results to make specific, experimentally testable predictions regarding the role of various neural structures in sequential learning (Robertson & Pascual-Leone, 2001). Our model (Fig. 5.5, see colour plate at www.cambridge.org/9780521114462). proposes that the sensory, guiding cue (and by extrapolation the sensory input) is central to the neural principles of sequence learning. Furthermore, the model proposes that the sensory cue provides the organizing structure for the prefrontal cortex, which is constituted by an array of modality specific parallel processing streams. This is in contrast to a pervading a ssumption that awareness of an underlying sequence determines the recruitment of cortical and subcortical areas, particularly of the prefrontal cortex, during sequence learning. Such an assumption persists despite recent studies, which suggest that it may be the functional coupling or connectivity between areas, which lies at the basis of awareness rather than the recruitment of specific cortical areas (for example, see Pascual-Leone & Walsh, 2001).

Prefrontal cortex: awareness vs. sensory modality

Recent studies have convincingly demonstrated that the prefrontal cortex makes a critical contribution to learning even without awareness of an underlying sequence. An inability to acquire a sequence has been observed in patients suffering from frontal lobe damage and following functional disruption with repetitive transcranial magnetic stimulation (rTMS) of the dorsolateral prefrontal cortex (Gomez Beldarrain et al., 1999; Pascual-Leone et al., 1995c, 1996). These studies are important for they demonstrate the critical contribution made by the prefrontal cortex during implicit sequence learning; however, they fail to offer much insight into the nature of this contribution. Recently, we explored this issue by contrasting the learning impairment resulting from rTMS across variations of the SRTT in which position, colour, or combined position and colour cues guide learning (Fig. 5.6(a), see colour plate at www.cambridge.org/9780521114462). These studies allow a dissociation between the general and the cue-specific components of sequence learning (Robertson et al., 2001). Sequence learning guided by spatial cues was prevented following rTMS of the dorsolateral prefrontal cortex, confirming earlier observations (Pascual-Leone et al., 1996); however, learning using colour as a cue was unaffected (Fig. 5.6(b), see colour plate at www.cambridge.org/9780521114462). When colour and position cues were combined, the normally augmented learning was reduced to a level commensurate with only the colour cue being available. This pattern of effects across the three SRTT tasks was specific to the dorsolateral prefrontal cortex because the same stimulation regime applied to the parietal cortex had no effect upon learning.

These observations are consistent not only with the organizing principles of our model but also with an important theory of prefrontal cortex function (Goldman-Rakic, 1987, 1998). This domain-specific theory suggests that segregation across the prefrontal cortex is based upon the type of sensory information being processed and in particular that the dorsolateral prefrontal cortex is dedicated to processing spatial information. Other prefrontal regions, perhaps the ventrolateral and ventromedial prefrontal cortex, are thought to perform an analogous function for non-spatial cues (Levy &

Goldmann-Rakic, 2000). The dissociation between dorsolateral and ventro-lateral functions of the prefrontal cortex for spatial vs. object information can be demonstrated using rTMS in studies of working memory (Mottaghy et al., 2002).

Hence, the underlying organizing principle for the critical contribution made by the prefrontal cortex during sequence learning appears to be related to the cue guiding learning and not an awareness of the sequence. Recently, we have examined this issue further using another modified version of the SRTT (Fig. 5.7(a), see colour plate section). We have developed a task, which allows two sequences to be acquired simultaneously. Each sequence is represented by a different component of a guiding stimulus. Initially, responses are dictated by the colour of the stimulus, while stimulus position is also changing across trials. Both of these components follow distinct and independent sequences. Although responses are initially dictated only by colour, we have also observed the simultaneous acquisition of the position sequence. This was demonstrated by skilful performance of the position sequence over a limited number of trials, when position rather than colour was responsible for dictating the correct response. Under normal circumstances this limited exposure would be insufficient for the development of skill. Thus this task allows the concurrent acquisition of two independent sequences represented by two distinct components of a stimulus. In a recent study we have allowed a component of this dual learning task to become explicit by giving declarative knowledge of the colour sequence, while the position sequence remains implicit (E.M. Robertson & A. Pascual-Leone, unpublished data). In this way it becomes possible to further explore the relationship between the sensory guiding cue and awareness.

Declarative knowledge of the colour sequence was acquired over a couple of days before the start of the experiment. However, the position sequence remained implicit. Critically, subjects also remained ignorant of the arbitrary visuomotor relationship between colour and response, so that they were unable to unintentionally acquire procedural knowledge of the sequence before the start of the experiment. Eight subjects were randomly allocated to receive rTMS over the dorsolateral or the ventrolateral prefrontal cortex with the primary motor cortex acting as the control site for both groups. The order of stimulation sites was counterbalanced across the subjects. Following 10 minutes of 1 Hz stimulation at 115% of motor threshold, each subject performed the dual task. These stimulation parameters are based on the observation that slow rTMS (1 Hz) of the motor cortex can decrease corticospinal excitability (Chen et al., 1997; Maeda et al., 2000), primarily by reducing corticocortical facilitation (Romero et al., 2002). These neurophysiological effects of rTMS can outlast the duration of the rTMS train, hence allowing application of the rTMS before starting a cognitive task, inducing a temporary disruption of cortical activity, and minimizing potential confounders of rTMS when applied during the behavioural task. In cognitive neuroscience, this so-called distal or 'off-line' TMS was first applied to investigate visual imagery (Kosslyn et al., 1999), and since then it has been applied in a stream of studies targeting different brain areas and behaviours and establishing the utility of the methodology (for example, see Hilgetag et al., 2001; Mottaghy et al., 2002; Robertson et al., 2001; Theoret et al., 2001). The first stage consisted of 300 trials sandwiched between two blocks of 100 random trials. Each of these cues had both a position and a colour, both following their own independent sequence; however, it was only the colour component, which dictated the response. In the final stage, of 150 trials sandwiched between two blocks of 100 random trials, the position of the cue determined the response. After waiting 20 minutes to allow the effects of stimulation to dissipate, the remaining site was disrupted. Therefore, in the initial stage of the experiment the implicit position sequence was only observed passively, while the previously explicitly learned colour sequence dictated the correct response. Thereafter, the position component of the stimulus was attended to, while the colour cue, although also following a sequence, was ignored.

Our observations (Fig. 5.7, see colour plate at www.cambridge.org/9780521114462). are consistent with the predictions of our model and strengthen the view that the fundamental organizing principle of prefrontal cortex contribution to sequence learning is related to the sensory modality of the guiding cue. Although rTMS over the dorsolateral prefrontal cortex prevented acquisition of the implicit position sequence, there was clear evidence of having acquired the explicit colour sequence. This situation was reversed for the ventrolateral prefrontal cortex, with no evidence of having acquired the explicit colour sequence following stimulation, but a clear demonstration of skill at performing the implicit position sequence. These observations, combined with our earlier exploration of the dorsolateral prefrontal cortex's contribution to implicit learning guided by both spatial and colour cues, offers a consistent perspective: guiding cue rather than awareness seems to determine the area of prefrontal cortex recruited during sequence learning.

An interesting pattern was also observed following stimulation over the primary motor cortex: acquisition of the explicit colour sequence was prevented but the implicit position sequence was learnt. We believe that this is related to the effector used to acquire the sequence. In the case of the explicit colour sequence, the effector was the hand; consequently, preventing learning following disruption over the hand area is perhaps not all that surprising. In contrast, the skill observed in the position dominant task could well have been acquired initially through eye movements and then transferred to the hand (so-called oculo-manual transfer). Potentially, this difference is reflected in the critical area of the primary motor cortex recruited during the performance of the position dominant task. These findings provide a critical expansion to our model, requiring introduction of frontal eye-fields and oculomotor control into the neural circuitry.

Representations and cue-dependence

A key concept of this model is for sequence acquisition to depend critically upon an interaction and co-operation between cue-dependent and -independent circuits. Cue-dependent regions lie upstream from the confluence site and are responsible for the short-term retention and manipulation of sensory cues. This information is then transformed into a common framework and used to drive sequence learning in downstream sites, regardless of the guiding cue. Inevitably, this scheme results in cues from a variety of different modalities being represented within the same downstream circuits. However, this does not imply that representations of identical sequences, which were guided by distinct sensory cues, are equivalent. Instead, these representations are thought likely to reflect the sensory cue responsible for guiding their acquisition. Thus an abstract representation of a sequence is not necessarily held within the generic downstream sites. Instead, the cue independence of these circuits is merely thought to reflect the use of a common neuronal circuit and algorithm for sequence acquisition, irrespective of the guiding sensory cues. This potential contrast between abstract representations divorced of guiding cue and the implementation of the sequence with those representations merely within cue-independent circuits has recently been explored in a couple of functional imaging studies.

The pattern of blood flow across the motor cortex has been shown to depend upon whether a spatial or non-spatial cue is guiding the performance of a sequence (Hazeltine et al., 1997). Thus, although exactly the same sequence was being performed, the neuronal representation, as reflected in the blood flow patterns, depends upon the guiding cue. An important principle may be that the history of how a movement was learnt is crucial in determining both the anatomical structures critical for learning and the nature of the final representation of an action. This feature has also been reflected in the neurophysiological evolution of awareness during sequence learning. Although exactly the same sequence can be performed with or without awareness, substantial changes in excitability across the motor cortex are associated with achieving awareness of the sequence (Pascual-Leone et al., 1994). During implicit learning, we found an enlargement of the motor cortical output maps that was selective for the representation of muscles involved in the task (Fig. 5.8). When the subjects became aware of the repeating nature of the stimuli, an explicit search strategy was likely engaged. Eventually, as the subjects learned the full repeating sequence of stimuli and performance became primarily driven by explicit knowledge, we found a rapid reduction of the motor cortical output maps towards the baseline (Fig. 5.8). A similar contrast in cortical excitability may be associated with acquiring the same sequence when guided by different cues.

Nevertheless, abstract representations of sequences may well be formed, potentially within areas of the neural substrate responsible for cue-independent sequence learning. A recent functional imaging study implicated area 40 of the parietal cortex in representing a sequence independent of its production (Grafton et al., 1998). Hence, this area may form an abstract representation of a sequence, but this may not be critical to sequence learning *per se*, consistent with our failing to observe a learning impairment following rTMS at this site (Robertson et al., 2001). Instead, this area might only supply a critical role when a skill has to be transferred to a novel environment. Potentially, abstract representations are a useful byproduct of sequence learning rather than being critical to the acquisition of a sequence.

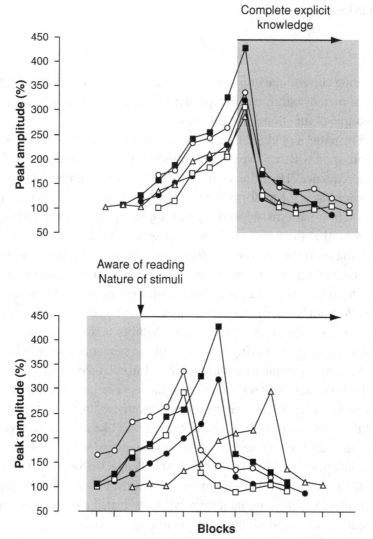

Fig. 5.8   Graph of the size of the motor output maps over time during performance of the SRTT and procedural acquisition of the sequence in five individual subjects. Note the consistency across subjects: the maps of all of them suddenly reverse towards baseline as soon as complete explicit knowledge of the sequence is attained (top). The time-point at which such explicit knowledge is reached varies from subject to subject hence supporting the notion that the changes in motor output maps are not related to amount of practice, but rather are due to a more fundamental, learning-related phenomenon. Recognition that there is a repeating organization to the stimuli (and hence initiating an explicit search strategy) is not sufficient to lead to the changes in motor output maps (bottom). (Modified from Pascual-Leone et al., 1994.)

Conclusions

TMS can be used in a variety of ways to study plasticity during skill learning (Pascual-Leone et al., 1999): (a) as a mapping tool to demonstrate plasticity during skill acquisition; (b) as a neurophysiological tool to investigate cortical excitability and provide insights into the mechanisms underlying such plasticity; and (c) as a method to transiently disrupt focal cortical function and hence address the casual role of a given brain area in a changing behaviour. In all these ways of applying TMS, the fundamental realization is that, at the heart of brain function, there is a lack of functional stability: the rate and efficacy of synaptic transmission can alter radically in only a matter of minutes, possibly even anatomical connections can come and go. While these changes are likely to be essential for individuals to adapt to their environment, and hence develop and learn throughout life, such instability presumably harbours grave dangers for the nervous system. This alternative side of plasticity remains under-explored even though it may be fundamental to the pathophysiology of neuropsychiatric disorders. In this context, our challenge is to understand the mechanisms of plasticity better, in order to guide them for the best functional outcome for each given individual: enhance plasticity when advisable or reduce it in instances of potential maladaptive change. Repetitive TMS, being able to modulate cortical excitability beyond the duration of the stimulation itself (Pascual-Leone et al., 1998b; Maeda et al., 2000), might be an ideally suited tool for this purpose of guiding plasticity.

Acknowledgements

Some of the work described in this manuscript was done in collaboration with Mark Hallett, Nguyet Dang, Leonardo Cohen, José María Tormos, Josep Valls-Solé, Terrance Sanger, Gottfried Schlaug, Fumiko Maeda, Daniel Tarsy, Jesus Pujol, and Jaume Roset-Llobet. It was supported in part by the General Clinical Research Center at Beth Israel Deaconess Medical Center (National Center for Research Resources MO1 RR01032) and grants from the National Institutes of Health (RO1MH57980, RO1EY12091), National Institute of Mental Health (MH57980, MH60734), the National Eye Institute (EY 12091), the Goldberg Foundation, a NARSAD Young Investigator award (EMR) and a Fellowship from the Canadian Institutes of Health Research (HT).

REFERENCES

Bara-Jimenez, W., Shelton, P., Sanger, T.D. & Hallett, M. (2000). Sensory discrimination capabilities in patients with focal hand dystonia. *Ann. Neurol.*, **43**: 377–380.

Chen, R., Classen, J., Gerloff, C. et al. (1997). Depression of motor cortex excitability by low-frequency transcranial magnetic stimulation. *Neurology*, **48**: 1398–1403.

Chollet, F. (2000). Plasticity of the adult human brain. In *Brain Mapping: The Systems*, ed. J.C. Mazziotta, A.W. Toga & R.S. Frackowiak, pp. 621–638. San Diego: Academic Press.

Chollet, F. & Weiller, C. (2000). Recovery of neurological function. In *Brain Mapping: The Disorders*, ed. J.C. Mazziotta, A.W. Toga & R.S. Frackowiak, pp. 587–597. San Diego: Academic Press.

Doyon, J., Owen, A.M., Petrides, M., Sziklas, V. & Evans, A.C. (1996). Functional anatomy of visuomotor skill learning in human subjects examined with positron emission tomography. *Eur. J. Neurosci.*, **8**: 637–648.

Doyon, J. (1997). Skill learning. *Int. Rev. Neurobiol.*, **41**: 273–294.

Doyon, J., Gaudreau, D., Laforce, R. Jr. et al. (1997). Role of the striatum, cerebellum, and frontal lobes in the learning of a visuomotor sequence. *Brain Cogn.*, **34**: 218–245.

Elbert, T., Pantev, C., Wienbruch, C., Rockstroh, B. & Taub, E. (1995). Increased cortical representation of the fingers of the left hand in string players. *Science*, **270**: 305–307.

Elman, J.L. (1990). Finding structure in time. *Cogn. Sci.*, **14**: 179–211.

Ferbert, A., Priori, A., Rothwell, J.C., Day, B.L., Colebatch, J.G. & Mardsen, C.D. (1992). Interhemispheric inhibition of the human motor cortex. *J. Physiol.* (*Lond.*), **453**: 525–546.

Fuster, J.M. (1995). Memory in the cerebral cortex. *An Empirical Approach to Neural Networks in the Human and Nonhuman Primate*. Cambridge, MA: The MIT Press.

Goldman-Rakic, P. (1987). Circuitry of primate prefrontal cortex and by representation of memory and the regulation of behaviour by representational memory. In *Handbook of Physiology*, ed. F. Plum & V. Mountcastle, vol. 5, pp. 373–417. Washington: American Physiological Society, Washington.

Goldman-Rakic, P. (1998). The prefrontal landscape: implications of functional architecture for understanding human mentation and the central executive. In *The Prefrontal Cortex: Executive and Cognitive Functions*, ed. A.C. Roberts, T.W. Robbins & L. Weiskrantz, pp. 87–102. Oxford: Oxford University Press.

Gomez-Beldarrain, M., Grafman, J., Pascaul-Leone, A. & Garcia-Monoco, J.C. (1999). Procedural learning is impaired in patients with prefrontal lesions. *Neurology*, **52**: 1853–1860.

Grafton, S.T., Mazziotta, J.C., Presty, S., Friston, K.J., Frackowiak, R.S. & Phelps, M.E. (1992). Functional anatomy of human procedural learning determined with regional cerebral blood flow and PET. *J. Neurosci.*, **12**: 2542–2548.

Grafton, S.T., Woods, R.P. & Tyszka, M. (1994). Functional imaging of procedural motor learning: relating cerebral blood flow with individual subject performance. *Hum. Brain Mapp.*, **1**: 221–234.

Grafton, S.T., Hazeltine, E. & Ivry, R. (1995). Functional anatomy of motor sequence learning in humans. *J. Cogn. Neurosci.*, **7**: 497–510.

Grafton, S.T., Hazeltine, E. & Ivry, R.B. (1998). Abstract and effector specific representations of motor sequences identified with PET. *J. Neurosci.*, **18**: 9420–9428.

Hazeltine, E., Grafton, S.T. & Ivry, R. (1997). Attention and stimulus characteristics determine the locus of motor-sequence encoding. A PET study. *Brain*, **120**: 123–140.

Hazeltine, E. (2001). Ipsilateral sensorimotor regions and motor sequence learning. *Trends Cogn. Sci.*, **5**: 281–282.

Hikosaka. O., Nakahara, H., Rand, M.K. et al. (1999). Parallel neural networks for learning sequential procedures. *Trends Neurosci.*, **22**: 464–471.

Hilgetag, C.C., Theoret, H. & Pascual-Leone, A. (2001). Enhanced visual spatial attention ispsilateral to rTMS induces 'virtual lesions' of human parietal cortex. *Nature Neurosci.*, **4**: 953–957.

Honda, M., Deiber, M.P., Ibanez, V., Pascual-Leone, A., Zhuang, P. & Hallett, M. (1998). Dynamic cortical involvement in implicit and explicit motor sequence learning. A PET study. *Brain*, **121**: 2159–2173.

Jordan, M.I. (1996). *Serial Order: A Parallel Distributed Processing Approach*. Hillside, NJ: Erlbum.

Kaas, J.H. (1997). *Functional Plasticity in Adult Cortex*, vol. 9. Orlando, FL: Academic Press.

Kaas, J.H. (2000). The reorganization of somatosensory and motor cortex after peripheral nerve or spinal cord injury in primates. *Prog. Brain Res.*, **128**: 173–179.

Karni, A. & Bertini, G. (1997). Learning perceptual skills: behavioural probes into adult cortical plasticity. *Curr. Opin. Neurobiol.*, **7**: 530–535.

Karni, A., Meyer, G., Jezzard, P., Adams, M.M., Turner, R. & Ungerleider, L.G. (1995). Functional MRI evidence for adult motor cortex plasticity during motor skill learning. *Nature*, **377**: 155–158.

Kiriakopoulos, E., Kauffman, T., Hamilton, R. & Pascual-Leone, A. (1999). Relationship between tactile acuity and cortical activation in early blind subjects. *Neuroimage*, **9**: S571.

Kosslyn, S.M., Pascual-Leone, A., Felician, O. et al. (1999). The role of area 17 in visual imagery: convergent evidence from PET and rTMS. *Science*, **284**: 167–170.

Kujirai, T., Caramia, M.D., Rothwell, J.C., Day, B.L., Thompson, B.D. & Ferbert, A. (1993). Cortico-cortical inhibition in human motor cortex. *J. Physiol.* (*Lond.*), **471**: 501–520.

Levy, R. & Goldmann-Rakic, P.S. (2000). Segregation of working memory function within the dorsolateral prefrontal cortex. *Exp. Brain Res.*, **133**: 23–32.

Maeda, F., Keenan, J.P., Tormos, J.M., Topka, H. & Pascual-Leone, A. (2000). Modulation of cortico-spinal excitability by repetitive transcranial magnetic stimulation. *Clin. Neurophysiol.*, **111**: 800–805.

Martin, T.A., Keating, J.G., Goodkin, H.P., Bastian, A.J. & Thach, W.T. (1996). Throwing while looking through prisms. II. Specificity and storage of multiple gaze throw calibrations. *Brain*, **119**: 1199–1211.

Mottaghy, F.M., Gangitano, M., Sparing, R., Krause, B.J. & Pascual-Leone, A. (2002). Segregation of areas related to visual working memory in the prefrontal cortex revealed by rTMS. *Cereb. Cortex*, in press.

Nissen, M.J. & Bullemer, P. (1987). Attentional requirements of learning: evidence from performance measures. *Cogn. Psychol.*, **19**: 1–32.

Pascual-Leone, A. (2001). The brain that plays music and is changed by it. In *Music and the Brain*, ed. R. Zatorre and I. Peretz. New York: New York Academy of Sciences.

Pascual-Leone, A. & Walsh, V. (2001). Fast backprojections from the motion to the primary visual area necessary for visual awareness. *Science*, **292**: 510–512.

Pascual-Leone, A., Cammarota, A., Wassermann, E.M., Brasil-Neto, J.P., Cohen, L.G. & Hallett, M. (1993). Modulation of motor cortical outputs to the reading hand of braille readers. *Ann. Neurol.*, **34**: 33–37.

Pascual-Leone, A., Grafman, J. & Hallett, M. (1994). Modulation of cortical motor output maps during development of implicit and explicit knowledge. *Science*, **263**: 1287–1289.

Pascual-Leone, A., Nguyet, D., Cohen, L.G., Brasil-Neto, J.P., Cammarota, A. & Hallett, M. (1995a). Modulation of muscle responses evoked by transcranial magnetic stimulation during the acquisition of new fine motor skills. *J. Neurophysiol.*, **74**: 1037–1045.

Pascual-Leone, A., Wassermann, E.M., Sadato, N. & Hallett, M. (1995b). The role of reading activity on the modulation of motor cortical outputs to the reading hand in braille readers. *Ann. Neurol.*, **38**: 910–915.

Pascual-Leone, A., Grafman, J. & Hallett, M. (1995c). Procedural learning and prefrontal cortex. *Ann. NY Acad. Sci.*, **769**: 61–70.

Pascual-Leone, A., Wassermann, E.M., Grafman, J. & Hallett, M. (1996). The role of the dorsolateral prefrontal cortex in implicit procedural learning. *Exp. Brain Res.*, **107**: 479–485.

Pascual-Leone, A., Hamilton, R., Tormos, J.M., Keenan, J. & Catala, M.D. (1998a). Neuroplasticity in the adjustment to blindness. *Neuroplasticity: Building a Bridge from the Laboratory to the Clinic*, ed. J. Grafman & Y. Christen, pp. 93–108. Munich & New York: Springer-Verlag.

Pascual-Leone, A., Tormos, J.M., Keenan, J., Tarazona, F., Canete, C. & Catala, M.D. (1998b). Study and modulation of human cortical excitability with transcranial magnetic stimulation. *J. Clin. Neurophysiol.*, **15**: 333–343.

Pascual-Leone, A., Tarazona, F. & Catalá, M.D. (1999). Applications of transcranial magnetic stimulation in studies on motor learning. In *Transcranial Magnetic Stimulation*, Supplement of Electroencephalography and Clinical Neurophysiology, EEG Suppl. 51, ed. W. Paulus, M. Hallett, P.M. Rossini & J.C. Rothwell.

Pearce, A.J., Thickbroom, G.W., Byrnes, M.L. & Mastaglia, F.L. (2000). Functional reorganisation of the corticomotor projection to the hand in skilled racquet players. *Exp. Brain Res.*, **130**: 238–243.

Poldrack, R.A. (2000). Imaging brain plasticity: conceptual and methodological issues – a theoretical review. *Neuroimage*, **12**: 1–13.

Pujol, J., Roset-Llobet, J., Rosines-Cubells, D. et al. (2000). Brain cortical activation during guitar-induced hand dystonia studied by functional MRI. *Neuroimage*, **12**: 257–267.

Rauch, S.L., Savage, C.R., Brown, H.D. et al. (1995). A PET investigation of implicit and explicit sequence learning. *Hum. Brain Mapp.*, **3**: 271–286.

Ridding, M.C., Brouwer, B. & Nordstrom, M.A. (2000). Reduced interhemispheric inhibition in musicians. *Exp. Brain Res.*, **133**: 249–253.

Robertson, E.M. & Miall, R.C. (1999). Visuomotor adaptation during inactivation of the dentate nucleus. *Neuroreport*, **10**: 1029–1034.

Robertson, E.M. & Pascual-Leone, A. (2001). Aspects of sensory guidance in sequence learning. *Exp. Brain Res.*, **137**: 336–345.

Robertson, E.M., Tormos, J.M., Maeda, F. & Pascual-Leone, A. (2001). The role of the dorsolateral prefrontal cortex during sequence learning is specific for spatial information. *Cereb. Cortex*, **11**: 628–635.

Romero, R., Anshel, D., Sparing, R., Gangitano, M. & Pascual-Leone, A. (2002). Subthreshold low frequency repetitive transcranial magnetic stimulation selectively decreases facilitation in the motor cortex. *Clin. Neurophysiol.*, **113**: 101–107.

Schacter, D.L. & Buckner, R.L. (1998). On the relations among priming, conscious recollection, and intentional retrieval: evidence from neuroimaging research. *Neurobiol. Learn. Mem.*, **70**: 284–303.

Schlaug, G., Jancke, L., Huang, Y., Staiger, J.F. & Steinmetz, H. (1995). Increased corpus callosum size in musicians. *Neuropsychologia*, **33**: 1047–1055.

Schnitzler, A., Kessler, K.R. & Benecke, R. (1996). Transcallosally mediated inhibition of interneurons within human primary motor cortex. *Exp. Brain Res.*, **112**: 381–391.

Theoret, H., Haque, J. & Pascual-Leone, A. (2001). Increased variability of paced finger tapping accuracy following repetitive magnetic stimulation of the cerebellum in humans. *Neursci. Lett.*, **306**: 29–32.

van Boven, R.W., Hamilton, R.H., Kauffman, T., Keenan, J.P. & Pascual-Leone, A. (2000). Tactile spatial resolution in blind braille readers. *Neurology*, **54**: 2230–2236.

van Mier H. (2000). Human learning. In *Brain Mapping: The Systems*, ed. J.C. Mazziotta, A.W. Toga & R.S. Frackowiak, pp. 605–620. San Diego: Academic Press.

Willingham, D.B., Nissen, M.J. & Bullemer, P. (1989). On the development of procedural knowledge. *J. Exp. Psychol. Learn. Mem. Cogn.*, **15**: 1047–1060.

6

Stimulation-induced plasticity in the human motor cortex

Joseph Classen[1] and Ulf Ziemann[2]

[1]Human Cortical Physiology and Motor Control Laboratory, Department of Neurology, Bayerische Julius-Maximilians Universität, Würzburg, Germany
[2]Clinic of Neurology, J.W. Goethe-University Frankfurt am Main, Germany

Introduction

Neuronal plasticity may be defined as any functional change within the nervous system outlasting an (experimental) manipulation. Plasticity, by this definition, does not comprise structural changes, such as those occurring during development or repair. Although there is no universally accepted lower limit of its duration, the term 'plasticity' is usually only applied when neuronal changes outlast the manipulation by more than a few seconds. In experimental animals, as well as in humans, plasticity is usually defined neurophysiologically by changes in the stimulus–response characteristics ('excitability').

Plasticity of the central nervous system has attracted much interest because it is thought to be related to the mechanisms underlying the formation of memories and the learning of new skills. Very likely, it is also involved in restoration of brain function after its initial loss as a consequence of brain injury. Neuronal plasticity may be induced internally, such as by practising movements (see Chapter 4), or externally, for instance, by limb amputation, spinal cord injury or cerebral stroke (see Chapter 8), or by repetitive electrical or magnetic neuronal stimulation, as reviewed here. Models of plasticity relying on external stimulation may be attractive because they allow best to control for experimental conditions. Human models of central nervous system plasticity may contribute particularly relevant information to the understanding of fundamental principles of plasticity. Additionally, the neuronal changes induced in human models of plasticity may themselves prove to be therapeutically useful.

Over the last decade, a number of human models have been described that lead to predictable changes of excitability. TMS protocols leading to nervous system plasticity may be divided into those that utilize a single route of manipulation and those that use a dual route. Among those that employ a single route there are some that operate by manipulating afferent input to the central nervous system and others that operate on manipulating the central nervous system directly, by cortical stimulation. Table 6.1 summarizes several of the protocols, published in recent years, that have been shown to produce plasticity. It is immediately clear that some protocols lead to depression while others lead to facilitation of excitability as judged by the size of MEPs evoked by TMS over the primary motor cortex.

It is, however, important to bear in mind that changes of MEP size may be influenced by effects at all possible levels of the motor system, i.e. at the motor cortex, subcortex, spinal cord, or a combination of those. Such effects need not be of the same sign. Whenever a protocol induces, e.g. depression of cortical excitability, it must be considered that, at the same time, facilitation at the level of the spinal cord may occur. Furthermore, it is important to note that MEP size evoked by single pulse TMS is but one measure of motor excitability. It is possible that MEP size increases following a particular stimulation protocol, while other parameters, such as short-latency paired-pulse inhibition, or silent period duration, indicate a change into the opposite direction, towards less excitability. Another point which has not always been fully appreciated is the dynamic nature of excitability changes following experimental manipulation. For instance, excitability may be unchanged or increased immediately following a certain manipulation, but may be decreased thereafter, with no further intervening stimulation.

Thus, the effects of a stimulation protocol cannot be described in a meaningful way unless, apart from the details of the stimulation protocol, the specific parameters and time of evaluation after the experimental manipulation are given.

Protocols

Repetitive TMS (rTMS)

Effects on motor system excitability

The first and most simple protocol by which excitability of the motor system was shown to be modifiable by external stimulation involves the repetitive

Table 6.1. Different protocols for stimulation-induced plasticity

Reference	Technique	Manipulation	Net direction of excitability change	Duration	Site	Additional tests
Pascual-Leone et al., 1994	rTMS (20 Hz, 150% RMT, 10 pulses)	Brain stimulation	Up	3–4 min	Unknown	–
Berardelli et al., 1998	rTMS (5 Hz, 120% RMT)		Up	900 ms	Cortical and spinal	H-reflex
Maeda et al., 2000	rTMS (90% RMT, 1–20 Hz, 240–1600 pulses)		Down/up	130 s		–
Modugno et al., 2001	rTMS (5–20 Hz, 100%–150% RMT, 1–13 pulses)		Down/up	1–2 min max	Cortical only	H-reflex, TES+H-reflex
Nitsche & Paulus, 2000, 2001	Cathodal/anodal direct current stimulation		Down/up	Several min up to 1 h	Unknown	–
Chen et al., 1997	rTMS (0.9 Hz, 115% RMT, 15 min)		Down	≥15 min	Unknown	–
Muellbacher et al., 2000	rTMS (1 Hz, 115% RMT, 15 min)		Down	>30 min	Unknown	RMT
Hamdy, 1998	Electrical pharyngeal stimulation (10 Hz, 10 min)	Somatic stimulation	Up	30 min	Cortical	TES, brainstem reflexes
Ridding et al., 2000	Electrical stimulation of the ulnar nerve		Up	≥15 min	Cortical	F-waves, TES
Struppler et al., 1996	Magnetic stimulation of the median nerve		Up	1–2 days	Unknown	–
Ziemann et al., 1998a,b	Ischemic nerve block+rTMS	Dual manipulation	Up	≥1 h	Cortical	Paired-pulse inhibition/ facilitation
Stefan et al., 2000	Paired associative stimulation		Up	>1 h	Cortical	F-waves/brainstem stimulation
Sandbrink et al., 2001	Paired associative stimulation		Down	>1 h	Cortical	F-waves/brainstem stimulation

application of TMS (rTMS) pulses directed to the primary motor cortex or other cortical regions of the brain (Pascual-Leone et al., 1994). This protocol, and its variations, continue to be of paramount importance because it remains the most extensively used protocol applied for therapeutic purposes by a large number of laboratories, in particular in the field of neuropsychiatry. Given its widespread use, it is somewhat surprising how little is known about its basic physiological properties and the mechanisms operative in altering excitability by rTMS. In their initial study, Pascual-Leone and coworkers showed that the excitability of the motor system following ten pulses of TMS at 20 Hz and 150% threshold intensity facilitated the response to a smaller (90% threshold) test stimulus for 3–4 min in relaxed subjects (Pascual-Leone et al., 1994). A multitude of partially interdependent variables have to be taken into account when reviewing the physiological effects of rTMS. Among those are stimulus frequency, stimulus intensity, the duration of the stimulus train, and the total number of stimuli. When trains of stimulus trains (i.e. the intertrain interval is reduced to the extent that the effect of a given train is influenced by the effect of preceding ones) or trains of stimulus pairs (Sommer et al., 2001) are employed, the number of variables and combinations increases even further.

Only few studies have addressed the question of whether the effects of rTMS on MEP size are due to effects originating at the cortical, subcortical or spinal level. In one study, H-reflexes and transcranial electrical stimulation (TES) were used to show that rTMS simultaneously facilitated cortical mechanisms and suppressed H-reflexes (Berardelli et al., 1998). Modugno and coworkers extended these studies by employing H-reflexes and, in addition, facilitation of H-reflexes by anodal TES (Modugno et al., 2001). With the specific rTMS parameters used by these authors, there was, however, no indication for a change of spinal excitability despite significant changes in MEP size.

Experiments that varied the frequency of stimulation have shown that higher frequencies tend to increase corticospinal excitability (Berardelli et al., 1998; Maeda et al., 2000; Pascual-Leone et al., 1994), whereas lower frequencies (less than 5 Hz) tend to depress excitability (Chen et al., 1997; Maeda et al., 2000; Muellbacher et al., 2000; Touge et al., 2001; Wassermann et al., 1996). Chen and coworkers showed that low-frequency rTMS (0.9 Hz; 115% resting motor threshold; 15 min) led to a decrease in MEP amplitude of on average 20% of the baseline amplitude (Chen et al., 1997). This decrease lasted for at least 15 minutes after the end of rTMS. These results were confirmed by Muellbacher and colleagues (Muellbacher et al., 2000). In addition, they showed that rTMS produced a significant increase in resting motor threshold (RMT) and a significant suppression of the MEP input–output curve. This effect persisted for 30 min. RMT may be viewed as a measure of neuronal membrane excitability because RMT is, to a certain extent, independent of acute alterations in neurotransmission by neuropharmacological manipulation but increases with blockade of voltage-dependent sodium channels (Ziemann et al., 1996a). Therefore, an increase in RMT suggests that alterations of membrane excitability may be involved in the depression of MEP size following 1 Hz rTMS (Muellbacher et al., 2000). This suppressive effect was restricted to the hand motor representation which was the primary target of the focal stimulation procedure, while there were no significant effects on the biceps representation (Muellbacher et al., 2000). In the study of Chen and coworkers (Chen et al., 1997), spread of excitation, which may be a warning sign for seizures (Pascual-Leone et al., 1994), occurred in one subject but this was not accompanied by an increase in MEP amplitude. This observation suggests that spread of excitation and MEP amplitude changes are different phenomena. It also indicates the need for adequate clinical and EMG monitoring, even when low-frequency rTMS protocols are used.

Touge and colleagues showed that, after 150–1500 TMS pulses applied to motor cortex at an intensity of 95% RMT, MEP size decreased for 2–10 min (Touge et al., 2001), confirming previous results (Chen et al., 1997). They also showed that the size of H-reflexes remained unchanged following rTMS, in keeping with the results of Modugno and coworkers (Modugno et al., 2001), but at variance with Berardelli and colleagues, who, however, used a rTMS protocol to induce an increase in MEP size (Berardelli et al., 1998). The fact that H-reflexes remained unchanged in the study of Touge and coworkers (Touge et al., 2001) is compatible with a cortical site of excitability changes. In addition, they observed that the suppression of MEPs occurred only when the target muscle was relaxed but not during voluntary activation. Therefore, the authors suggested that depression of neuronal transmission in synaptic connections to pyramidal cells activated by the test TMS pulse was an unlikely mechanism for the MEP suppression in the resting condition. However, because voluntary activation may lead to (recurrent) activation of inhibitory intracortical circuits, which may stabilize the output from the primary motor cortex, such an activation of inhibitory circuits may mask rTMS-induced changes in synaptic transmission. Therefore, the role of modulation of the strength of synaptic transmission in modulating MEP size following rTMS has not been finally clarified.

Only recently, the influence of stimulation intensity was studied. Low intensity stimuli tended to produce post-train MEP suppression, even if applied at frequencies >5 Hz, while suprathreshold stimuli produced MEP facilitation (Modugno et al., 2001). Similar effects occurred with variation of the duration of the stimulus train. A short train (four stimuli) at 5 Hz and 130% of motor threshold produced post-train MEP inhibition, while a longer train (20 stimuli) with otherwise identical stimulus settings produced MEP facilitation (Modugno et al., 2001). These results are consistent with the idea that inhibition and facilitation build up gradually during the course of a stimulation train, with inhibition reaching its maximum after a lower 'dose' of stimulation than facilitation.

Excitability at the level of the motor cortex can be assessed more specifically by a short interstimulus interval paired-pulse protocol (Kujirai et al., 1993). Peinemann and colleagues demonstrated that paired-pulse inhibition was reduced following 1250 pulses of 5 Hz rTMS at 90% of RMT over the primary motor cortex (Peinemann et al., 2000). Similar observations were made by Wu and coworkers using rTMS at 120% RMT (Wu et al., 2000). Following a TMS train of 30 paired-pulses at frequencies of 5 and 15 Hz, paired-pulse inhibition was reduced for 3.2 min and paired-pulse facilitation was enhanced for 1.5 min, whereas amplitudes of MEPs evoked by single TMS were increased in the first 30 s only (Wu et al., 2000). The different time course of the effects confirms the notion that the interneuronal apparatus generating paired-pulse inhibition differs from that generating paired-pulse facilitation (Ziemann et al., 1996b) and that rTMS may exert differential effects on either one of these circuits, which are again at least partly distinct from the one generating the MEP evoked by single-pulse TMS. No reports have examined so far intracortical excitability in the paired-pulse protocol if single-pulse MEP were depressed by low-frequency rTMS.

Remote effects

Recently, considerable experimental evidence has accumulated suggesting that rTMS of the primary motor cortex induces effects in remote, non-stimulated brain areas. Depression of excitability in the homologous non-stimulated motor cortex occurred with rTMS (15 min, suprathreshold intensity) applied at 1 Hz over the other primary motor cortex (Wassermann et al., 1998). Similarly, excitability of the primary somatosensory cortex, as measured by somatosensory-evoked potential amplitude, is depressed following 100 pulses of rTMS (1 Hz; 110% RMT) over the primary motor cortex of the same hemisphere (Enomoto et al., 2001). This effect was long-lasting (>100 min) and specific for a coil position over the motor cortex, while it did not emerge when the coil was held over the primary somatosensory cortex. It is likely that corticocortical pathways between the motor and somatosensory cortex mediated this effect (Enomoto et al., 2001). Functional neuroimaging studies showed that rTMS over the primary motor cortex may induce lasting changes of excitability in several brain regions in addition to the homologous contralateral motor cortex or the ipsilateral somatosensory cortex, for instance, in the supplementary motor cortex (Siebner et al., 2001).

Finally, rTMS of brain areas other than the primary motor cortex, e.g. the premotor and other frontal areas, even at intensities below the resting motor threshold, induced lasting alterations of brain activity in remote brain areas including the ipsilateral primary motor cortex (Gerschlager et al., 2001; Münchau et al., 2002; Paus et al., 2001; Rollnik et al., 2000). In addition, rTMS may induce not only remote cortical, but also subcortical effects, for example, at the level of the basal ganglia (Strafella et al., 2001).

Direct current (DC) stimulation

Nitsche and Paulus, building on earlier observations by Creutzfeldt (Creutzfeldt et al., 1962) and by Birbaumer and coworkers (Jaeger et al., 1987), showed that robust excitability changes of up to 40% compared to the baseline MEP amplitude can be induced by the sustained application of DC electric current flowing between electrodes attached to frontal and central skull regions overlying the primary motor cortex (Nitsche & Paulus, 2000, 2001). The changes in MEP amplitude lasted several minutes after the end of DC stimulation. Anodal DC stimulation (i.e. anode over motor cortex) resulted in MEP facilitation, while cathodal DC stimulation resulted in MEP depression (Nitsche & Paulus, 2000, 2001). By varying the intensity and duration of DC stimulation, the strength and duration of the after-effects could be controlled. When DC stimulation was applied for 13 min, MEP changes lasted for 60 min or more (Nitsche & Paulus, 2001).

Little is known about the mechanisms involved. Because the sign of excitability changes could be controlled by the direction of current flow, it is most likely that the effects were induced by a modification of membrane polarization.

Repetitive afferent stimulation

Prolonged, repetitive mixed nerve stimulation (trains of 10 Hz) induced an increase in MEP amplitude in the primary motor cortex contralateral to afferent stimulation (Ridding et al., 2000). The MEP increase was specific for the muscles innervated by the nerve being stimulated, suggesting input specificity and ruling out unspecific (e.g. arousal) effects (Kaelin-Lang et al., 2002; Ridding et al., 2000). Control experiments employing TES, electrical brainstem stimulation, F-waves and M-waves provided no evidence for a spinal or peripheral origin of the excitability changes (Kaelin-Lang et al., 2002; Ridding et al., 2000). Follow-up experiments showed that, in addition to an increase in MEP size, the maps of motor representations in the primary motor cortex shifted by afferent stimulation, suggesting that this form of experimental manipulation does not only result in an increase in excitability but also in changes in topographic distribution (Ridding et al., 2001). Similar results were obtained by Hamdy and coworkers, who showed that repetitive (10 Hz) pharyngeal stimulation over a period of 10 min induced a lasting (30–60 min) increase of MEP amplitude in pharyngeal muscles (Hamdy et al., 1998). This increase was accompanied by a decrease of MEP amplitudes in oesophageal muscles. This suggests that the cortical representation of pharyngeal muscles had increased at the expense of the representation of oesophageal muscles. The MEP increase in pharyngeal muscles was not observed when the MEP were elicited by TES, or when pharyngeal reflex response was elicited by trigeminal or vagal nerve stimulation, suggesting that the effects of repeated electrical pharyngeal stimulation took place at the level of the motor cortex (Hamdy et al., 1998).

Models of long-term potentiation (LTP) in human motor cortex

Of several candidate mechanisms for cortical plasticity, persistent changes of synaptic efficacy have attracted considerable attention because they are believed by many to underlie learning and memory (Buonomano & Merzenich, 1998; Donoghue et al., 1996; Sanes & Donoghue, 2000). LTP has been produced by a number of different stimulation protocols in vitro in animal preparations of neocortical slices derived from virtually any cortical region. Recently, two protocols of stimulation-induced plasticity in humans have been published whose principles of design were shaped to generate conditions known to produce LTP in animal studies.

Stimulation-induced plasticity in motor cortex during reduced cortical inhibition

LTP is characterized by four basic properties (Bliss & Collingridge, 1993).

Co-operativity   This describes the existence of an intensity threshold for induction.

Associativity   A single afferent input is not sufficient for induction, but LTP occurs if the subthreshold input is coupled with a separate but convergent and coincident input.

Input-specificity   LTP occurs only along pathways activated by stimulation, but not in others not active during the stimulation procedure.

Involvement of NMDA and GABA receptors   Cortical LTP is N-methyl-D-aspartate (NMDA) receptor dependent and frequently requires reduction of gamma-aminobutyric acid (GABA) related local inhibition. The experiments of the following subchapters test some of these basic properties of LTP in models of stimulation-induced plasticity in the human motor cortex.

Experiment I: Co-operativity of stimulation-induced plasticity (Ziemann et al., 1998a)

Six healthy subjects were tested in three different interventions: ischemic nerve block (INB alone) of one hand; repetitive transcranial magnetic stimulation (rTMS alone); rTMS during INB (rTMS+INB). INB was accomplished by inflating a cuff at the proximal forearm to a suprasystolic blood pressure level for about 40 minutes. INB leads to a rapid increase in MEP of the biceps muscle elicited from the motor cortex contralateral to INB (Brasil-Neto et al., 1992). This MEP increase is very likely caused by a rapid decrease in GABA related inhibition, as shown by multimetabolite MR spectroscopy (Levy et al., 2002). rTMS was set to a rate of 0.1 Hz and an intensity of 120% of RMT in the biceps muscle, and applied to the optimal position to elicit MEP in the biceps. These particular rTMS parameters were chosen because previous experiments had shown no effect on motor cortex excitability when this low-rate rTMS was delivered in the absence of INB (Chen et al., 1997). Therefore, rTMS+INB is the crucial condition of the present experiments, to test whether rTMS that does not induce plasticity when given in the absence of INB is capable of inducing plasticity when delivered in the presence of INB. If so, this would suggest the existence of co-operativity. Plasticity of the motor cortex ARM representation was evaluated by measuring motor threshold, MEP size and paired-pulse intracortical inhibition and facilitation of the biceps muscle before and after experimental manipulation, using focal TMS.

The main result is shown in Fig. 6.1. INB alone resulted in a mild increase in biceps MEP size. rTMS in the absence of INB did not change

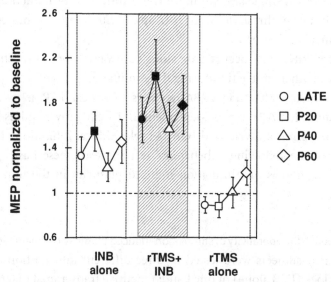

Fig. 6.1   Changes in MEP size in the biceps muscles (means of six subjects) produced by the different interventions given on the x-axis. Data are expressed as values normalized to the pre-intervention baseline that has been assigned a value of 1. Different symbols refer to time points late into intervention (circles), and 20 minutes (squares), 40 minutes (triangles) and 60 minutes (diamonds) after the end of intervention. The grey column shows the test intervention (rTMS during INB). Filled symbols indicate time-points that were significantly different from baseline ($P < 0.05$). Note that rTMS (0.1 Hz, 120% of biceps motor threshold) that did not produce a change in biceps MEP size when given in the absence of INB, produced a significant increase in MEP size when given in the presence of INB (modified from Ziemann et al., 1998a, with permission.)

MEP size. In contrast, rTMS in the presence of INB led to a significant and long-lasting (>60 min) increase in MEP size beyond the changes induced by INB alone. Figure 6.2 shows even more impressive results for paired-pulse intracortical inhibition and facilitation. These measures test synaptic excitability of inhibitory and excitatory neural circuits specifically at the level of the motor cortex (Di Lazzaro et al., 1998; Kujirai et al., 1993; Ziemann, 1999; Ziemann et al., 1996b). While INB alone and rTMS alone exerted no significant effects, rTMS+INB resulted in a significant long-lasting (>60 min) decrease of inhibition and increase of facilitation. Motor threshold was not affected by intervention. In summary, these findings are suggestive of the presence of co-operativity because low-rate rTMS is capable of producing a long-lasting enhancement of the motor cortex arm representation only when applied during reduced inhibition of the stimulated motor cortex.

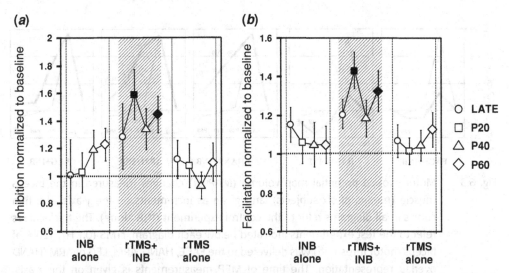

Fig. 6.2   Changes in (*a*) intracortical inhibition and (*b*) facilitation (means of six subjects) produced by the different interventions given on the *x*-axis. Data are expressed as values normalized to a pre-intervention baseline that has been assigned a value of 1. Otherwise, conventions and arrangement are as described in Fig. 6.1. Note that a significant decrease of intracortical inhibition (i.e. values > 1) and a significant increase in intracortical facilitation were produced by rTMS+INB only. (Modified from Ziemann et al., 1998a, with permission.)

Experiment II: Input specificity of stimulation-induced plasticity (Ziemann et al., 2002)   Six healthy subjects were tested in six different experimental conditions. rTMS (0.1 Hz, 120% of biceps RMT) was delivered in the presence of INB to either the ARM, HAND, FACE, LEG or ARM/HAND overlap representation, using focal TMS. If input specificity applied to this model of plasticity, it would be expected that an enhancement of the ARM representation, as measured by MEP size of the biceps muscle, does occur only, if the ARM representation was stimulated by rTMS.

Figure 6.3 shows the main results. MEP size (here given as MAP volume, i.e. the sum of MEP sizes across a map of the ARM representation) briefly increased in the INB alone condition (control experiment). ARM and ARM/HAND stimulation resulted in a significant and long-lasting (>40 min) prolongation of this enhancement of the ARM representation. In contrast, stimulation of the laterally adjacent HAND and FACE representations produced a significant depression of the short-lasting enhancement observed

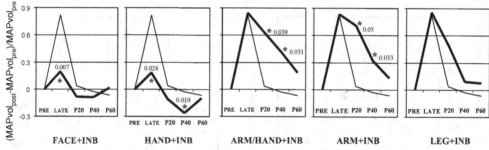

Fig. 6.3   Motor evoked potential map volume (MAPvol) changes measured in the biceps muscle (means of six subjects), and given as increments on the y-axis. The thin curves in all diagrams refer to the control experiment (INB alone). The thick curves refer to the test experiments indicated below each diagram. rTMS (0.1 Hz, 120% of biceps motor threshold) was delivered to the FACE, HAND, ARM, LEG or ARM/HAND overlap representation. The time of MEP measurements is given on the x-axis. Asterisks indicate significant differences between the two curves in a given diagram. P values (paired two-tailed t tests) are also shown. Note that INB alone resulted in only a transient enhancement of MAPvol, while ARM/HAND+INB and ARM+INB led to a long-lasting enhancement. In contrast, FACE+INB and HAND+INB produced a suppression of the transient enhancement seen with INB alone, and HAND+INB even resulted in a long-lasting suppression. LEG+INB was not significantly different from INB alone. (Modified from Ziemann et al., 2002.)

with INB alone. LEG stimulation was not different from INB alone. Two important conclusions can be drawn from these findings: (a) the long-lasting enhancement of the ARM representation displays input-specificity because the enhancement was induced only when the ARM representation was effectively stimulated; (b) the HAND and FACE representations have a depressive effect on the excitability of the ARM representation. While the mechanisms of this depressive effect are unknown, it may be pointed out that a competitive interaction between the FACE and the ARM/HAND representations in the motor cortex was described in several previous TMS studies in patients with facial palsy (Rijntjes et al., 1997), facial hemispasm (Liepert et al., 1999) and upper limb amputees (Karl et al., 2001). For example, in patients with facial palsy, TMS mapping demonstrated an enlargement and lateral shift of the HAND representation towards the FACE representation (Rijntjes et al., 1997). It therefore appears that activity-dependent processes may foster large-scale across-representation plasticity in human motor cortex. The present experiments show that this can occur rapidly, within minutes of stimulation in the presence of reduced cortical inhibition.

Experiment III: Cancellation of stimulation-induced plasticity by blockade of NMDA receptors or stimulation of GABA-A receptors (Ziemann et al., 1998b)   Six healthy subjects participated in six experiments. In each experiment, rTMS (0.1 Hz, 120% of biceps RMT) was applied to the ARM representation in the presence of INB as above (see rTMS+INB condition in Experiment I). In the different experiments, subjects were either pre-treated with no drug (control 1 and control 2), 150 mg of the non-competitive NMDA receptor antagonist dextromethorphan (DMO), 2 mg of the GABA-A receptor agonist lorazepam (LZP), 300 mg of the voltage-gated sodium channel blocker lamotrigine (LTG), or one-night sleep deprived (SLD) in order to control for the sedative side effects common to all three drugs. If it were correct that the stimulation-induced long-lasting enhancement of the ARM representation in the present plasticity model is similar to LTP, it would be expected that the pre-treatment with DMO and LZP leads to a suppression of this form of stimulation-induced plasticity.

The main results are presented in Figs. 6.4 and 6.5. LZP and LTG led to a significant reduction of the rTMS+INB-induced increase in biceps MEP size (Fig. 6.4) while DMO and SLD had no effect. However, all three drugs

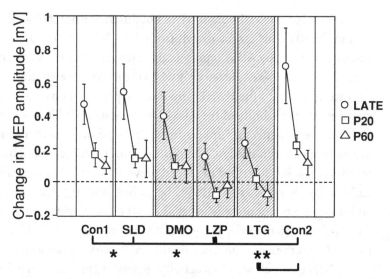

Fig. 6.4   Effect of intervention on the increase in MEP size (means of six subjects) induced by rTMS+INB (Con1 and Con2). Intervention is given on the x-axis. SLD, One-night sleep deprivation; DMO, pre-treatment with 150 mg of dextromethorphan; LZP, pre-treatment with 2 mg of lorazepam; LTG, pre-treatment with 300 mg of lamotrigin. Changes in MEP size measured late into intervention (circles), and 20 minutes (squares) and 60 minutes (triangles) after the end of intervention are given as differences (ΔmV) from the values before intervention, which were assigned a value of 0 (y-axis). Grey boxes indicate the drug experiments. Note that LZP and LTG led to suppression of the rTMS+INB-induced increase in MEP size. * $P < 0.05$; $^{**}P < 0.01$. (Modified from Ziemann et al., 1998b, with permission.)

suppressed the rTMS+INB-induced long-lasting decrease in intracortical inhibition seen in the control and SLD conditions (Fig. 6.5). In summary, these findings show that (a) the rTMS+INB-induced long-lasting enhancement of the ARM representation can be disrupted if GABA-related inhibition is increased by pretreatment with a GABA-A receptor agonist; (b) the rTMS+INB-induced long-lasting decrease in intracortical inhibition, a measure of excitability of inhibitory neural transmission in motor cortex can be disrupted by pre-treatment with a NMDA receptor antagonist. Both findings are compatible with the proposition that the rTMS+INB-induced enhancement of the ARM representation reflects plasticity that is similar to LTP.

In conclusion, the findings of Experiments I–III demonstrate that the stimulation-induced enhancement of the ARM representation in human

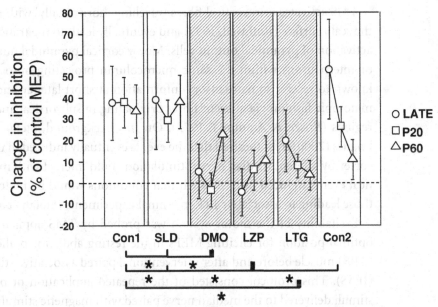

Fig. 6.5   Effect of intervention on the decrease in intracortical inhibition (means of six subjects) induced by rTMS+INB (Con1 and Con2). Interventions on the x-axis as in Fig. 6.4. Intracortical inhibition measured late into intervention (circles), and 20 minutes (squares) and 60 minutes (triangles) after the end of intervention are given as differences from the values before intervention (in Δ%). Differences > 0% indicate a decrease in intracortical inhibition. Note that DMO, LZP and LTG led to significant suppression of the rTMS+INB-induced decrease in intracortical inhibition. *P < 0.05. (Modified from Ziemann et al., 1998b, with permission.)

motor cortex displays co-operativity, input-specificity and disruption by pharmacological blockade of NMDA receptors or stimulation of GABA-A receptors. All characteristics are compatible with the basic properties of LTP as usually defined in slice preparations of animal neocortex or hippocampus.

Interventional paired associative stimulation (IPAS)-induced plasticity

LTP is called associative or Hebbian, if the postsynaptic cell is depolarized synchronously with the afferent input from another cell, or if two independent afferent signals reach the same cell in synchrony (Buonomano & Merzenich, 1998). Associative LTP in the motor cortex displays several distinct features which may allow operation of this cellular mechanism to be identified even at a systems physiological level.

TMS activates intracortical fibres travelling 'horizontally' with respect to the scalp surface (Rothwell, 1997) and eventually leads to the trans-synaptic activation of pyramidal output cells. Motor cortical pyramidal output cells, or interneurons within the same microcolumn projecting onto them are known to receive somatosensory information at short latency and in a somatotopic fashion via afferent fibres originating in subcortical and cortical regions (Rosen & Asanuma, 1972). On this background, Stefan and colleagues (2000) hypothesized that the events eventually induced in the motor cortex by afferent median nerve stimulation could interact with motor cortical events induced by TMS such that conditions would be matched with those leading to associative LTP in animal experiments (Stefan et al., 2000).

Excitability of the motor system was probed by TMS applied over the optimal position for eliciting MEPs in the resting abductor pollicis brevis (APB) muscle before and after interventional paired associative stimulation (IPAS). This protocol consisted of the repeated application of peripheral stimuli delivered to the median nerve paired with magnetic stimuli over the contralateral motor cortex (optimal position for APB muscle). The interval between peripheral nerve stimulation and TMS was 25 ms. Likely, at this interval, the afferent signal would reach the motor cortex nearly in synchrony with the application of the TMS pulse. Ninety stimulus pairs were applied at an interpair interval of 20 s. This IPAS led to an increase of APB MEP amplitude, amounting to approximately 50% of the baseline value (Stefan et al., 2000).

The timing of the TMS pulse with respect to the afferent pulse was critical to produce this effect. The increase in resting MEP amplitude was induced only at an interstimulus interval of 25 ms (termed here $IPAS_{25\,ms}$), but not when the interstimulus interval was 100 ms or longer (Stefan et al., 2000). When the interstimulus interval between median nerve stimulation and TMS was shortened to 10 ms ($IPAS_{10\,ms}$), the resting MEP amplitude was decreased following IPAS (Fig. 6.6) (Sandbrink et al., 2001). The opposite effects of $IPAS_{25\,ms}$ and $IPAS_{10\,ms}$ may be explained by the fact that, with $IPAS_{25\,ms}$, the motor cortex output neurons fire an TMS-induced action potential after the arrival of the afferent conditioning stimulus, while with $IPAS_{10\,ms}$ the order of events is reversed. This may be similar to animal experiments where the time between action potential firing and depolarization of the cell by afferent stimulation is critical to induce either LTP or long-term

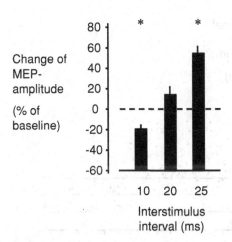

Fig. 6.6   Effect of different intervals between afferent conditioning stimulation at the right median nerve, and magnetic stimulation over the left motor cortex during IPAS on cortical excitability. Changes of cortical excitability were assessed by comparing the amplitude of the motor evoked potential (MEP) in the resting APB elicited by TMS before and after IPAS. MEP amplitudes ($n = 40$ experiments) increased when using an interstimulus interval of 25 ms, and decreased ($n = 10$) when using an interval of 10 ms. Asterisks indicate significant changes compared to baseline ($P < 0.05$).

depression (LTD) (Bi & Poo, 1998; Markram et al., 1997; van Rossum et al., 2000).

Two different approaches were used to demonstrate that the observed changes in MEP amplitudes were located cortically. F-waves were not changed significantly following IPAS at the same time when MEP amplitudes were increased (IPAS$_{25\,ms}$, Stefan et al., 2000), or decreased (IPAS$_{10\,ms}$, Sandbrink et al., 2001). Similarly, when electrical brainstem stimulation was employed, which excites the cortical output elements downstream from the cortex, and, thus, downstream of the influence of intracortical circuits, resting amplitudes remained unchanged while amplitudes of TMS-evoked MEPs increased (IPAS$_{25\,ms}$, Stefan et al., 2000), or decreased (IPAS$_{10\,ms}$, Sandbrink et al., 2001).

The increase of resting MEP amplitudes after IPAS$_{25\,ms}$ lasted longer than 30 min in 11 subjects and outlasted 1 hour in two subjects (Fig. 6.7). However, resting MEP amplitudes measured 24 h after IPAS$_{25\,ms}$ were similar as before the intervention, indicating that this effect was fully reversible. Similarly, the decrease of MEP amplitude with IPAS$_{10\,ms}$ lasted longer than 90 min

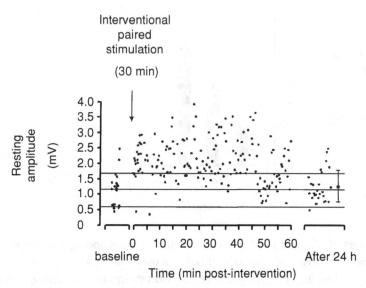

Fig. 6.7   Duration of increase in MEP size induced by IPAS$_{25\,ms}$. Example from one subject.
Note persistence of increased MEP for 60 min and return to baseline at 24 h
after IPAS$_{25\,ms}$. Thick horizontal line designates mean resting MEP amplitude in trials
recorded before IPAS$_{25\,ms}$ ('baseline'). Thin lines above and below show one standard deviation of baseline data. Filled square and error bars show mean $\pm$ S.D. of
resting MEP obtained after 24 h.

and returned to near the baseline level after 2 h (Sandbrink et al., 2001). In
addition, the increase of cortical excitability (IPAS$_{25\,ms}$) was topographically
specific. The increase in MEP size was confined to muscles represented in the
IPAS-targeted hemisphere receiving a dual and synchronous input from TMS
and afferent stimulation. MEP of other muscles (i.e. supplied by peripheral
nerves that were not stimulated during IPAS) in the same or in the opposite
hemisphere as the target APB remained unchanged.

It may be hypothesized that changes of GABA$_A$ receptor-mediated cortical
inhibition contributed to the increase in MEP induced by IPAS. Intracortical
inhibition has been proposed to represent one of the principal candidate
mechanisms underlying changes of cortical excitability (Donoghue et al.,
1996; Jones, 1993). The intracortical GABA$_A$ receptor-mediated inhibition
can be probed by a conditioning-test protocol (Kujirai et al., 1993). Following
IPAS$_{25\,ms}$, Stefan and colleagues (Stefan et al., 2002) found intracortical inhibition to be decreased (Fig. 6.8), when using the same test stimulus intensity as

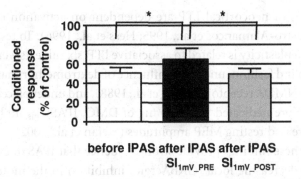

Fig. 6.8   Paired-pulse inhibition following IPAS$_{25\,ms}$. Paired-pulse inhibition was assessed before (open bars) and after (black and grey) IPAS$_{25\,ms}$. Stimulus intensity was SI$_{1\,mV\_PRE}$ (open and black bars), or SI$_{1\,mV\_POST}$ (grey bars). Following IPAS$_{25\,ms}$, the mean paired-pulse inhibition decreased when using a conditioning stimulus intensity of 70% of resting motor threshold and a test stimulus intensity of SI$_{1\,mV\_PRE}$. With the test stimulus set to SI$_{1\,mV\_POST}$, the paired-pulse inhibition matched that measured prior to IPAS$_{25\,ms}$. Asterisks indicate significant differences of paired-pulse inhibition obtained pre-(SI$_{1\,mV\_PRE}$) vs. post-IPAS$_{25\,ms}$ (SI$_{1\,mV\_PRE}$) and post-IPAS$_{25\,ms}$ (SI$_{1\,mV\_PRE}$) vs. post-IPAS$_{25\,ms}$(SI$_{1\,mV\_POST}$). Data are from six subjects. Columns and bars are means ± S.D.

before IPAS. At first sight, this would support the concept of disinhibition as a mechanism underlying the IPAS-induced increase in MEP amplitude. However, intracortical inhibition, as measured by the double-pulse protocol, depends on the intensity of both the conditioning and the test stimulus (Kujirai et al., 1993). Control experiments showed that, when the test stimulus intensity was lowered after IPAS, to account for the increased efficacy of the test stimulus and to match the magnitude of the unconditioned test MEP to the baseline MEP before IPAS, intracortical inhibition remained unchanged when compared to the baseline (Fig. 6.8). Further control experiments showed that the efficacy of the conditioning magnetic pulse was not changed by IPAS (Stefan et al., 2002).

The intracortical inhibition induced by somatosensory afferent input (Di Lazzaro et al., 2000; Tokimura et al., 2000) is far less well characterized than the paired-pulse intracortical inhibition (Kujirai et al., 1993). There was no indication for a decrease of this type of inhibition after IPAS (Stefan et al., 2002, data not shown). Thus, when appropriate corrections are applied, there is no evidence that intracortical inhibition is changed by IPAS.

Most forms of neocortical LTP are dependent on activation of NMDA receptors (Castro-Alamancos et al., 1995; Hess et al., 1996). To test whether IPAS-induced plasticity is related to associative LTP, six subjects were studied in a double-blind fashion, under the influence of dextromethorphan (DMO) which blocks NMDA receptors (Wong et al., 1988), and under placebo. When subjects were premedicated with 150 mg of DMO, $IPAS_{25\,ms}$ no longer resulted in increased resting MEP amplitudes (Stefan et al., 2002).

Together, these findings provide strong evidence that IPAS does not alter MEP size by decreasing local (GABAergic) inhibition in the motor cortex. Therefore, IPAS-induced plasticity probably relies on other cellular mechanisms. Because of the principle of stimulation design, and the physiological and pharmacological properties, these experiments suggest that IPAS-induced cortical plasticity may exclusively depend on alteration of synaptic efficacy.

Common mechanisms

Although the exact mechanism(s) underlying stimulation-induced cortical excitability changes are not known in any of the paradigms, it is safe to assume that there is no single mechanism in any particular paradigm and even if there is a mixture of mechanisms, its composition is likely to differ in the various examples of stimulation-induced plasticity. Furthermore, while molecular biology teaches us that successful induction of neuronal plasticity requires the completion of a multitude of steps in a chain of events, the concept of cortical plasticity as a multistep process is only beginning to shape in systems physiology.

However, if one summarizes the above INB and IPAS experiments, the following common lines appear:

(a) A reduction of GABAergic inhibition in the stimulated motor cortex is permissive for the development of significant and long-lasting rTMS effects (Stefan et al., 2002; Ziemann et al., 1998a). In the INB experiments, this reduction of cortical inhibition was produced by ischemic nerve block of a contralateral limb. The associated decrease in GABA content in the deprived motor cortex was demonstrated by magnetic resonance spectroscopy (Levy et al., 2002). In the IPAS experiments, the afferent stimulation resulted in a short-lasting reduction in paired-pulse inhibition (Stefan et al., 2002). The permissive role of cortical disinhibition is underlined by experiments that explored the effects of pretreatment with GABAergic drugs; 2 mg of lorazepam, a GABA-A receptor agonist, cancelled the rTMS-induced MEP increase in the INB experiments (Ziemann et al., 1998b). Similarly, lorazepam blocked the increase in MEP amplitude following repetitive stimulation of somatosensory afferents (Kaelin-Lang et al., 2002).

(b) The reduction of GABA-related inhibition is not, by itself, the mechanism of the induced increase in MEP amplitude. This was demonstrated by the dissociation of increase in MEP amplitude and no change in paired-pulse intracortical inhibition (Kaelin-Lang et al., 2002; Ridding & Taylor; 2001 Stefan et al., 2002).

(c) Converging evidence supports the idea that the nature of the rTMS induced increase (or decrease) of MEP amplitude is LTP (or LTD)-like. Similar to cortical LTP, the rTMS-induced changes in motor cortical excitability reported here depend on reduced cortical inhibition (Ziemann et al., 1998a); Stefan et al., 2002), are input specific (Stefan et al., 2000; Ziemann et al., 2002), and rely on NMDA receptor activation (Ziemann et al., 1998b; Stefan et al., 2002).

Functional relevance of induced plasticity

Cortical excitability is altered in a number of neurological and psychiatric disorders, although a causal link between altered excitability and a particular symptom has hardly been established. Conceivably, stimulation-induced plasticity should be an attractive tool for future therapeutic use. Investigations into the functional, in particular behavioural, consequences of stimulation-induced plasticity will therefore prove particularly important in the future.

Stimulation-induced plasticity in healthy subjects

Although repetitive TMS has already been used in a number of therapeutic settings, very little is known about its functional consequences in healthy subjects.

At a cognitive level it seems that a single session of suprathreshold rTMS at various cortical stimulation sites does not interfere with performance on such tasks as story recall, word fluency or naming (Pascual-Leone et al., 1993). Recent studies showed that analogic reasoning was enhanced by subthreshold 5 Hz rTMS of the left dorsolateral prefrontal cortex (Boroojerdi et al., 2001), and picture naming by 20 Hz stimulation over Wernicke's area (Mottaghy et al., 1999).

Similarly, in the motor domain, evidence is scarce that rTMS induces a measureable change in performance. A slight facilitation of the finger tapping rate was observed early (<1 h) after 1 Hz rTMS in the hand contralateral to the stimulated motor cortex (Wassermann et al., 1996). By contrast, Rossi and coworkers did not find a change in tapping performance after rTMS at 1 Hz for 15 min over the motor cortex (Rossi et al., 2000). However, in that study the Bereitschaftspotential was decreased over a topographically defined brain region, indicating that movement-related activation of the motor cortex was altered by rTMS. Muellbacher and colleagues explored the effects of low-frequency rTMS (1 Hz; 15 min; 115% of RMT) of the primary motor cortex on motor excitability and basic motor behaviour in humans (Muellbacher et al., 2000). Changes in motor behaviour were studied by the maximal and mean peak force between thumb and index finger during a pincer grip, and the peak acceleration of ballistic thumb flexion and fifth finger abduction movements. Replicating previous studies (Chen et al., 1997), low-frequency rTMS produced a suppression of MEP input–output curves and an increase in RMT, lasting for 30 min. In the presence of these effects, peak force and peak acceleration were not affected by rTMS (Muellbacher et al., 2000). It is not known if DC-induced cortical plasticity has behavioural consequences in the motor domain. However, a recent study on DC-induced plasticity in the visual cortex showed that static and dynamic contrast sensitivities were reduced during, and immediately after, 7 min of cathodal DC stimulation of the visual cortex (Antal et al., 2001).

The failure of rTMS to induce behavioural consequences in the studies by Muellbacher et al. (2000) and Rossi et al. (2000) can be explained by two alternatives. (a) The behavioural measures of motor performance were not sensitive enough to detect changes following experimental manipulation. (b) The functional consequences of stimulation-induced plasticity are not on motor performance *per se*, but on the capacity of the motor cortex to undergo further plastic changes such as during motor learning. The latter view is supported by findings investigating DC-induced effects on plasticity of kinematic cortical movement representations. Training of a thumb movement in the opposite direction of a TMS-evoked thumb movement induces a transient directional change of post-training TMS-evoked thumb movements towards the trained direction (Classen et al., 1998). Rosenkranz and coworkers applied DC stimulation to the motor cortex while subjects performed a training of repetitive thumb movements (Rosenkranz et al., 2000). DC stimulation of either anodal or cathodal polarity significantly reduced the training-induced directional change of thumb movements during a 10 min post-training interval, indicating that DC stimulation interfered with rapid training-induced plasticity. However, precisely what are the mechanisms by which this interference occurred is unknown. Because modulation of synaptic efficacy may be involved in training-induced plasticity (Bütefisch et al., 2000), it is conceivable that DC stimulation interacted with this mechanism, either directly, e.g. by saturating synaptic efficacy, or indirectly, by interfering with one of the intermediate steps necessary for altering synaptic efficacy.

The view that motor cortex stimulation may interfere particularly with motor learning is supported by another recent rTMS study that showed that the early consolidation of motor practice (increase in peak acceleration between thumb and index finger in a pincer grip) was significantly and specifically disturbed by 1 Hz rTMS over the primary motor cortex contralateral to the task hand (Muellbacher et al., 2002). At the same time, basic motor behaviour (peak acceleration and peak force) remained unaffected by rTMS (Muellbacher et al., 2000, 2002).

Event-related MRI was used as a first approach to the question of whether the neuronal activation induced by voluntary movements is changed after IPAS. If a significant change in the motor cortical voluntary activation pattern could be demonstrated, this would be a hint as to a behavioural relevance of IPAS. Six subjects performed 25 thumb abduction movements at a pace of one movement every 20 s. Ten images were acquired for each movement and the haemodynamic response was modelled. $IPAS_{25\,ms}$ led to an increase of the size of MEP amplitudes and the number of voxels activated by thumb abductions. Control experiments using IPAS at an interstimulus interval of 10 000 ms did not show an enlargement of cortical activation with voluntary activation (Stefan et al., 2001). While these preliminary findings support the conclusion that modulation of cortical excitability by IPAS may affect the pattern of activation evoked by voluntary activation, the evidence is indirect, and the effects of IPAS on motorcortical function have yet to be shown more directly by studying motor behaviour itself.

Clinical applications of stimulation-induced plasticity in the motor cortex

Stimulation-induced plasticity, in particular following rTMS, has been applied with a therapeutic intention in several neurological and psychiatric disorders. A full account on rTMS-induced effects in neuropsychiatry is given in Chapter 10.

Abnormalities in motor cortical excitability have been recognized in several studies that explored the cortical pathophysiology of movement disorders (Ridding et al., 1995a,b). Therefore, researchers and clinicians were prompted to modulate motor cortical excitability externally by applying various protocols of stimulation-induced plasticity. Although promising results have been obtained, there is as yet no consensus that one protocol or another may be regarded as unequivocally beneficial. Siebner and coworkers showed that bradykinesia (Siebner et al., 1999a) and the UPDRS motor score (Siebner et al., 2000) improved after 5 Hz subthreshold rTMS over the motor hand area in non-medicated patients with Parkinson's disease. Clinically significant effects were also observed by Shimamoto and coworkers who performed a double-blind study in nine patients with Parkinson's disease (Shimamoto et al., 2001). Two months after rTMS, patients having previously received rTMS over frontal areas (30 pulses, 0.2 Hz, one session per week over 2 months) improved in several clinical and functional scales of motor behaviour. However, these positive results were not obtained by others (Ghabra et al., 1999; Tergau et al., 1999b). In patients with writers' cramp, low-frequency rTMS (1 Hz) reduced writing pressure and motor disturbance (Siebner et al., 1999b).

Stimulation-induced plasticity has also been used as a treatment strategy in medically refractory patients with various forms of epilepsy. In a preliminary study on nine patients, Tergau and colleagues observed a significant drop of seizure frequency following low-frequency (0.33 Hz; 2×500 pulses daily, 5 days) rTMS (Tergau et al., 1999a). The effect lasted for 6–8 weeks. These findings await confirmation in a controlled study design in a larger population of patients. Similarly, preliminary data showed a reduction in cortical myoclonus after low-frequency rTMS (Wedegaertner et al., 1997).

Finally, several reports demonstrated a positive effect of rTMS applied to the motor cortex in patients with severe central pain (Lefaucheur et al., 2001a,b; Migita et al., 1995). Lefaucheur and colleagues showed that this therapeutic effect was sensitive to stimulation frequency (positive effect with 10 Hz, no effect with 0.5 Hz) (Lefaucheur et al., 2001a), and long lasting (up to 8 days after the intervention) (Lefaucheur et al., 2001b).

Conclusions

Stimulation-induced plasticity, defined as any change in neuronal excitability or synaptic efficacy outlasting the stimulation, may serve as an experimental model to study the capacity of the brain to undergo alteration. In addition, stimulation-induced plasticity in the nervous system may be of interest because of its therapeutic potential.

Of several protocols of stimulation-induced plasticity, the most simple one involves the repetitive application of single TMS pulses (rTMS). This protocol has been used with a wide range of different stimulation intensities, frequencies, train durations and total number of stimuli. rTMS over the primary motor cortex may induce facilitation or depression of amplitudes of motor-evoked potential (MEP), when MEPs elicited prior to and after rTMS are compared. The available evidence suggests that rTMS induces multiple effects of variable duration simultaneously at several sites within the nervous system while relatively little is known about the exact mechanisms involved. Stimulation-induced plasticity can also be obtained by the application of direct electric current (DC) flowing between electrodes attached to frontal and central skull regions overlying the primary motor cortex. The sign of DC-induced plasticity, i.e. MEP facilitation or depression, is entirely determined by the current direction (anodal or cathodal stimulation). Other protocols involve the repetitive stimulation of afferent input to the cortex. Finally, two protocols involve the combined action of rTMS over the primary motor cortex and manipulation of afferent input. The mechanisms underlying the plasticity induced by these protocols are discussed in detail and may be related to modulation of intracortical inhibition and to long-term potentiation of synaptic efficacy in the human primary motor cortex.

The functional consequences of stimulation-induced plasticity and some of the potential therapeutic applications of rTMS are discussed.

Acknowledgements

This work was supported by Deutsche Forschungsgemeinschaft Cl 95/3-1, and Zi 542/1-1 and Zi 542/2-1.

REFERENCES

Antal, A., Nitsche, M.A. & Paulus, W. (2001). External modulation of visual perception in humans. *Neuroreport*, **12**: 3553–3555.

Berardelli, A., Inghilleri, M., Rothwell, J.C. et al. (1998). Facilitation of muscle evoked responses after repetitive cortical stimulation in man. *Exp Brain Res*, **122**: 79–84.

Bi, G.Q. & Poo, M.M. (1998). Synaptic modifications in cultured hippocampal neurons: dependence on spike timing, synaptic strength, and postsynaptic cell type. *J. Neurosci.*, **18**: 10464–10472.

Bliss, T.V. & Collingridge, G.L. (1993). A synaptic model of memory: long-term potentiation in the hippocampus. *Nature*, **361**: 31–39.

Boroojerdi, B., Phipps, M., Kopylev, L., Wharton, C.M., Cohen, L.G. & Grafman, J. (2001). Enhancing analogic reasoning with rTMS over the left prefrontal cortex. *Neurology*, **56**: 526–528.

Brasil-Neto, J.P., Cohen, L.G., Pascual-Leone, A., Jabir, F.K., Wall, R.T. & Hallett, M. (1992). Rapid reversible modulation of human motor outputs after transient deafferentation of the forearm: a study with transcranial magnetic stimulation. *Neurology*, **42**: 1302–1306.

Buonomano, D.V. & Merzenich, M.M. (1998). Cortical plasticity: from synapses to maps. *Annu. Rev. Neurosci.*, **21**: 149–186.

Bütefisch, C.M., Davis, B.C., Wise, S.P. et al. (2000). Mechanisms of use-dependent plasticity in the human motor cortex. *Proc. Natl Acad. Sci., USA*, **97**: 3661–3665.

Castro-Alamancos, M.A., Donoghue, J.P. & Connors, B.W. (1995). Different forms of synaptic plasticity in somatosensory and motor areas of the neocortex. *J. Neurosci.*, **15**: 5324–5333.

Chen, R., Classen, J., Gerloff, C. et al. (1997). Depression of motor cortex excitability by low-frequency transcranial magnetic stimulation. *Neurology*, **48**: 1398–1403.

Classen, J., Liepert, J., Wise, S.P., Hallett, M. & Cohen, L.G. (1998). Rapid plasticity of human cortical movement representation induced by practice. *J. Neurophysiol.*, **79**: 1117–1123.

Creutzfeldt, O.D., Fromm, G.H. & Kapp, H. (1962). Influence of transcortical dc currents on cortical neuronal activity. *Exp. Neurol.*, **5**: 436–452.

Di Lazzaro, V., Restuccia, D., Oliviero, A. et al. (1998). Magnetic transcranial stimulation at intensities below active motor threshold activates intracortical inhibitory circuits. *Exp. Brain Res.*, **119**: 265–268.

Di Lazzaro, V., Oliviero, A., Profice, P. et al. (2000). Muscarinic receptor blockade has differential effects on the excitability of intracortical circuits in human motor cortex. *Exp. Brain Res.* **135**: 455–461.

Donoghue, J.P., Hess, G. & Sanes, J.N. (1996). Substrates and mechanisms for learning in motor cortex. In *Acquisition of Motor Behavior in Vertebrates*, ed. J. Bloedel, T. Ebner & S.P. Wise, pp. 363–386. Cambridge, MA: MIT Press.

Enomoto, H., Ugawa, Y., Hanajima, R. et al. (2001). Decreased sensory cortical excitability after 1 Hz rTMS over the ipsilateral primary motor cortex. *Clin. Neurophysiol.*, **112**: 2154–2158.

Gerschlager, W., Siebner, H.R. & Rothwell, J.C. (2001). Decreased corticospinal excitability after subthreshold 1 Hz rTMS over lateral premotor cortex. *Neurology*, **57**: 449–455.

Ghabra, M.B., Hallett, M. & Wassermann, E.M. (1999). Simultaneous repetitive transcranial magnetic stimulation does not speed fine movement in PD. *Neurology*, **52**: 768–770.

Hamdy, S., Rothwell, J.C., Aziz, Q., Singh, K.D. & Thompson, D.G. (1998). Long-term reorganization of human motor cortex driven by short-term sensory stimulation. *Nature Neurosci.*, **1**: 64–68.

Hess, G., Aizenman, C.D. & Donoghue, J.P. (1996). Conditions for the induction of long-term potentiation in layer II/III horizontal connections of the rat motor cortex. *J. Neurophysiol.*, **75**: 1765–1778.

Jaeger, D., Elbert, T., Lutzenberger, W. & Birbaumer, N. (1987). The effects of externally applied transcephalic weak direct currents on lateralization in choice reaction tasks. *J. Psychophysiol.*, **1**: 127–133.

Jones, E.G. (1993). GABAergic neurons and their role in cortical plasticity in primates. *Cereb. Cortex*, **3**: 361–372.

Kaelin-Lang, A., Luft, A.R., Sawaki, L., Burstein, A.H., Sohn, Y.H. & Cohen, L.G. (2002). Modulation of human corticomotor excitability by somatosensory input. *J. Physiol.*, **540**: 623–633.

Karl, A., Birbaumer, N., Lutzenberger, W., Cohen, L.G. & Flor, H. (2001). Reorganization of motor and somatosensory cortex in upper extremity amputees with phantom limb pain. *J. Neurosci.*, **21**: 3609–3618.

Kujirai, T., Caramia, M.D., Rothwell, J.C. et al. (1993). Corticocortical inhibition in human motor cortex. *J. Physiol. (Lond.)*, **471**: 501–519.

Lefaucheur, J.P., Drouot, X., Keravel, Y. & Nguyen, J.P. (2001a). Pain relief induced by repetitive transcranial magnetic stimulation of precentral cortex. *Neuroreport*, **12**: 2963–2965.

Lefaucheur, J.P., Drouot, X. & Nguyen, J.P. (2001b). Interventional neurophysiology for pain control: duration of pain relief following repetitive transcranial magnetic stimulation of the motor cortex. *Neurophysiol. Clin.*, **31**: 247–252.

Levy, L.M., Ziemann, U., Chen, R. & Cohen, L.G. (2002). Rapid modulation of GABA in sensorimotor cortex induced by acute deafferentiation. *Ann. Neurol.*, **52**: 755–761.

Liepert, J., Oreja-Guevara, C., Cohen, L.G., Tegenthoff, M., Hallett, M. & Malin, J-P. (1999). Plasticity of cortical hand muscle representation in patients with hemifacial spasm. *Neurosci. Lett.*, **272**: 33–36.

Maeda, F., Keenan, J.P., Tormos, J.M., Topka, H. & Pascual-Leone, A. (2000). Modulation of corticospinal excitability by repetitive transcranial magnetic stimulation. *Clin. Neurophysiol.*, **111**: 800–805.

Markram, H., Lubke, J., Frotscher, M. & Sakmann, B. (1997). Regulation of synaptic efficacy by coincidence of postsynaptic APs and EPSPs. *Science*, **275**: 213–215.

Migita, K., Uozumi, T., Arita, K. & Monden, S. (1995). Transcranial magnetic coil stimulation of motor cortex in patients with central pain. *Neurosurgery*, **36**: 1037–1039; discussion 1039–1040.

Modugno, N., Nakamura, Y., MacKinnon, C.D. et al. (2001). Motor cortex excitability following short trains of repetitive magnetic stimuli. *Exp. Brain Res.*, **140**: 453–459.

Mottaghy, F.M., Hungs, M., Brugmann, M. et al. (1999). Facilitation of picture naming after repetitive transcranial magnetic stimulation. *Neurology*, **53**: 1806–1812.

Muellbacher, W., Ziemann, U., Boroojerdi, B. & Hallett, M. (2000). Effects of low-frequency transcranial magnetic stimulation on motor excitability and basic motor behavior. *Clin. Neurophysiol.*, **111**: 1002–1007.

Muellbacher, W., Ziemann, U., Wissel, J. et al. (2002). Early consolidation in human primary motor cortex. *Nature*, **415**: 640–644.

Münchau, A., Orth, M., Rothwell, J.C. et al. (2002). Intracortical inhibition is reduced in a patient with a lesion in the posterolateral thalamus. *Mov. Disord.*, **17**: 208–212.

Nitsche, M.A. & Paulus, W. (2000). Excitability changes induced in the human motor cortex by weak transcranial direct current stimulation. *J. Physiol.*, **527**: 633–639.

Nitsche, M.A. & Paulus, W. (2001). Sustained excitability elevations induced by transcranial DC motor cortex stimulation in humans. *Neurology*, **57**: 1899–1901.

Pascual-Leone, A., Houser, C.M., Reese, K. et al. (1993). Safety of rapid-rate transcranial magnetic stimulation in normal volunteers. *Electroencephalogr. Clin. Neurophysiol.*, **89**: 120–130.

Pascual-Leone, A., Valls-Sole, J., Wassermann, E.M. & Hallett, M. (1994). Responses to rapid-rate transcranial magnetic stimulation of the human motor cortex. *Brain*, **117**: 847–858.

Paus, T., Castro-Alamancos, M.A. & Petrides, M. (2001). Cortico-cortical connectivity of the human mid-dorsolateral frontal cortex and its modulation by repetitive transcranial magnetic stimulation. *Eur. J. Neurosci.*, **14**: 1405–1411.

Peinemann, A., Lehner, C., Mentschel, C., Munchau, A., Conrad, B. & Siebner, H.R. (2000). Subthreshold 5-Hz repetitive transcranial magnetic stimulation of the human primary motor cortex reduces intracortical paired-pulse inhibition. *Neurosci. Lett.*, **296**: 21–24.

Ridding, M.C., Brouwer, B., Miles, T.S., Pitcher, J.B. & Thompson, P.D. (2000). Changes in muscle responses to stimulation of the motor cortex induced by peripheral nerve stimulation in human subjects. *Exp. Brain Res.*, **131**: 135–143.

Ridding, M.C., Inzelberg, R. & Rothwell, J.C. (1995a). Changes in excitability of motor cortical circuitry in patients with Parkinson's disease. *Ann. Neurol.*, **37**: 181–188.

Ridding, M.C., McKay, D.R., Thompson, P.D. & Miles, T.S. (2001). Changes in corticomotor representations induced by prolonged peripheral nerve stimulation in humans. *Clin. Neurophysiol.*, **112**: 1461–1469.

Ridding, M.C., Sheean, G., Rothwell, J.C., Inzelberg, R. & Kujirai, T. (1995b). Changes in the balance between motor cortical excitation and inhibition in focal, task specific dystonia. *J. Neurol. Neurosurg. Psychiatry*, **59**: 493–498.

Ridding, M.C. & Taylor, J.L. (2001). Mechanisms of motor-evoked potential facilitation following prolonged dual peripheral and central stimulation in humans. *J. Physiol.*, **537**: 623–631.

Rijntjes, M., Tegenthoff, M., Liepert, J. et al. (1994). Cortical reorganization in patients with facial palsy. *Ann. Neurol.*, **41**: 621–630.

Rollnik, J.D., Schubert, M. & Dengler, R. (2000). Subthreshold prefrontal repetitive transcranial magnetic stimulation reduces motor cortex excitability. *Muscle Nerve*, **23**: 112–114.

Rosen, I. & Asanuma, H. (1972). Peripheral afferent inputs to the forelimb area of the monkey motor cortex: input-output relations. *Exp. Brain Res.*, **14**: 257–273.

Rosenkranz, K., Nitsche, M.A., Tergau, F. & Paulus, W. (2000). Diminution of training-induced transient motor cortex plasticity by weak transcranial direct current stimulation in the human. *Neurosci. Lett.*, **296**: 61–63.

Rossi, S., Pasqualetti, P., Rossini, P.M. et al. (2000). Effects of repetitive transcranial magnetic stimulation on movement-related cortical activity in humans. *Cereb. Cortex*, **10**: 802–808.

Rothwell, J.C. (1997). Techniques and mechanisms of action of transcranial stimulation of the human motor cortex. *J. Neurosci. Methods*, **74**: 113–122.

Sandbrink, F., Stefan, K., Wolters, A., Kunesch, E., Benecke, R. & Classen, J. (2001). Induktion von Longterm-Depression im menschlichen Motorkortex durch assoziative Paarstimulation [abstract]. *Klin. Neurophysiol.*, **32**: 194.

Sanes, J.N. & Donoghue, J.P. (2000). Plasticity and primary motor cortex. *Annu. Rev. Neurosci.*, **23**: 393–415.

Shimamoto, H., Takasaki, K., Shigemori, M., Imaizumi, T., Ayabe, M. & Shoji, H. (2001). Therapeutic effect and mechanism of repetitive transcranial magnetic stimulation in Parkinson's disease. *J. Neurol.*, **248**: III48–52.

Siebner, H.R., Mentschel, C., Auer, C. & Conrad, B. (1999a). Repetitive transcranial magnetic stimulation has a beneficial effect on bradykinesia in Parkinson's disease. *Neuroreport*, **10**: 589–594.

Siebner, H.R., Peller, M., Takano, B. & Conrad, B. (2001). Neue Einblicke in die Hirnfunktion durch Kombination von transkranieller magnetischer Kortexstimulation und funktioneller zerebraler Bildgebung. *Nervenarzt*, **72**: 320–326.

Siebner, H.R., Rossmeier, C., Mentschel, C., Peinemann, A. & Conrad, B. (2000). Short-term motor improvement after sub-threshold 5-Hz repetitive transcranial magnetic stimulation of the primary motor hand area in Parkinson's disease. *J. Neurol. Sci.*, **178**: 91–94.

Siebner, H.R., Tormos, J.M., Ceballos-Baumann, A.O. et al. (1999b). Low-frequency repetitive transcranial magnetic stimulation of the motor cortex in writer's cramp. *Neurology*, **52**: 529–537.

Sommer, M., Tergau, F., Wischer, S. & Paulus, W. (2001). Paired-pulse repetitive transcranial magnetic stimulation of the human motor cortex. *Exp. Brain Res.*, **139**: 465–472.

Stefan, K., Binkofski, F., Shah, N.J., Seitz, R. & Classen, J. (2001). Rekrutierung neuer neuronaler Elemente im menschlichen Motorkortex nach Induktion von LTP. Eine kombinierte fMRI- und TMS-Studie [abstract]. *Klin. Neurophysiol.*, **32**: 198.

Stefan, K., Kunesch, E., Benecke, R., Cohen, L.G. & Classen, J. (2002). Mechanisms of enhancement of human motor cortical excitability induced by interventional paired associative stimulation. *J. Physiol.*, **543**: 699–708.

Stefan, K., Kunesch, E., Cohen, L.G., Benecke, R. & Classen, J. (2000). Induction of plasticity in the human motor cortex by paired associative stimulation. *Brain*, **123**: 572–584.

Strafella, A.P., Paus, T., Barrett, J. & Dagher, A. (2001). Repetitive transcranial magnetic stimulation of the human prefrontal cortex induces dopamine release in the caudate nucleus. *J. Neurosci.*, **21**: RC157.

Struppler, A., Jakob, C., Müller-Barna, P. et al. (1996). New method for ealry rehabilitation in extremities palsies of central origin by magnetic stimulation. *Z. EEG–EMG*, **27**: 151–157.

Tergau, F., Naumann, U., Paulus, W. & Steinhoff, B.J. (1999a). Low-frequency repetitive transcranial magnetic stimulation improves intractable epilepsy [letter]. *Lancet* **353**: 2209.

Tergau, F., Wassermann, E.M., Paulus, W. & Ziemann, U. (1999b). Lack of clinical improvement in patients with Parkinson's disease after low and high frequency repetitive transcranial magnetic stimulation. *Electroencephalogr. Clin. Neurophysiol. Suppl.*, **51**: 281–288.

Tokimura, H., Di Lazzaro, V., Tokimura, Y. et al. (2000). Short latency inhibition of human hand motor cortex by somatosensory input from the hand. *J. Physiol.*, **523**: 503–513.

Touge, T., Gerschlager, W., Brown, P. & Rothwell, J.C. (2001). Are the after-effects of low-frequency rTMS on motor cortex excitability due to changes in the efficacy of cortical synapses? *Clin. Neurophysiol.*, **112**: 2138–2145.

van Rossum, M.C., Bi, G.Q. & Turrigiano, G.G. (2000). Stable Hebbian learning from spike timing-dependent plasticity. *J. Neurosci.*, **20**: 8812–8821.

Wassermann, E.M., Grafman, J., Berry, C. et al. (1996). Use and safety of a new repetitive transcranial magnetic stimulator. *Electroencephalogr. Clin. Neurophysiol.*, **101**: 412–417.

Wassermann, E.M., Wedegaertner, F.R., Ziemann, U., George, M.S. & Chen, R. (1998). Crossed reduction of human motor cortex excitability by 1-Hz transcranial magnetic stimulation. *Neurosci. Lett.*, **250**: 141–144.

Wedegaertner, F., Garvey, M., Cohen, L.G., Hallett, M. & Wassermann, E.M. (1997). Low frequency repetitive transcranial magnetic stimulation can reduce action myoclonus [abstract]. *Neurology*, **48**: A119.

Wong, B.Y., Coulter, D.A., Choi, D.W. & Prince, D.A. (1988). Dextrorphan and dextromethorphan, common antitussives, are antiepileptic and antagonize *N*-methyl-D-aspartate in brain slices. *Neurosci. Lett.*, **85**: 261–266.

Wu, T., Sommer, M., Tergau, F. & Paulus, W. (2000). Lasting influence of repetitive transcranial magnetic stimulation on intracortical excitability in human subjects. *Neurosci. Lett.*, **287**: 37–40.

Ziemann, U. (1999). Intracortical inhibition and facilitation in the conventional paired TMS paradigm. *Electroencephalogr. Clin. Neurophysiol. Suppl.*, **51**: 127–136.

Ziemann, U., Lönnecker, S., Steinhoff, B.J. & Paulus, W. (1996a). Effects of antiepileptic drugs on motor cortex excitability in humans: a transcranial magnetic stimulation study. *Ann. Neurol.*, **40**: 367–378.

Ziemann, U., Rothwell, J.C. & Ridding, M.C. (1996b). Interaction between intracortical inhibition and facilitation in human motor cortex. *J. Physiol. (Lond.)*, **496**: 873–881.

Ziemann, U., Corwell, B. & Cohen, L.G. (1998a). Modulation of plasticity in human motor cortex after forearm ischemic nerve block. *J. Neurosci.*, **18**: 1115–1123.

Ziemann, U., Hallett, M. & Cohen, L.G. (1998b). Mechanisms of deafferentation-induced plasticity in human motor cortex. *J. Neurosci.*, **18**: 7000–7007.

Ziemann, V., Wittenberg, G.F. & Cohen, L.G. (2002). Stimulation-induced within-representation and across-representation plasticity in human motor cortex. *J. Neurosci.*, **22**: 5563–5571.

7

Lesions of cortex and post-stroke 'plastic' reorganization

Paolo M. Rossini[1,2,3] and Joachim Liepert[4]

[1]Clinica Neurologica Università Campus Bio-Medico, Rome, Italy
[2]AFaR, Dept. Neuroscience, Ospedale Fatebenefratelli, Isola Tiberina, Rome, Italy
[3]IRCCS Centro S. Giovanni di Dio, Brescia, Italy
[4]Department of Neurology, University of Hamburg, Germany

General introduction

Stroke is still the third cause of death and the first cause of chronic, highly disabling disease because of the frequent neurological sequelae affecting sensorimotor integration, movement programming and execution, walking, language, balance, mood and sensory perception. It is a well-accepted notion that, following the acute ischemic block of blood perfusion, there is a central core of dead neurons circumscribed by a shell of so-called *ischemic penumbra*, where the neurons adjacent to the damaged core are functionally blocked but still alive, because of the suboptimal flow from arterioles and capillaries and collaterals from the bed of vessels in the lesional periphery. This situation is of relatively brief duration (from hours to few days) and is followed either by a full recovery of the non-functioning, but still living, neurons (with a rapid, partial or total restoration of the lost functions) or by a complete loss of the perilesional contingent of brain cells with consequent stabilization of the clinical picture, i.e. the presence of more or less severe deficits. Several mechanisms contribute to the final volume of the lesioned tissue; from what can be inferred from the ischemia/reperfusion animal model, they include: 'inflammatory-like' reactions in which cytokines (mainly interleukin-1 and tumour necrosis factor) attract polymorphonuclear leukocytes, which create mechanical obstruction to erythrocytes' circulation by adherence to corresponding endothelial cell ligands, as well as becoming a source of oxygen free radicals (including nitric oxide, superoxide and peroxynitrite; del Zoppo & Garcia, 1995); later, a platelet activating factor induces platelets aggregation in the damaged area of microcirculation; in the core of the ischemic area, neuronal death may be mediated by the effects of excitatory neurotransmitters, e.g. glutamate which promotes calcium influx in the injured cells, and the accumulation of lactic acid as the result of a metabolic switch to anaerobiosis (Garcia et al., 1994). Delayed neuronal death also occurs in focal cerebral ischemia models, due to the fact that cell damage can develop not only via direct insult to cell body but also via axonal degeneration either anterograde or retrograde; both types of degeneration can additionally induce transneuronal changes across a synapse presumably because the lack of stimulation and of some trophic substance released by the synaptic terminals of the dead neuron (Kelly, 1985). Hyperglycaemia and hyperthermia can badly influence the amount and timing of the cascade of damaging factors on brain neurons, while several predisposing factors have been investigated and identified, including atrial fibrillation, cardiac valvular disease, collagenopathies, hypertension, hyperdyslipidaemias, diabetes, smoking and drinking habits. The heat shock and immediate–early genes families, such as *hsp 70, c-fos* and *jun B* are induced in the ipsilateral thalamus after experimental middle cerebral artery (MCA) occlusion, showing that gene expression can be changed in regions remote from brain infarction (Kinouchi et al., 1994).

Poststroke recovery of hand sensorimotor function has been ascribed to several phenomena, not mutually exclusive, but often overlapping, which include: the reabsorption of perilesional oedema, the interindividual variability of the territory of the MCA perfusion and, more important, the amount and extent of collaterals and neuronal pools receiving blood supply from adjacent arteries, the multiple representations of the same muscles in separate clusters of cortical motoneurons in primary motor cortex (MI), the presence and amount of ipsilateral corticospinal fibres (Rossini, 2001).

It is, however, a common experience that a slow, but consistent recovery of the apparently stabilized neurological deficits takes place in the weeks and months following a stroke (Twitchell, 1951). This can be of little or great functional impact even in patients with apparently identical clinical pictures in the early stroke stages. At the present time, despite several reports in the past claiming the possibility of predicting final outcome, there is no clinical or technological mean to prognosticate correctly as to whether and to which extent a given patient will recover from stabilized, poststroke deficits.

Brain plasticity is a somewhat controversial term, which in its general assumption embraces all the mechanisms of self-repair and/or of reorganization of neural connections, including the use of alternative pathways functionally homologous but anatomically distinct from the damaged ones (i.e. corticospinal pathways different from the pyramidal tract), synaptogenesis, dendritic arborization, and experience-based reinforcement of previous existing, but functionally silent, synaptic connections (Wall & Egger, 1971, 1980). All such mechanisms are strongly influenced by complex interactions coming from the remote effects, termed diaschisis, provoked by the loss of excitatory/inhibitory modulation from the damaged area on adjacent or distant brain centres via cortico-cortical and/or transcallosal connections. The cortico-cortical inputs to MI are dominated by those from the supplementary motor area, premotor cortex and primary sensory cortices 1, 2 and 5, where egocentric and allocentric spatiotemporal maps are processed in register, allowing the integration of proprioceptive, tactile and visual cues necessary for manual actions (Rossini, 2000).

Voluntary motor activity in humans requires sensory feedback from the moving part, as is clearly shown by functional imaging with PET (Seitz et al., 1995; Pantano et al., 1996); this explains why patients with poor or no post-stroke improvement of the hand motor control show a severe metabolic depression in the thalamus (Fries et al., 1993; Binkofski et al., 1996). An appropriate sensory feedback from the paretic hand, therefore, seems to play a pivotal role in long-term motor recovery, also by favouring neuronal reorganization beyond the limits of the usual sensorimotor areas (Stepniewska et al., 1993). Moreover, corollary discharges in primary somatosensory cortex (SI) are fired by MI output, probably providing the 'efferent copy' of a motor programme, with which the sensory feedback should be matched (Blakemore et al., 1998, 1999; Rossi et al., 1998).

Functional brain imaging: technological issues and review of findings in stroke

Nowadays, modern magnetic resonance imaging (MRI) technologies allow precise reconstruction of brain structure, including the location and volume of a lesion. Moreover, functional MRI (fMRI), single photon emission computerized tomography (SPECT) and positron emission tomography (PET) allow evaluation of baseline and task-related function of the relevant brain areas. Such methodologies have superb space discrimination, but rather poor time discrimination, i.e. they scarcely disentangle a hierarchical organization, if any in the neural network activated by a given task. Also, they do not allow distinction between excitatory and inhibitory phenomena or 'functional' importance of given activated brain regions. Finally, 'natural' types of activation including movement tasks (i.e. finger tapping) reflex mixed outflow/inflow informational processing of the brain, including corollary discharges in linked brain areas and feedback from the moving part (Rossini, 2000; Gosh et al., 1987). In this respect neurophysiological techniques, including advanced EEG, magnetoencephalography (MEG), transcranial magnetic stimulation (TMS), provide an excellent time discrimination of the examined function down to fractions of milliseconds, appreciate excitatory and inhibitory contributions and provide an indirect measure of the strength of the contributing brain generators in a given circuitry. Advanced EEG methods, via Laplacian transforms and an appropriate number of scalp electrodes, makes it possible to eliminate the contribution of volume currents, in order to obtain reference-free recordings and to disentangle locoregional, rhythmic or transient neuronal activities produced by both tangential and radially oriented generators from discrete brain areas underlying the exploring electrode (Nunez et al., 1997). MEG, because of its physical properties, is blind to the influence of extracerebral layers (skull, meninges, etc.). It can localize and measure the intracellular currents in a shallow brain region exactly below the recording sensor without any contribution from volume currents, but is only sensitive to the tangential component of the active dipoles (Romani, 1990). It localizes a neural generator with extremely high precision (better than the EEG; Hari et al., 1993; Nakasato et al., 1994) and is not distorted by nearness of lesioned tissue. TMS activates cortical cells, subcortical fibres and cortico-cortical connections immediately via brief, painless magnetic pulses that induce transcranial currents, which circulate within the brain underlying the stimulating coil with an orientation opposite to that of the current circulating in the coil (Cohen et al., 1990; Fuhr et al., 1991a; Pascual-Leone et al., 1994). Figure-of-eight coils with an appropriate orientation on the scalp make it possible to stimulate restricted brain regions and, when repeatedly applied on a properly designed multiple points grid, to map out the scalp representation of a given 'function' (i.e. the motor representation of one or more muscles; Rossini & Pauri, 2000). It is therefore conceivable that the combined and integrated use of different types of structural and functional imaging of the brain should allow the best and most reliable view of 'plastic' post-lesional changes of brain function (Rossini et al., 1998a).

Today, various imaging techniques allow reorganization of neuronal networks in the human brain in vivo to be identified. Evidence of reorganizational capacities does not only improve our understanding of how the brain works but, even more importantly, could have major implications for the development of adequate therapeutic strategies.

The degree to which brain areas can be recruited for reorganization after an infarction is probably influenced by numerous factors, e.g. site and extent of the lesion, remote lesion-induced effects in structurally intact areas ('diachisis'), and pre-stroke organization of motor areas (e.g. amount of ipsilateral uncrossed corticospinal fibres) (see later; Weiller, 1998).

Studies on sensorimotor reorganization after stroke show a number of congruencies, but also several substantial differences. In most fMRI or PET studies involving active or passive movements, a widespread network of neurons was activated in both hemispheres. The areas included frontal and parietal cortices, sometimes also basal ganglia and cerebellum. They are in accordance with the finding that various brain areas are devoted to motor control and motor activity (Rizzolatti et al., 1998). In particular, (ipsilateral) premotor cortex, SMA, anterior parts of the insula/frontal operculum and bilateral inferior parietal cortices, are commonly found to be activated (Cao et al., 1998; Chollet et al., 1991; Dettmers et al., 1997; Marshall et al., 2000; Nelles et al., 1999a,b; Pantano et al., 1996; Seitz et al., 1998; Weiller et al., 1992). These results suggest that sensorimotor functions are represented in extended, variable, probably parallel processing, bilateral networks (Weiller & Rijntjes, 1999). Some of these areas (e.g. SMA, lateral premotor cortex) are supposed to be mainly involved in planning, preparation and initiation of movements. However, these additional motor areas contribute substantial numbers of fibres to the corticospinal tract (Dum & Strick, 1991) and could therefore functionally substitute damaged fibres.

During finger movements, stroke patients usually show stronger activations compared to healthy controls. This could reflect a greater effort to perform the movement (Price et al., 1994). Alternative explanations might be a lesion-induced disinhibition (Liepert et al., 2000a–d; Witte, 1998) through impairment of transcallosal fibres or a compensatory mechanism of the brain by the attempt to enhance excitability through reduction of intracortical inhibition.

Another common finding is activation of areas in the undamaged hemisphere. Again, interpretation of this result is not trivial. In some, but not all, studies these activations could be related to the occurrence of associated movements of the unaffected hand. Therefore, these results can only be interpreted if motor behaviour and EMG activity is recorded during scanning. TMS results (see below) suggest that, in some patients, ipsilateral corticospinal projections may be of major importance for motor recovery (Caramia et al., 1996; Alagona et al., 2001). In most PET and fMRI studies stroke patients are enrolled after a substantial recovery of function. This makes an interpretation even more difficult, as it remains unclear whether the activations represent a correlate of recovery or if they are an epiphenomenon. To evaluate the contribution of the undamaged hemisphere, studies are needed that correlate activations in specific brain areas with a change in motor performance. This can be done by repetition of measurements during spontaneous recovery, as detailed in the later part of this chapter (Cicinelli et al., 1997a,b; Nelles et al., 1999b; Traversa et al., 1997; Wikström et al., 2000) or after a particular therapeutic intervention (Kopp et al., 1998; Liepert et al., 1998a,b, 2000a,b). Nelles et al. (1999a,b) demonstrated with repeated PET measurements (two measurements within 12 weeks after subcortical stroke) a complex pattern of increases of regional cerebral blood flow in both hemispheres. Early after stroke, many more areas showed activation. The ipsilateral premotor cortex was the only area that was solely activated at the second measurement. The authors concluded that this brain area is critical for reorganization of sensory and motor pathways.

By conducting such a brief review, it was shown that the vast majority of studies that focused on neuronal reorganization following stroke, deal particularly with the brain sensorimotor areas devoted to hand control; this is because of the large hand representation, which makes it easier to disentangle even minor changes in the topography of the homuncular hand, and because of the paramount importance of hand control in daily activities. In particular, MEG and TMS have shown a remarkable percentage of subjects in whom sensorimotor hand somatotopy had asymmetrically reorganized following stroke in the affected hemisphere (for a review, see Rossini & Pauri, 2000). In this respect, the pivotal observation was that, in healthy humans, most of the neurophysiological characteristics of the hand sensorimotor primary areas are quite symmetrical in the two hemispheres; this is somewhat different from posterior parietal areas devoted to sensory integration and from uni- vs. bimanual sensory perception (Oliveri et al., 1999, 2000). For the motor output, the parameters that have been found symmetrical on the two hemispheres include: number and location of the excitable scalp sites with respect to anatomical landmarks, centre of gravity of the motor maps, threshold of excitability in complete relaxation, latency of motor evoked potentials (MEPs) in the hand 'target' muscles (Cicinelli et al., 1997b) as well as central conduction time along the pyramidal tract and recovery curves to paired stimuli reflecting intracortical facilitatory (ICF) and inhibitory (ICI) mechanisms (Kujirai et al., 1993; Shimizu et al., 1999; Cicinelli et al., 2000). For the sensory input they include: location, depth, latency and strength of the dipoles responsible for responses in the 50 ms post-stimulus epoch (mainly around 20 and 30 ms) from SI after median nerve, or little and thumb finger stimulation, the hand extension measured as the euclidean distance between the fifth and thumb finger baricentres of the equivalent current dipoles (ECD), waveshape analysis via cross-correlation coefficient (Tecchio et al., 2000). Such symmetrical organization was found both with respect to skull (nasion, inion, vertex, preauricular points) and brain (Ω- or ε-shaped knob of the central sulcus) anatomical landmarks (Pizzella et al., 1999). The measured parameters were also stable when repeated in time in the same subject (an observation of paramount importance whenever follow-up recordings are needed; Cicinelli et al., 1997a; Tecchio et al., 1998). The intersubject variability of the interhemispheric differences of such parameters was relatively little different from that observed for their absolute values. In other words, if a subject, because of personal characteristics, has a more or less latero/medial shift of the sensorimotor brain areas, this is also reflected as a 'mirror image' in the opposite hemisphere. Therefore, the absolute values of the measured parameters vary widely from subject to subject, while their interhemispheric differences remain relatively stable (Rossini et al., 1994, 1998a, 2001; Wikstrom et al., 1997). A roughly symmetrical organization of sensorimotor hand areas in the right and left hemispheres has been found in healthy humans by different methods of functional brain imaging, including positron emission tomography (PET) and fMRI, particularly during stimuli on median nerve and fingers identical to those employed for MEG recordings (Puce et al., 1995; Del Gratta et al., 2000).

On this solid basis it was relatively easy to predict that an acute monohemispheric lesion like a stroke affecting the hand sensorimotor areas when followed by any 'plastic' reorganization should remarkably affect such a strong interhemispheric symmetry of the sensorimotor hand areas of the brain as seen in the healthy. It is worth remembering that the spatial sensory coordinates of the fingers ECDs are consistent with the known sensory homunculus somatotopy with the little finger more medial and posterior, the thumb more lateral and anterior and median nerve in between (Tecchio et al., 1997); moreover, they are strictly adjacent to the knob of the central sulcus containing the hand motor area (Yousry et al., 1997; Pizzella et al., 1999). Meanwhile, the hand extension in the healthy is ranging between 12 and 17 mm for the N20 and P30 components, respectively (Tecchio et al., 1997). The hand motor output area shows an average of 3.5 excitable sites during TMS on each hemisphere (Cicinelli et al., 1997a).

The morphology of brain responses to peripheral stimuli roughly reflect the cerebral circuitries and relays devoted to processing of the incoming stimulus, which shape-up the final response in time (peak latency), firing rate and number of synchronously firing neurons (peak amplitude) and excitatory/inhibitory net effect (peak polarity). Absolute waveforms are extremely variable across different subjects, mainly in wave polarity and shape. However, intrasubject interhemispheric differences are extremely low with a correlation coefficient which, in the healthy, is invariably higher than 0.83 (1 means shape identity; Fig. 7.1; Tecchio et al., 2000).

TMS as an early predictor of functional outcome

After a stroke it is desirable to know as soon as possible to what extent motor recovery can be expected. This knowledge is important for assessment of prognosis and for an early determination of rehabilitation procedures. In numerous studies TMS has been used as a predictor of outcome after stroke. However, results are not consistent. For example, Timmerhuis et al. (1996) found that only MEPs measured in the acute stage had predictive value. In contrast, Arac et al. (1994) reported that, irrespective of presence or

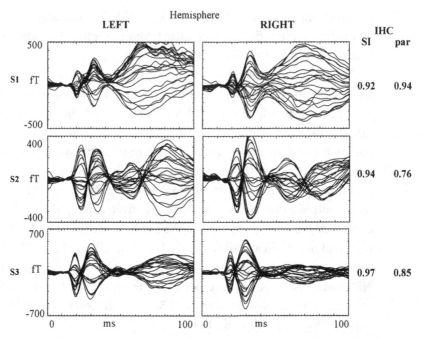

Fig. 7.1   Superimposition of all recording channels in left/right parietal regions (respectively, left/right columns) in the 100 ms post-stimulus period. SEFs of three paradigmatic subjects are presented, to show different SEF morphologies (compare S1, S2, S3 in one hemisphere) in this time interval. By comparing SEF from left vs. right hemisphere for each subject, the intrasubject interhemispheric shape similarity is appreciable. (From Tecchio et al., 2000.)

absence of MEPs in the acute stage patients had the same motor function 3–6 months later. Catano et al. (1996) suggested that motor threshold determination 30 days after stroke had the best correlation with outcome. However, Di Lazzaro et al. (1999) found motor thresholds within the first 8 hours after stroke to be a reasonable predictor of outcome. In most studies TMS was performed within the first few days (e.g. Escudero et al., 1998; Heald et al., 1993; Pennisi et al., 1999; Péréon et al., 1995; Vang et al., 1999) or even hours (Di Lazzaro et al., 1999) after stroke. Results obtained by TMS were compared with overall functional outcome, measured by Barthel index or Rankin scale, or to motor recovery. Outcome evaluation was usually performed 2 to 12 months after stroke. Some studies repeated TMS to compare electrophysiological follow-up with clinical progress (Catano et al., 1996;

Cruz Martinez et al., 1999; D'Olhaberriague et al., 1997; Hendricks et al., 1997; Pennisi et al., 1999; Péréon et al., 1995; Rapisarda et al., 1996; Timmerhuis et al., 1996). In most studies patients were subdivided into groups according to the TMS results. Patients with existing MEPs were usually compared with those without MEPs. Other investigators defined patient groups according to their clinical symptoms (D'Olhaberriague et al., 1997). In some papers patients were not grouped, but a statistical analysis was performed to discriminate the most important variables for predicting outcome results (e.g. Feys et al., 2000). Patient populations were quite different: in some studies the number of severely affected patients with poor recovery was particularly high, and in most studies cortical and subcortical infarctions as well as ischemic and haemorrhagic lesions were mixed. The above-mentioned different methods probably contribute substantially to the different results that are encountered (Rossini, 2000).

However, the majority of studies supports the following statements:

1. Patients in whom MEPs can be elicited in the paretic limb early after stroke have a significantly better clinical outcome than patients without MEPs at early stage (Dominkus et al., 1990).
2. Presence or absence of an MEP is a more important variable than a differentiation between normal and delayed central motor conduction times (CMCT) (Catano et al., 1995; Heald et al., 1993; Rapisarda et al., 1996).
3. TMS should not only be performed while the target muscle is relaxed but also during facilitation (contraction of the target muscle or, if impossible, innervation of the homologous contralateral muscle). Patients without MEPs at rest but with MEPs during facilitation have a substantially better prognosis than patients who have no MEPs during facilitation (Heald et al., 1993; Catano et al., 1995).
4. The inability to obtain MEPs early after stroke is associated with a poor recovery (Escudero et al., 1998; Rapisarda et al., 1996; Vang et al., 1999).
5. Motor thresholds are often elevated after stroke (particularly in subcortical strokes). They tend to decrease in the subsequent months. The best predictive value was found when determining motor threshold 30 days after stroke (Catano et al., 1996) but even threshold evaluation within the first 8 hours after stroke may predict outcome (Di Lazzaro et al., 1999).

Several studies have compared the prognostic value of motor-evoked potentials with somatosensory evoked potentials (SSEPs) in stroke (Macdonell et al., 1989; Abbruzzese et al., 1991; Péréon et al., 1995; Timmerhuis et al., 1996; Hendricks et al., 1997; Feys et al., 2000). In most studies the authors found MEPs to be more sensitive in the prediction of outcome (Macdonell et al., 1989; Abbruzzese et al., 1991; Péréon et al., 1995; Timmerhuis et al., 1996; Hendricks et al., 1997). Feys et al. (2000) concluded from their data that, in the acute phase, a combination of a motor score and SSEP results had the best prognostic value, whereas 2 months after stroke the combination of motor score and MEPs was best for predicting the long-term outcome.

In studies that exclusively included patients with brainstem lesions, TMS abnormalities were closely related to the degree of paresis (Ferbert et al., 1992), and absent MEPs were highly correlated with presence of persisting motor deficit 3 months later (Schwarz et al., 2000).

A still debated issue is the contribution to recovery of ipsilateral uncrossed fibres. In most functional imaging studies using PET or fMRI activations in the ipsilateral non-lesioned hemisphere were observed during passive or active movements of the paretic hand (Cao et al., 1998; Chollet et al., 1991; Dettmers et al., 1997; Marschall et al., 2000; Nelles et al., 1999a,b; Pantano et al., 1996; Seitz & Freund, 1997; Weiller et al., 1992). Some of these studies did not control for mirror movements performed with the unaffected hand. Thus it remained unclear whether or not the brain activations were exclusively related to movements with the paretic hand. Moreover, the results did not allow deciding if ipsilateral activations are clinically relevant for motor function or if they are mere epiphenomena.

In normal subjects high-intensity TMS can produce ipsilateral MEPs (iMEPS) during strong muscle contraction (Wassermann et al., 1994; Ziemann et al., 1999; Alagona et al., 2001). As iMEP amplitudes could be modulated by neck rotations, it was suggested that these iMEPs are mediated through corticoreticulospinal or corticopropriospinal pathways (Ziemann et al., 1999). Palmer et al. (1992) were unable to stimulate ipsilateral pathways in stroke patients and concluded that ipsilateral corticospinal connections do not contribute to motor recovery. In other studies with stroke patients, iMEPs could either be elicited by TMS over the non-lesioned hemisphere (Turton et al., 1996; Hendricks et al., 1997; Netz et al., 1997; Caramia et al., 1996; 2000, Trompetto et al., 2000) or over the affected hemisphere (Fries et al., 1991; Trompetto et al., 2000; Alagona et al., 2001). In these patients iMEPs were usually obtained by stimulating anteriorly and medially to the primary motor cortex. This probably indicates that corticospinal pathways originating from premotor areas were activated.

Those patients who had iMEPs when stimulating the non-affected hemisphere still had a variable outcome: some authors (Caramia et al., 1996, 2000; Trompetto et al., 2000) found a correlation between iMEPs and motor recovery, while other investigators described an association between the occurrence of iMEPS and a poor outcome (Turton et al., 1996; Netz et al., 1997; Hendricks et al., 1997). It remains unclear if clinical, pathophysiological or methodological differences are responsible for these different observations. In any case iMEPs described by Caramia et al. (1996) and Trompetto et al. (2000) seem to differ from those reported by Turton et al. (1996) in some electrophysiological features: iMEPS in Caramia's and Trompetto's patient group had rather low excitability thresholds and rather large amplitudes, while in Turton's patients only small iMEPs could be elicited with high stimulation intensities.

Therefore, it seems possible that two different patient groups exist: probably one small group with a larger portion of ipsilateral, uncrossed corticospinal fibres, which contribute to a quick recovery. However, the majority of patients probably has less ipsilateral corticospinal connections. They may become accessible but may not support restitution of function substantially.

Alagona et al. (2001) found an association between iMEPs produced by stimulation of the affected hemisphere and bimanual dexterity 6 months after stroke. Results suggested that the existence of these iMEPs indicates a hyperexcitability of premotor areas in the affected hemisphere.

The study of intracortical inhibition and facilitation (Kujirai et al., 1993) in stroke patients early after the event allows the suggestion of some mechanisms of brain plasticity. In patients with hemiplegia, due to a large infarction in the territory of the middle cerebral artery, the contralateral, non-lesioned hemisphere was studied with single- and paired-pulse TMS, and recordings were taken from the unaffected first dorsal interosseous muscle. A decrease of ICI was found 2 weeks after stroke (Liepert et al., 2000c). This finding corresponds with results obtained in animal studies (Buckremer-Ratzmann et al., 1996, 1997; Reinecke et al., 1999). In rats the disinhibition was associated with down-regulation of GABA (A) receptors and enhancement of glutamatergic activity (Que et al., 1999a,b). As changes of ICI are supposed to be modulated by GABAergic activity (Chen et al., 1998; Ziemann et al., 1996), the decreased ICI in the non-lesioned hemisphere of patients with large territorial infarctions may indicate a down-regulation of GABA activity in this hemisphere. Two main mechanisms could be responsible: a damage of transcallosal fibres, which could lead to a loss of physiological intercortical inhibition (Boroojerdi et al., 1996; Ferbert et al., 1992; Leocani et al., 2000, Liepert et al., 2001) or an enhanced use of the unaffected arm in all daily activities as ICI is modified in a task- and use-dependent manner (Liepert et al., 1998a). The idea of a disinhibition in the non-lesioned hemisphere is also supported by others who found enlarged MEP amplitudes when stimulating the unaffected hemisphere after stroke (Cicinelli et al., 1997b; Trompetto et al., 2000).

In another study ICI and ICF were studied in a subgroup of stroke patients with a mean interval of 8.7 days after the event. This group consisted of patients who either had a small motor deficit at onset of symptoms or who underwent a rapid (spontaneous) motor recovery. Thus, the patients had almost recovered at the time of electrophysiological evaluation. In this group, a loss of intracortical inhibition was observed in the affected hemisphere. In contrast, ICI in the unaffected hemisphere was not different from that in an age-matched control group (Liepert et al., 2000d). This result corresponds to animal studies which described a loss of GABAergic inhibition in the area around a cortical lesion (Schiene et al., 1996) and suggests that the rapid clinical improvement of the stroke patients might be induced by motor cortical disinhibition.

Another parameter which has proved to be helpful in detecting subclinical deficits after stroke is the silent period (SP). This phenomenon, the interruption of voluntary muscle activity by a TMS pulse, is attributed to activation of spinal and cortical inhibitory circuits (Cantello et al., 1992; Fuhr et al., 1991b; Roick et al., 1993; Triggs et al., 1993). SP duration shows a high interindividual variability. However, intraindividual interhemispheric differences are small (Cicinelli et al., 1997a; Fritz et al., 1997; Haug et al., 1992), which makes SP measurements particularly useful for evaluation of unilateral abnormalities. Early after stroke the SP is prolonged on the paretic side (Ahonen et al., 1998; Braune & Fritz, 1995; Classen et al., 1997; Faig & Busse, 1996; Haug et al., 1992; Kukowski & Haug, 1992; Liepert et al., 1995). SP abnormalities occurred more often than prolongations of central motor latencies, indicating that SP is a more sensitive parameter. Von Giesen et al. (1994) pointed out that small lesions within the primary sensorimotor cortex were associated with a reduction of SP duration, whereas patients with subcortical infarcts or lesions in premotor, parietal and temporal areas showed SP prolongations on the affected side. Classen et al. (1997) reported a close association between SP duration and motor performance. Patients with motor disturbances that resembled motor neglect had particularly prolonged SPs.

Spasticity was associated with a shortening of SP duration (Catano et al., 1997a; Cruz Martinez et al., 1998; Liepert et al., 1995), thus reflecting a decreased activity of inhibitory circuits. A SP shortening during a high level of voluntary contraction (as compared to SP duration during low force contractions) predicted the eventual occurrence of spasticity (Catano et al., 1997b). In conclusion, SP evaluation can be a valuable additional tool in stroke patients, particularly in those with normal MEPs and normal central motor latencies.

Intervention-induced changes of motor cortex excitability

Plastic changes after stroke may occur due to different conditions, e.g. (a) as a passive adaptation of the brain to the lesion and the impairment of neuronal networks; (b) as a reorganization of the brain due to spontaneous recovery of (partially) damaged brain tissue; (c) as a reorganization induced by behavioural consequences of the lesion, e.g. learned non-use of a formerly paretic limb or (d) as a reorganization of the brain evoked by specific therapeutic interventions. As well as findings reported in the section of the previous chapter, specific approaches can be applied to distinguish between them. Four different study designs are particularly well-known: (a) the 'AB design' (A: observation period; B: intervention period); (b) the withdrawal design which consists of first observation period–intervention period–second observation period; (c) the multiple baseline design which extends the classic AB format by varying the length of the baseline phase across subjects or settings; (d) the alternating treatment design which compares the effects of two or more treatment conditions (Backman et al., 1997).

Another way to specifically examine intervention-induced reorganization is to study patients in the chronic stage of their illness. In that phase the probability of spontaneous recovery is negligible (Liepert et al., 1998b, 2000a). Still another possibility is to study the effects of short-term interventions (e.g. within a single day). Behavioural or electrophysiological changes observed after a single therapeutic session are much more likely to be due to the intervention itself than to spontaneous improvements of motor performance.

As stroke patients can differ in many respects (e.g. site and extent of the lesion, cognitive and motivational aspects, degree of paresis), it is not easy to find homogeneous patient groups. Therefore, it is generally preferable to examine intraindividual rather than interindividual changes/differences (single subject research).

Intervention-induced effects on motor reorganization have been studied in a limited number of studies. Several investigators chose constraint-induced movement therapy (CIMT) (Taub et al., 1993) and applied different techniques to demonstrate plastic changes (Kopp et al., 1999; Levy et al., 2001; Liepert et al., 1998; 2000a). TMS was used to demonstrate changes of motor excitability (Liepert et al., 1998b; 2000a), MEG was employed to identify shifts of movement-related cortical potentials (Kopp et al., 1999), and in a pilot study with two patients (one stroke, one brain tumour) functional MRI was performed (Levy et al., 2001). In the TMS studies a mapping technique with a focal figure-of-eight coil was used. Using two baseline measurements it was shown that stroke patients in the chronic stage of their illness (>6 months after the event) had highly reproducible results, indicating that neither electrophysiologically nor clinically spontaneous recovery occurred. Prior to CIMT, the patients had higher motor thresholds and smaller motor output maps in the lesioned hemisphere. After therapy, motor output maps in the affected hemisphere had increased by approximately 40% while those in the non-affected hemisphere had non-significantly decreased. Thus, the cortical representation area in the affected hemisphere had become larger than the cortical map in the non-affected hemisphere. Both changes presumably reflect use-dependent mechanisms: the increased amount of use of the paretic hand during the training period and the decreased use of the immobilized non-affected hand. These electrophysiological changes were paralleled by a large improvement of motor function (Fig. 7.2). Motor thresholds remained identical after CIMT. As motor thresholds are determined in the centre of the cortical representation area, it was concluded that enlargements of the motor output map were due to increases of excitability at the borders of the representation area. One of the mechanisms involved in these map changes could be a GABA-dependent modulation of horizontal intracortical inhibitory

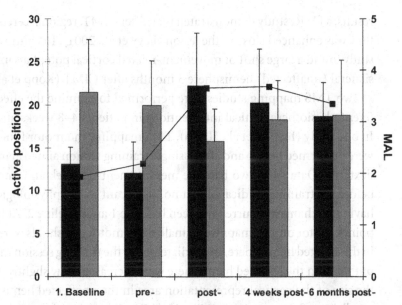

Fig. 7.2   Number of active TMS positions in the infarcted (black bars) and non-infarcted (grey bars) hemispheres 2 weeks and 1 day pre-treatment and 1 day, 4 weeks and 6 months post-treatment. Black squares indicate the corresponding motor activity log (MAL) data for the paretic limb. $P < 0.05$ (From Liepert et al., 2000a.)

circuits, which strongly influence the size of a representation area (Jacobs & Donoghue, 1991).

After CIMT, the amplitude-weighted centres of the motor output maps (centre of gravity, CoG) had shifted significantly more in the affected than in the non-affected hemisphere. These shifts were mainly observed in the medio-lateral axis. The authors suggested that CoG shifts indicated an intervention-induced recruitment of additional brain areas that were adjacent to the areas excitable prior to therapy. Similar results have also been reported in monkey studies (Nudo et al., 1996; Rouiller et al., 1998). In the subsequent 6 months after CIMT the motor output map sizes equalized (the area size in the affected hemisphere decreased somewhat, and the map in the non-affected hemisphere increased somewhat), while motor performance remained unchanged. The electrophysiological changes were interpreted as an indicator of increased effective connectivity between neuronal populations, which allows reducing the excitability level while maintaining the same level of performance (Liepert et al., 2000a). Similar to the TMS results, a fMRI study demonstrated that, after CIMT, regional cerebral blood flow was enhanced close to the lesion (Levy et al., 2001). In contrast, a MEG study found a large shift of movement-related cortical potentials into the ipsilateral (unaffected) hemisphere 3 months after CIMT (Kopp et al., 1999).

Two TMS mapping studies were performed to examine the effects of different physiotherapeutical interventions in patients 4–8 weeks after stroke. In one study (Liepert et al., 2000b), TMS mapping and motor function tests were performed before and after a single training session aimed at improving dexterity. Data from two baseline measurements (1 week and immediately before the training) indicated that no significant electrophysiological or behavioural changes occurred between baseline 1 and baseline 2. At both time points, motor output maps were smaller and motor thresholds were elevated in the affected hemisphere. Immediately after the training session motor output maps in the lesioned hemisphere were increased, now slightly exceeding the size of the cortical representation area in the unaffected hemisphere. In parallel, performance in the Nine Hole Peg Test, a test that predominantly measures dexterity, was significantly improved. Motor thresholds remained unchanged. One day after the training, some patients still had improvements of dexterity and enlarged representation areas while in other patients values had returned to baseline (Liepert et al., 2000b). It is noteworthy that, in contrast to the 2-week period of CIMT, the single treatment session did not induce CoG shifts.

In another study, 1 week of conventional physiotherapy was compared with 1 week of conventional physiotherapy combined with forced-use therapy. The forced use basically consisted of immobilization of the unaffected hand (Wolf et al., 1989). Similarly to the studies mentioned above, patients had smaller motor output maps and elevated motor thresholds in the affected hemisphere prior to therapy. This difference persisted after the first week of physiotherapy. In contrast, the motor output map in the affected hemisphere was significantly enlarged after forced-use therapy. This increase in motor cortex excitability was accompanied by a significant improvement of dexterity. Across the 2 treatment weeks, medio-lateral CoG shifts in the affected hemisphere were significantly stronger than in the non-affected hemisphere, suggesting the recruitment of adjacent brain areas. Thus, similarly to the study in chronic patients participating in CIMT, this study indicates that increases of motor cortex excitability are closely related to the amount of use of the target muscle. Comparable results were reported from healthy subjects (Pascual-Leone et al., 1995). Hummelsheim & Hauptmann (1999) used TMS to examine the facilitatory effects of different interventions in stroke patients. They reported that contraction of the target muscle exceeded all other facilitatory techniques, such as preinnervation of proximal muscles or contralateral homologous muscles and passive cutaneous stimulation. These results support the finding that increased or repetitive use has facilitatory effects and improves motor performance (Bütefisch et al., 1995).

A single training session also enhances corticospinal excitability. However, in a majority of patients effects from a single treatment had disappeared 24 hours later. It remains to be clarified whether TMS results obtained after one training session allow prediction of the long-term functional outcome of individual patients, and if TMS mapping allows distinction between patients who need daily training and those who might also improve with a lower treatment frequency.

Interhemispheric asymmetries in stabilized stroke

TMS of the MI area controlling the ADM muscle was carried out in patients at 2 and 4 months following monohemispheric stroke (Traversa et al., 1997). From the affected hemisphere (AH) several parameters were found significantly abnormal, including: increased excitability threshold, increased MEP latency, increased asymmetry of the motor maps with a lower number of excitable sites on the AH. This last parameter, in particular, was significantly modified during follow-up, with an increase at the fourth month control (Fig. 7.3; Traversa et al., 1997; Cicinelli et al., 1997b).

In a limited number of studies, integrated methods of functional brain imaging have been used. In a paradigmatic case, fMRI, TMS and MEG were all showing an asymmetrical enlargement and posterior shift of the sensorimotor areas of the AH (Rossini et al., 1998a,b). Quite recently, four patients previously submitted to MEG analysis with a clear-cut asymmetrical reorganization of the AH have been investigated via fMRI during median nerve stimulation and the execution of the 'finger tapping' task. They showed a relatively good correspondence between fMRI and MEG findings (Rossini et al., 2001, unpublished data).

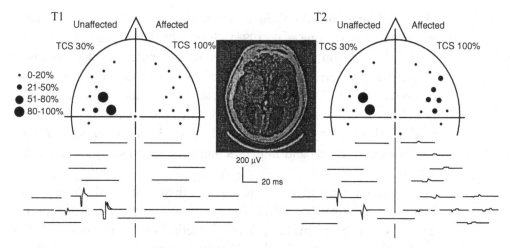

Fig. 7.3   CF, male 62 years, mainly cortical lesion. Tracings and CT scan showed in T1 (2 months after the stroke) the inexcitability of the AH, even with maximal intensity of the stimulator output. In T2 (4 months after the stroke, 8 weeks of neurorehabilitation) several responsive sites were identified on the AH, even if it was not possible to recognize a clear-cut 'hot spot'. Clinical recovery of hand functionality was relatively good. (From Cicinelli et al., 1997b.)

When following up the characteristics of motor output of stroke patients in an apparently clinically stabilized situation, interesting observations were obtained. Five recording sessions were distributed in a time epoch spanning from about 40 to 200 days from stroke. Recovery slopes of the various neurophysiological and clinical parameters were identified (Figs. 7.4, 7.5) and correlated with each other. In particular, the excitability threshold progressively decreased during the follow-up only on the AH, while MEP amplitudes and latencies tended toward normality, but more in the resting than in the contracted condition (Fig. 7.4). The steepest parts of the recovery slopes were concentrated in the 40 to 80 days post-stroke epoch (Traversa et al., 2000).

When another group of patients with similar characteristics was investigated via MEG recordings, the following was observed (Rossini et al., 2001): a group with cortical (C) stroke consisted of four patients, and a group with subcortical (S) stroke consisted of ten patients, respectively. In all cases, MRI was performed a few days after the MEG session: the thalamus was involved in two patients in association with internal capsule, basal ganglia

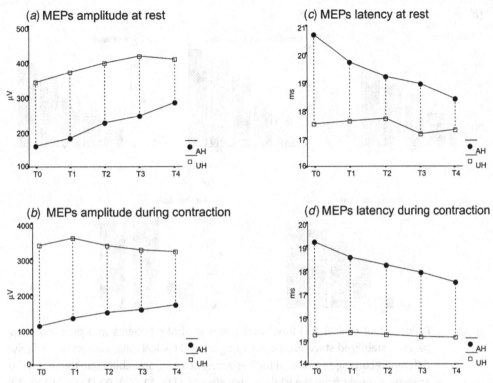

Fig. 7.4   Mean motor evoked potentials (MEPs) amplitude (*a*) at rest and (*b*) during contraction and mean MEPs latency (*c*) at rest and (*d*) during contraction as a function of time and hemisphere (AH-affected; UH-unaffected). Neurophysiological data were recorded in five different recording sessions: at the beginning of a neurorehabilitation treatment (T0, at about 5 weeks from the ictal events), after 15 (T1), 42 (T2) 90 (T3) and 120 (T4) days from T0. (From Traversa et al., 2000.)

and internal capsule were selectively involved in three and two cases, respectively, while both were lesioned in three patients. In 13 out of the 14 patients with recordable SEF from the AH, both the M20 and M30 components were reliably identified from all the stimulated districts (nerve and digits). In the remaining case, the entire SEFs were missing on the AH during finger stimulation.

Latencies of brain responses

Latencies of M20 and M30 peaks were always normal on the UH. On the other hand, the mean percentage of latency alterations on the AH was 23%

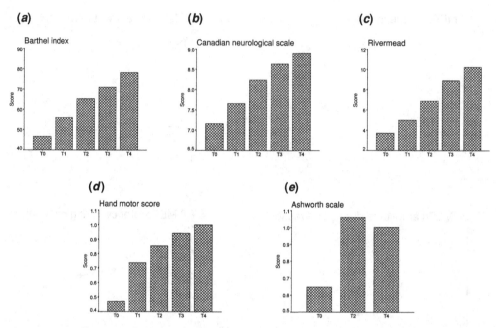

Fig. 7.5   Follow-up of clinical and functional scales in stroke patients in a post-acute, apparently stabilized stage. Neurophysiological and clinical data were recorded in five different recording sessions: at the beginning of a neurorehabilitation treatment (T0, at about 5 weeks from the ictal events), after 15 (T1), 42 (T2), 90 (T3) and 120 (T4) days from T0. (From Traversa et al., 2000.)

after an S lesion, and 13% after a C lesion. When analysing ECD latencies with respect to the clinical outcome, the mean percentage of delayed ECDs was slightly, but not significantly, larger in patients without clinical recovery.

Strengths of generator sources

Eleven out of the 14 patients with reliable SEFs from the AH showed an excessive interhemispheric asymmetry of signal strength at least for one stimulated district, and a total of 21 ECD pairs from homologous districts (=25%) had asymmetries exceeding the normative limits, with similar incidence in C and S patients. All ECD pairs with excessive asymmetries always had the strongest ECD in the AH after a C lesion, whereas this was the case in only a quarter of cases following an S lesion. When considering absolute values of ECD strength in the UH, in only one patient did they result in larger values than in the normal population. When considering strength data in relation with the clinical outcome this parameter was more frequently abnormal in patients with clinical recovery; it is worth noting that all ECDs excessively stronger in AH with respect to UH, belonged to this group.

Waveshape of SEFs

An excessive asymmetry of this parameter was found in nine patients out of 14, and was more frequent in patients with S than with C lesions (70% and 50%, respectively); this finding was also combined with a clear-cut spatial shift of the ECD toward an area outside the normative limits. In relation to the clinical outcome, abnormal waveshapes were observed in 75% and 50% of patients with, and without, clinical recovery, respectively.

Locations of generator sources

Thumb and little finger ECDs were always positioned according to the classical homunculus topography (i.e. little finger more medial and posterior). When present, the hand area enlargement was explained by a medial shift of the little finger ECD. Therefore, reorganization of the hand area, as reflected by enlargement of the 'hand area' parameter, took place at the expense of the forearm more than at the face of the homuncular representation. All ECDs were localized outside the area of structural lesion, as evaluated by MEG/MRI integration. In relation with the clinical outcome, the mean number of altered locations was slightly, but not significantly, larger in the patients with clinical recovery.

Concerning the 'hand area', the mean percentage of altered parameters was 20% of S and 13% of C patients. This alteration was due to an enlargement in the AH. The mean 'hand area' length in the abnormal cases was 39 ± 7 mm in the S group and 27 mm in the C patients (vs. 16 ± 5 mm in healthy controls). The hand area enlargement was not significantly combined with clinical outcome. Such findings demonstrate that SI and adjacent brain areas following a vascular insult undergo a remarkable amount of reorganization, mainly within the AH but also in the UH. This is witnessed by both the significant topographical shift of the generator sources and the enlargement of sensory hand representation, as well as by modifications of reactivity to the incoming impulses. The amount of reorganization was higher in the cases affected by subcortical lesions than in patients with cortical lesions. It is worth remembering that sensory hand area that is tracked via MEG methods roughly overlaps the metabolic activation seen via fMRI, both in controls and in stroke patients (Rossini et al., 1998). By matching MEG results with the clinical outcome, patients with sensory and/ or motor recovery of hand function showed ECDs more asymmetrical in strength, in spatial characteristics and in morphology than in patients with no recovery. These alterations in ECD parameters possibly reflect the cortical reorganization of the hand sensory area as a mechanism underlying the functional recovery. Otherwise, unilateral latency prolongation in the AH reflected a stabilized deficit of hand sensory and motor control. This result suggests that the reorganization of neural circuitries subtending primary sensory processing from the paretic hand favour functional recovery. However, when considering the clinical status at the time of the MEG examination, regardless of the eventual improvement from the symptoms' onset condition, it is worth mentioning that patients with the worse hand scores were characterized by larger MEG asymmetries. Therefore, when the damage is affecting the core of the sensorimotor areas for sensory processing, reorganization is absolutely crucial for functional recovery; meanwhile, reorganization outside the usual SI cortex boundaries never reaches the functional efficiency of the original circuitries. When integration with MRI was carried out, a statistical correlation with MEG abnormalities and the lesion location was found. In the acute stage the lesional burden as measured on MRI did not significantly correlate with the clinical outcome at 3 months, while several MEG parameters appeared to be good predictors of clinical outcome (Rossini et al., 2001). Interhemispheric asymmetries on MEG parameters were more frequently encountered in the S than in the C type of lesions (49% vs. 22%); this was particularly valid for the 'hand extension parameter' due to a medial shift of the little finger representation, combined with a frontal shift (Rossini et al., 1998). It is noteworthy that larger than normal amplitudes of evoked responses with an asymmetrical waveshape modification were found quite frequently from the AH, especially following a C lesion (Fig. 7.6; Wikström et al., 2000; Rossini et al., 2001). A somewhat similar pattern of abnormality was seen in patients showing larger than normal active MEPs during TMS of the unaffected hemisphere; this was usually combined with absent response from the AH and was a bad prognostic index; whenever improvement at follow-up was seen, a progressive balancing between the two hemispheres was observed; that is an increment of the response amplitude from AH and a decrement

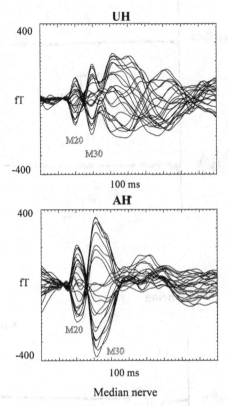

Fig. 7.6   Ischemic stroke involving the parietal lobe; partial motor recovery. Notice the remarkable amplitude increase, especially for the M30 component, of the responses
after median nerve stimulation in the AH (bottom box) respect to the UH. Waveshape analysis in this case gave a similarity between the two hemispheres of 0.71
(out of normality range). (From Rossini et al., 2001.)

of the 'giant' response from the UH (Fig. 7.7; Traversa et al., 1998). Such an
asymmetrical and unbalanced hyperreactivity of the AH and UH has been
ascribed to transient or permanent loss of transcallosal fibres modulation;
whether, and at which extent, this has to do with clinical recovery, plastic
reorganization and post-stroke epilepsy remains to be elucidated (Traversa
et al., 1998; Wikström et al., 2000; Rossini et al., 2001). For instance, hyperexcitability in UH is due to the loss of transcalilosal, mainly inhibitory,
fibres from the AH and has been considered a sign of recovery linked to
plastic reorganization phenomena (Glassman & Malamut, 1976; Buchkremer-
Ratzmann et al., 1996).

'Unbalancing'

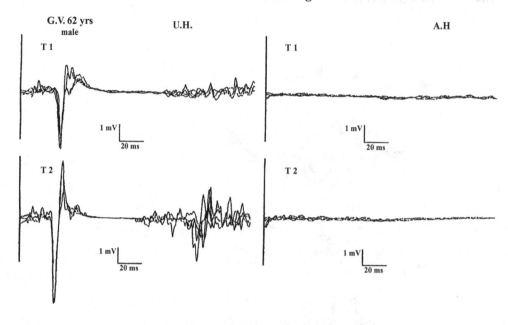

'Balancing'

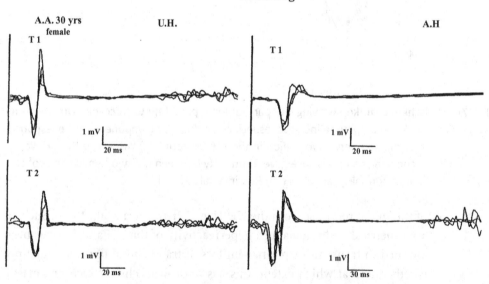

Fig. 7.7   Top: 'Unbalancing': contracted-motor evoked potentials (MEPs) from G.V., 62-year-old, hemiplegic patient with a left subcortical lesion. No evident clinical recovery between T1 and T2 was observed. MEPs from the affected hemisphere (AH) were absent both in T1 and T2. On the other hand, MEPs from the unaffected hemisphere (UH) were increasingly larger than normal both in T1 and T2 together with a decrement of the silent period duration. Same intensity of stimulation in T1 and T2 (45% of the stimulator output). Bottom: 'Balancing': contracted-MEPs

Conclusions and final remarks

As far as pyramidal fibres are concerned, much of the functional recovery is linked to the contingent of preserved axons mediating within-system recovery, while the role of substitution by non-pyramidal efferents is still unclear (Seitz & Freund, 1997).

It is unknown, even by the most sophisticated PET and fMRI studies, as to what degree the functional recovery parallels the 'awakening' of neurons in the perilesional zone of functional penumbra (Heiss & Graf, 1994; Maclin et al., 1994), or by plastic reorganization of the surviving brain tissue. For the sensory modality, ECD location shift from SI cortex, as a whole, suggest that brain areas, which are not usually reached by a dense input from hand and finger sensory receptors, can act as somatosensory 'hand' centres when the 'usual' ones are functionally disconnected. Whether such anomalous responses rely on newly established or on previously existing neural circuitries and synaptic connections, even if partly or entirely functionally silent (i.e. undergoing inhibitory modulation from the 'normal' areas within the lesional core), cannot be reliably defined by the present evidence. Newly established connections might be less direct than normal, due to the different amount and 'safety' of synaptic interruptions. It might be speculated that the longer latencies of SEFs, which often combine with ECD spatial displacements and morphological interhemispheric differences, might actually reflect a higher than normal number of synaptic relays on the route from the hand to sensory cortex. Besides the ECD shift in space, post-lesional neuronal reorganization also could end in receptive fields enlargement. In such a case an increase in ECD strength, as well as a deepening of the resulting baricentres could be seen (Okada, 1985). Short-latency activation of non-primary districts, as demonstrated both by MEG and TMS, was mainly concentrated in frontal areas adjacent to the central sulcus. In non-human primates, direct and indirect connections reach primary and non-primary motor cortices of

Fig. 7.7 (cont.) from a 30-year-old, right hemiparetic patient with a cortical lesion. Clinical improvement between T1 and T2 (Canadian scale from 8 to 10) as also shown by the increased amplitude of the amount of background EMG activity. Notice that MFPs amplitudes from UH (decreasing) and AH (increasing) are going in the opposite direction during follow-up. (Partially modified from Traversa et al., 1998.)

the frontal lobes from thalamic relays, as well as from areas 2 and 1 of the postcentral sensory cortex, respectively. Moreover, most motor cortex neurons concerned with movements of the hand and fingers are responsive to natural stimuli, such as joint rotation, muscle palpation, hair displacement and skin pressure (Rosen & Asanuma, 1972; Lemon & Porter, 1976). Sensory input to motor cortex is pivotal for tactile exploratory behaviour via independent finger movements (Darian-Smith et al., 1985; Jones, 1986; Holsapple et al., 1990). Heterosynaptic long-term potentiation-like mechanisms might be candidates for chronic changes in somatosensory receptive fields topography within the numerous alternative circuitries (Jones et al., 1986; Rossini et al., 1998 a,b).

The potential for reorganization in the adult brain has been largely underestimated in the past and we are now just at the beginning of a new era in which technologies become progressively available to document and understand the pathophysiology of brain 'plasticity' as involved in functional recovery. Moreover, it remains to be discovered at which extent aberrant 'plasticity' is inhibiting functional recovery. Finally, as the most important step, we aim to understand which is the molecular and neurochemical mechanism that drives the perilesional reorganization of neuronal circuitries toward 'good' or 'aberrant' plasticity and their chronological sequence. This would have a profound impact in managing post-stroke patients with appropriately timed pharmacological and rehabilitative treatments. A systematic follow-up study of stroke patients from the acute to the stabilized conditions is required, possibly using several methods of functional brain imaging in order to discriminate beween real spontaneous or induced plastic reorganization, redundancy and the timing and correlation of such changes with progressive recovery of the lost function. This would allow delineation of what is 'good' and what is 'aberrant plasticity' and avoidance of labelling any change of brain responsiveness as being due to 'plastic reorganization'.

In conclusion, the 'remodelling' of sensorimotor hand somatotopy and/or an enlargement of the hand representation often takes place following a monohemispheric stroke. The UH also undergoes a reorganizing process, even if to a much minor degree, which is also due to use-dependent structural events linked with overuse of the unaffected limbs (Jones & Shallert, 1994; Taub et al., 1994; Rossini et al., 1998a,b). Thus, the interhemispheric asymmetry of the sensorimotor areas seems to represent a clinically relevant probe in tracking brain reorganization following a monohemispheric lesion (Cicinelli et al., 1997a, 2000; Traversa et al., 1997; Wikstrom et al., 1997, 2000; Rossini et al., 1999; Liepert et al., 2000a, Tecchio et al., 2000). Future studies are needed to validate its usefulness in following up medical, as well as rehabilitative, procedures.

Acknowledgements

Paolo M Rossini acknowledges the pivotal role of Drs P. Cicinelli, C. Del Gratta, P. Pasqualetti, F. Pauri, V. Pizzella, G.L. Romani, F. Tecchio, R. Traversa for clinical records and data analysis.

REFERENCES

Abbruzzese, G., Morena, M., Dall' Agata, D., Abbruzzese, M. & Favale, E. (1991). Motor evoked potentials (MEPs) in lacunar syndromes. *Electroencephalogr. Clin. Neurophysiol.*, **81**: 202–208.

Ahonen, J.P., Jehkonen, M., Dastidar, P., Molnár, G. & Häkkinen, V. (1998). Cortical silent period evoked by transcranial magnetic stimulation in ischemic stroke. *Electroencephalogr. Clin. Neurophysiol.*, **109**: 224–229.

Alagona, G., Delvaux, V., Gérard, P. et al. (2001). Ipsilateral motor responses to focal transcranial magnetic stimulation in healthy subjects and acute-stroke patients. *Stroke*, **32**: 1304–1309.

Andrews, R.J., Bringas, J.R., Alonzo, G., Salamat, M.S., Khoshyomn, S. & Gluck, D.S. (1993). Corpus collosotomy effects on cerebral blood flow and evoked potentials (transcallosal dischisis). *Neurosci. Lett.*, **154**: 9–12.

Andrews, R.J. (1991). Transhemispheric diaschisis. *Stroke*, **22**: 943–949.

Arac, N., Sagduyu, A., Binai, S. & Ertekin, C. (1994). Prognostic value of transcranial magnetic stimulation in acute stroke. *Stroke*, **25**: 2183–2186.

Backman, C.L., Harris, S.R., Chisholm, J-A.M. & Monette, A. (1997). Single-subject research in rehabilitation: a review of studies using AB, withdrawal, multiple baseline, and alternating treatment designs. *Arch. Phys. Med. Rehabil.*, **78**: 1145–1153.

Binkofski, F., Seitz, R.J., Arnold, S., Classen, J., Benecke, R. & Freund, H.J. (1996). Thalamic metabolism and corticospinal tract integrity determine motor recovery in stroke. *Ann. Neurol.*, **39**: 460–470.

Blakemore, S.J., Goodbody, S.J. & Wolpert, D.M. (1998). Predicting the consequences of our own actions: the role of sensorimotor context estimation. *J. Neurosci.*, **18**: 7511–7518.

Blakemore, S.J., Frith, C.D. & Wolpert, D.M. (1999). Spatio-temporal prediction modulates the perception of self-produced stimuli. *J. Cogn. Sci.*, **11**: 551–559.

Bornschlag, M. & Asanuma, H. (1987). Importance of the projection from the sensory to the motor cortex for recovery of motor function following partial thalamic lesion in the monkey. *Brain Res.*, **437**: 121–30.

Braune, H.J. & Fritz, C. (1995). Transcranial magnetic stimulation-evoked inhibition of voluntary muscle activity (silent period) is impaired in patients with ischemic hemispheric lesion. *Stroke*, **26**: 550–553.

Buchkremer-Ratzmann, I. & Witte, O.W. (1997). Extended brain disinhibition following small photothrombotic lesions in rat frontal cortex. *Neuroreport*, **8**: 519–522.

Buchkremer-Ratzmann, I., August, M., Hagemann, G. & Witte, O.W. (1996). Electrophysiological transcortical diaschisis after acute photothrombosis in rat brain. *Stroke*, **27**: 1005–1111.

Bütefisch, C., Hummelsheim, H., Denzler, P. & Mauritz, K-H. (1995). Repetitive training of isolated movements improves the outcome of motor rehabilitation of the centrally paretic hand. *J. Neurol. Sci.*, **130**: 59–68.

Cantello, R., Gianelli, M., Civardi, C. & Mutani, R. (1992). Magnetic brain stimulation: the silent period after the motor evoked potential. *Neurology*, **42**: 1951–1959.

Cao, Y., D'Olhaberriague, L., Vikingstad, E.M. et al. (1998). Pilot study of functional MRI to assess cerebral activation of motor function after poststroke hemiparesis. *Stroke*, **29**: 112–122.

Caramia, M.D., Iani, C. & Bernardi, G. (1996). Cerebral plasticity after stroke as revealed by ipsilateral responses to magnetic stimulation. *Neuroreport*, **7**: 1756–1760.

Caramia, M.D., Palmieri, M.G., Giacomini, P., Iani, C., Dally, L. & Silvestrini, M. (2000). Ipsilateral activation of the unaffected motor cortex in patients with hemiparetic stroke. *Clin. Neurophysiol.*, **111**: 1990–1996.

Catano, A., Houa, M., Caroyer, J.M., Ducarne, H. & Noel, P. (1995). Magnetic transcranial stimulation in non-haemorrhagic sylvian strokes: interest of facilitation for early functional prognosis. *Electroencephalogr. Clin. Neurophysiol.*, **97**: 349–354.

Catano, A., Houa, M., Caroyer, J.M., Ducarne, H. & Noel, P. (1996). Magnetic transcranial stimulation in acute stroke: early excitation threshold and functional prognosis. *Electroencephalogr. Clin. Neurophysiol.*, **101**: 233–239.

Catano, A., Houa, M. & Noel, P. (1997a). Magnetic transcranial stimulation: dissociation of excitatory and inhibitory mechanisms in acute strokes. *Electroencephalogr. Clin. Neurophysiol.*, **105**: 29–36.

Catano, A., Houa, M. & Noel, P. (1997b). Magnetic transcranial stimulation: clinical interest of the silent period in acute and chronic stages of stroke. *Electroencephalogr. Clin. Neurophysiol.*, **105**: 290–296.

Chen, R., Corwell, B., Yaseen, Z., Hallett, M. & Cohen, L.G. (1998). Mechanisms of cortical reorganization in lower-limb amputees. *J. Neurosci.*, **18**: 3443–3450.

Chollet, F., DiPiero, V., Wise, R.J., Brooks, D.J., Dolan, R.J. & Frackowiak, R.S. (1991). The functional anatomy of motor recovery after stroke in humans: a study with positron emission tomography. *Ann. Neurol.*, **29**: 63–71.

Cicinelli, P., Traversa, R., Bassi, A., Scivoletto, G. & Rossini, P.M. (1997a). Interhemispheric differences of hand muscle representation in human motor cortex. *Muscle Nerve*, **20**: 535–542.

Cicinelli, P., Traversa, R. & Rossini, P.M. (1997b). Post-stroke reorganization of brain motor output to the hand: a 2–4 month follow-up with focal magnetic transcranial stimulation. *Electroencephalogr. Clin. Neurophysiol.*, **105**: 438–450.

Cicinelli, P., Traversa, R., Oliveri, M. et al. (2000). Intracortical excitatory and inhibitory phenomena to paired transcranial magnetic stimulation in healthy subjects: differences between the right and left hemisphere. *Neurosci. Lett.*, **288**: 171–174.

Classen, J., Schnitzler, A., Binkowski, F. et al. (1997). The motor syndrome associated with exaggerated inhibition within the primary motor cortex of patients with hemiparetic stroke. *Brain*, **120**: 605–619.

Cohen, L.G., Roth, B.J., Nilsson, J. et al. (1990). Effects of coil design on delivery of focal magnetic stimulation. Technical considerations. *Electroencephalogr. Clin. Neurophysiol.*, **75**: 350–357.

Cruz Martinez, A., Munoz, J. & Palacios, F. (1998). The muscle inhibitory period by transcranial magnetic stimulation. Study in stroke patients. *Electromyogr. Clin. Neurophysiol.*, **38**: 189–192.

Cruz Martinez, A., Tejada, J. & Dietz Tejedor, E. (1990). Motor hand recovery after stroke. Prognostic yield of early transcranial magnetic stimulation. *Electromyogr. Clin. Neurophysiol.*, **39**: 405–410.

Darian-Smith, I., Goodwin, A., Sugitami, M. & Heywood, J. (1985). Scanning a texture surface with the fingers: events in sensorimotor cortex. In *Hand Function and the Neocortex*, ed. A.W. Goodwin & I. Darian-Smith, pp. 17–43. Berlin: Springer. EBR suppl. 10.

Del Gratta, C., Della Penna, S., Tartaro, A. et al. (2000). Topographic organisation of the human primary and secondary somatosensory areas: an fMRI study. *Neuroreport*, **26**: 2035–2043.

del Zoppo, G.J. & Garcia, J.H. (1995). PMN leukocyte adhesion in cerebrovascular ischemia. In *Physiology and Pathophysiology of Leukocyte Adhesion*, ed. D.N. Granger & G. Schimdt-Schonbein, pp. 408–433. New York: Oxford University Press.

Dettmers, C., Stephan, K.M., Lemon, R.N. & Frackowiak, R.S.J. (1997). Reorganization of the executive motor system after stroke. *Cerebrovasc. Dis.*, **7**: 187–200.

Di Lazzaro, V., Oliviero, A., Profice, P., Saturno, E., Pilato, F. & Tonali, P. (1999). Motor cortex excitability changes within 8 hours after ischemic stroke may predict the functional outcome. *Eur. J. Emerg. Med.*, **6**: 119–121.

D'Olhaberriague, L., Espadaler Gamissans, J.M., Marrugat, J. et al. (1997). Transcranial magnetic stimulation as a prognostic tool in stroke. *J. Neurol. Sci.*, **147**: 73–80.

Dominkus, M., Grisold, W. & Jelinek, V. (1990). Transcranial electrical motor evoked potentials as a prognostic indicator for motor recovery in stroke patients. *J. Neurol. Neurosurg. Psychiatry*, **53**: 745–748.

Dum, R.P.R. & Strick, P.L. (1991). The origin of corticospinal projections from the premotor areas in the frontal lobe. *J. Neurosci.*, **11**: 667–689.

Escudero, J.V., Sancho, J., Bautista, D., Escudero, M. & Lopez-Trigo, J. (1998). Prognostic value of motor evoked potential obtained by transcranial magnetic brain stimulation in motor function recovery in patients with acute ischemic stroke. *Stroke*, **29**: 1854–1859.

Faig, J. & Busse, O. (1996). Silent period evoked by transcranial magnetic stimulation in unilateral thalamic infarcts. *J. Neurol. Sci.*, **142**: 85–92.

Ferbert, A., Vielhaber, S., Meincke, U. & Buchner, H. (1992). Transcranial magnetic stimulation in pontine infarction: correlation to degree of paresis. *J. Neurol. Neurosurg. Psychiatry*, **55**: 294–299.

Feys, H., Van Hees, J., Bruyninckx, F., Mercelis, R. & De Weerdt, W. (2000). Value of somatosensory and motor evoked potentials in predicting arm recovery after a stroke. *J. Neurol. Neurosurg. Psychiatry*, **68**: 323–331.

Fries, W., Daneck, A. & Witt, T.N. (1991). Motor responses after transcranial electrical stimulation of cerebral hemispheres with degenerated pyramidal tract. *Ann. Neurol.*, **29**: 646–649.

Fries, W., Danek, A., Scheidtnann, K. & Hamburger, C. (1993). Motor recovery following capsular stroke. Role of descending pathways from multiple motor areas. *Brain*, **116**: 369–382.

Fritz, C., Braune, H.J., Pylatiuk, C. & Pohl, M. (1997). Silent period following transcranial magnetic stimulation: a study of intra- and inter-examiner reliability. *Electroncephalogr. Clin. Neurophysiol.*, **105**: 235–240.

Fuhr, P., Cohen, L.G., Roth, B.J. & Hallett, M. (1991a). Latency of motor evoked potentials to focal transcranial stimulation varies as a function of scalp positions stimulated. *Electroencephalogr. Clin. Neurophysiol.*, **81**: 81–89.

Fuhr, P., Agostino, R. & Hallett, M. (1991b). Spinal motor neuron excitability during the silent period after cortical stimulation. *Electroencephalogr. Clin. Neurophysiol.*, **81**: 257–262.

Garcia, J.H., Liu, K.F., Yoshida, Y., Lian, J., Chen, S. & del Zoppo, G.J. (1994). Influx of leukocytes and platelets in an evolving brain infarct (Wistar rat). *Am. J. Pathol.*, **144**: 188–199.

Glassman, R.B. & Malamut, B.L. (1976). Recovery from electroencephalographic slowing and reduced evoked potentials after somatosensory cortical damage in cats. *Behav. Biol.*, **17**: 333–354.

Hari, R. & Ilmoniemi, R.J. (1986). Cerebral magnetic fields. *CRC Critical Rev. Biomed. Eng.*, **14**: 93126.

Hari, R., Hämäläinen, M., Ilmoniemi, R. & Lounasmaa, O.V. (1991). MEG versus EEG localization test (Letter to the Editor). *Ann. Neurol.*, **30**: 222–224.

Hari, R., Karhu, J., Hamalainen, M. et al. (1993). Functional organization of the human first and second somatosensory cortices: a neuromagnetic study. *Eur. J. Neurosci.*, **5**: 724–734.

Haug, B.A., Schönle, P.W., Knobloch, C. & Köhne, M. (1992). Silent period measurement revives as a valuable diagnostic tool with transcranial magnetic stimulation. *Electroencephalogr. Clin. Neurophysiol.*, **85**: 158–160.

Heald, A., Bates, D., Cartlidge, N.E., French, J.M. & Miller, S. (1993). Longitudinal study of central motor conduction time following stroke. 2. Central motor conduction measured within 72 h after stroke as a predictor of functional outcome at 12 months. *Brain*, **116**: 1371–1385.

Heiss, W.D. & Graf, R. (1994). The ischemic penumbrae. *Curr. Opin. Neurol.*, **7**: 11–19.

Hendricks, H.T., Hageman, G. & van Limbeek, J. (1997). Prediction of recovery from upper extremity paralysis after stroke by measuring evoked potentials. *Scand. J. Rehabil. Med.*, **29**: 155–159.

Holsapple, J.W., Preston, J.B. & Strick, P.L. (1990). Origin of thalamic inputs to the 'hand' representation in the primary motor cortex. *Soc. Neurosci. Abstr.*, **16**: 425.

Hummelsheim, H. & Hauptmann, B. (1999). Transcranial magnetic stimulation and motor rehabilitation. *Electroencephalogr. Clin. Neurophysiol. Suppl.*, **51**: 221–232.

Jacobs, K.M. & Donoghue, J.P. (1991). Reshaping the cortical motor map by unmasking latent intracortical connections. *Science*, **251**: 944–947.

Jones, E.G. (1986). Connectivity of the primate sensory-motor cortex. In *Cerebral Cortex*, ed. E.G. Jones & A. Peters, vol. 5, pp. 113–183. New York: Plenum.

Jones, T.A. & Schallert, T. (1994). Use-dependent growth of pyramidal neurons after neocortical damage. *J. Neurosci.*, **14**: 2140–2152.

Jones, E.G., Coulter, J.D. & Hendry, S.H.C. (1978). Intracortical connectivity of architectonic fields in the somatic sensory motor and parietal cortex of monkeys. *J. Comp. Neurol.*, **181**: 291–348.

Kelly, J.P. (1985). In *Principles of Neural Science*. ed. E.R. Kandel & J.H. Schwartz 2nd. edn, pp. 187–195. New York: Elsevier.

Kinouchi, H., Sharp, F.R., Chan, P.H. et al. (1994). MK-801 inhibits the induction of immediate early genes in cerebral cortex, thalamus, and hippocampus, but not in substantia nigra following middle cerebral artery occlusion. *Neurosci. Lett.*, **179**: 111–114.

Kopp, B., Kunkel, A., Muehlnickel, W., Villringer, K., Taub, E. & Flor, H. (1999). Plasticity in the motor system related to therapy-induced improvement of movement after stroke. *Neuroreport*, **10**: 807–810.

Kujirai, T., Caramia, M.D., Rothwell, J.C. et al. (1993). Corticocortical inhibition in human motor cortex. *J. Physiol.*, **471**: 501–519.

Kukowski, B. & Haug, B. (1992). Quantitative evaluation of the silent period, evoked by transcranial magnetic stimulation during sustained muscle contraction, in normal man and in patients with stroke. *Electromyogr. Clin. Neurophysiol.*, **32**: 373–378.

Lemon, R.H. & Porter, R. (1976). Afferent input to movement-related precentral neurones in conscious monkey. *Proc. R. Soc. Lond. Ser. B*, **194**: 313–339.

Levy, C.E., Nichols, D.S., Schmalbrock, P.M., Keller, P. & Chakerss, D.W. (2001). Functional MRI evidence of cortical reorganization in upper-limb stroke hemiplegia treated with constraint-induced movement therapy. *Am. J. Phys. Med. Rehabil.*, **80**: 4–12.

Liepert J. Tegenthoff, M. & Malin, J-P.(1995). Changes of postexcitatory inhibition after transcranial magnetic stimulation in the course of hemiparesis. *Neurol. Psychol. Brain Res.*, **4**: 1–6.

Liepert, J., Classen, J., Cohen, L.G. & Hallett, M. (1998a). Task-dependent changes of intracortical inhibition. *Exp. Brain Res.*, **118**: 421–426.

Liepert, J., Miltner, W.H.R., Bauder, H. et al. (1998b). Motor cortex plasticity during constraint-induced movement therapy in stroke patients. *Neurosci. Lett.*, **250**: 5–8.

Liepert, J., Bauder, H., Miltner, W.H.R., Taub, E. & Weiller, C. (2000a). Treatment-induced cortical reorganization after stroke in humans. *Stroke*, **31**: 1210–1216.

Liepert, J., Gräf, S., Uhde, I., Leidner, O. & Weiller, C. (2000b). Training-induced changes of motor cortex representations in stroke patients. *Acta Neurol. Scand.*, **101**: 321–326.

Liepert, J., Hamzei, F. & Weiller, C. (2000c). Motor cortex disinhibition of the unaffected hemisphere after acute stroke. *Muscle Nerve*, **23**: 1761–1763.

Liepert, J., Storch, P., Fritsch, A. & Weiller, C. (2000d). Motor cortex disinhibition in acute stroke. *Clin. Neurophysiol.*, **111**: 671–676.

Liepert, J., Uhde, I., Gräf, S., Leidner, O. & Weiller, C. (2001). Motor cortex plasticity during forced use therapy in stroke patients. *J. Neurol.*, **248**: 315–321.

Macdonell, R.A., Donnan, G.A. & Bladin, P.F. (1989). A comparison of somatosensory evoked and motor evoked potentials in stroke. *Ann. Neurol.*, **25**: 68–73.

Maclin, E.L., Rose, D.F., Knight, J.E., Orrison, W.W. & Davis, L.E. (1994). Somatosensory evoked magnetic fields in patients with stroke. *Electroencephalogr. Clin. Neurophysiol.*, **91**: 468–475.

Marshall, R.S., Perera, G.M., Lazar, R.M. et al. (2000). Evolution of cortical activation during recovery from corticospinal tract infarction. *Stroke*, **31**: 656–661.

Mauguiere, F., Merlet, I., Forss, N. et al. (1997). Activation of a distributed somatosensory cortical network in the human brain. A dipole modeling study of magnetic fields evoked by median nerve stimulation. Part I: Location and activation timing of SEF sources. *Electroencephalogr. Clin. Neurophysiol.*, **104**: 281–289.

Nakasato, N., Levesque, M.F., Barth, D.S., Baumgartner, C., Rogers, R.L. & Sutherling, W.W. (1994). Comparisons of MEG, EEG, and ECoG source localization in neocortical partial epilepsy in humans. *Electroencephalogr. Clin. Neurophysiol.*, **91**: 171–178.

Nelles, G., Spiekermann, G., Jueptner, M. et al. (1999a). Reorganization of sensory and motor systems in hemiplegic stroke patients. A positron emission tomography study. *Stroke*, **30**: 1510–1516.

Nelles, G., Spiekermann, G., Jueptner, M. et al. (1999b). Evolution of functional reorganization in hemiplegic stroke: a serial positron emission tomographic activation study. *Ann. Neurol.*, **46**: 901–909.

Netz, J., Lammers, T. & Hömberg, V. (1997). Reorganization of motor output in the non-affected hemisphere after stroke. *Brain*, **120**: 1579–1586.

Nudo, R.J., Wise, B.M., SiFuentes, F. & Milliken, G.W. (1996). Neural substrates for the effects of rehabilitative training on motor recovery after ischemic infarct. *Science*, **272**: 1791–1794.

Nunez, P.L., Srinivasan, R., Westdorp, A.F. et al. (1997). EEG coherency. I: Statistics, reference electrode, volume conduction, Laplacians, cortical imaging, and interpretation at multiple scales. *Electroencephalogr. Clin. Neurophysiol.*, **103**: 499–515.

Okada, Y. (1985). Discrimination of localized and distributed current dipole sources and localized single and multiple sources. In *Biomagnetism: Applications and Theory*, ed. H. Weinberg, G. Stroink & T. Katila, pp. 266–272. New York: Pergamon Press.

Oliveri, M., Rossini, P.M., Pasqualetti, P. et al. (1999). Interhemispheric asymmetries in the perception of unimanual and bimanual cutaneous stimuli. A study using transcranial magnetic stimulation. *Brain*, **122**: 1721–1729.

Oliveri, M., Caltagirone, C., Filippi, M.M. et al. (2000). Paired transcranial magnetic stimulation protocols reveals a pattern of inhibition and facilitation in the human parietal cortex. *J. Physiol.*, **529**: 461–468.

Palmer, E., Ashby, P. & Hajek, V.E. (1992). Ipsilateral fast corticospinal pathways do not account for recovery in stroke. *Ann. Neurol.*, **32**: 519–525.

Pantano, P., Formisano, R., Ricci, M. et al. (1996). Motor recovery after stroke. Morphological and functional brain alterations. *Brain*, **119**: 1849–1857.

Pascual-Leone, A., Cohen, L.G., Brasil-Neto, J.P., Valls-Sole, J. & Hallett, M. (1994). Differentiation of sensorimotor neuronal structures responsible for induction of motor evoked potentials, attenuation in detection of somatosensory stimuli, and induction of sensation of movement by mapping of optimal current directions. *Electroencephalogr. Clin. Neurophysiol.*, **93**: 230–236.

Pascual-Leone, A., Dang, N., Cohen, L.G., Brasil-Neto, J.P., Cammarota, A. & Hallett, M. (1995). Modulation of muscle responses evoked by transcranial magnetic stimulation during the acquisition of new fine motor skills. *J. Neurophysiol.*, **74**: 1037–1045.

Pennisi, G., Rapisarda, G., Bella, R. et al. (1999). Absence of response to early transcranial magnetic stimulation in ischemic stroke patients: prognostic value for hand motor recovery. *Stroke*, **30**: 2666–2670.

Péréon, Y., Aubertin, P. & Guihenuc, P. (1995). Prognostic significance of electrophysiological investigations in stroke patients: somatosensory and motor evoked potentials and sympathetic skin response. *Neurophysiol. Clin.*, **25**: 146–157.

Pizzella, V., Tecchio, F., Romani, G.L. & Rossini, P.M. (1999). Functional localization of the sensory hand area with respect to the motor central gyrus knob. *Neuroreport*, **16**: 3809–3814.

Price, C.J., Wise, R.J., Watson, J.D. et al. (1994). Brain activation during reading. The effects of exposure duration and task. *Brain*, **117**: 1255–1269.

Puce, A., Constable, R.T., Luby, M.L. et al. (1995). Functional magnetic resonance imaging of the sensory and motor cortex: comparison with electrophysiological localization. *J. Neurosurg.*, **83**: 262–270.

Que, M., Schiene, K., Witte, O.W. & Zilles, K. (1999a). Widespread up-regulation of N-methyl-D-aspartate receptors after focal photothrombotic lesion in rat brain. *Neurosci. Lett.*, **273**: 77–80.

Que, M., Witte, O.W., Neumann-Haefelin, T., Schiene, K., Schroeter, M. & Zilles, K. (1999b). Changes in GABA (A) and GABA (B) receptor binding following cortical photothrombosis: a quantitative receptor autoradiographic study. *Neuroscience*, **93**: 1233–1240.

Rapisarda, G., Bastings, E., Maertens de Noordhout, A., Pennisi, G. & Delwaide, P.J. (1996). Can motor recovery in stroke patients be predicted by early transcranial magnetic stimulation? *Stroke*, **27**: 2191–2196.

Reinecke, S., Lutzenburg, M., Hagemann, G., Bruehl, C., Neumann-Haefelin, T. & Witte, O.W. (1999). Electrophysiological transcortical diachisis after middle cerebral artery occlusion (MCAO) in rats. *Neurosci. Lett.*, **261**: 85–88.

Rizzolatti, G., Luppino, G. & Matelli, M. (1998). The organization of the cortical motor system: new concepts. *Electroencephalogr. Clin. Neurophysiol.*, **106**: 283–296.

Roick, H., von Giesen, H.J. & Benecke, R. (1993). On the origin of the postexcitatory inhibition seen after transcranial magnetic brain stimulation in awake human subjects. *Exp. Brain Res.*, **94**: 489–498.

Romani, G.L. (1990). Advances in neuromagnetic topography and source localization. *Brain Topogr.*, **3**: 95–102.

Rosen, I. & Asanuma, H. (1972). Peripheral afferent inputs to the forelimb area of the monkey motor cortex: input–output relations. *Exp. Brain Res.*, **14**: 257–273.

Rossi, S., Pasqualetti, P., Tecchio, F., Sabato, A. & Rossini, P.M. (1998). Modulation of corticospinal output to human hand muscles following deprivation of sensory feedback. *Neuroimage*, **8**: 163–175.

Rossini, P.M. (2000). Is transcranial magnetic stimulation of the motor cortex a prognostic tool for motor recovery after stroke? *Stroke*, **31**: 1463–1464.

Rossini, P.M. (2001). Brain redundancy: responsivity or plasticity? *Ann. Neurol.*, **48**: 128–129.

Rossini, P.M. & Pauri, F. (2000). Neuromagnetic integrated methods tracking human brain mechanisms of sensorimotor areas 'plastic' reorganisation. *Brain Res. Rev.*, **33**: 131–154.

Rossini, P.M., Narici, L., Martino, G. et al. (1994). Analysis of interhemispheric asymmetries of somatosensory evoked magnetic fields to right and left median nerve stimulation. *Electroencephalogr. Clin. Neurophysiol.*, **91**: 476–482.

Rossini, P.M., Caltagirone, C., Castriota-Scandenberg, A. et al. (1998a). Hand motor cortical areas reorganization in stroke: a study with fMRI, MEG and TCS maps. *Neuroreport*, **9**: 2141–2146.

Rossini, P.M., Tecchio, F., Pizzella, V. et al. (1998b). On the reorganization of sensory hand areas after monohemispheric lesion: a functional (MEG)/anatomical (MRI) integrative study. *Brain Res.*, **782**: 153–166.

Rossini, P.M., Tecchio, F., Pizzella, V., Lupoi, D., Cassetta, E. & Pasqualetti, P. (2001). Interhemispheric differences of sensory hand areas after monohemispheric stroke: MEG/MRI integrative study. *Neuroimage*, **14**: 474–485.

Rouiller, E.M., Yu, X.H., Moret, V., Tempini, A., Wiesendanger, M. & Liang, F. (1998). Dexterity in adult monkeys following early lesion of the motor cortical hand area: the role of cortex adjacent to the lesion. *Eur J. Neurosci.*, **10**: 729–740.

Schiene, K., Bruehl, C., Zilles, K. et al. (1996). Neuronal hyperexcitability and reduction of GABAA-receptor expression in the surround of cerebral photothrombosis. *J. Cereb. Blood Flow Metab.*, **16**: 906–914.

Schwarz, S., Hacke, W. & Schwab, S. (2000). Magnetic evoked potentials in neurocritical care patients with acute brainstem lesions. *J. Neurol. Sci.*, **172**: 30–37.

Seitz, R.J. & Freund, H.J. (1997). Plasticity of the human motor cortex. *Adv. Neurol.*, **73**: 321–333.

Seitz, R.J., Binkofski, F., Stephan, K.M., Benecke, R. & Freund, H.J. (1995). Prolonged muscular flaccidity. *Electroncephalogr. Clin. Neurophysiol.*, **97**: S230.

Seitz, R.J., Hoflich, P., Binkofski, F. et al. (1998). Role of the premotor cortex in recovery from middle cerebral artery infarction. *Arch. Neurol.*, **55**: 1081–1088.

Shimizu, T., Filippi, M.M., Palmieri, M.G. et al. (1999). Modulation of intracortical excitability for different muscles in the upper extremity: paired magnetic stimulation study with focal versus non-focal coils. *Clin. Neurophysiol.*, **110**: 575–581.

Stepniewska, I., Preuss, T.M. & Kaas, J. (1993). Architectonics, somatotopic organization, and ipsilateral cortical connections of the primary motor area (M1) of Owl monkey. *J. Comp. Neurol.*, **330**: 238–271.

Taub, E., Miller, N.E., Novack, T.A. et al. (1993). Technique to improve chronic motor deficit after stroke. *Arch. Phys. Med. Rehabil.*, **74**: 347–354.

Taub, E., Crago, J.E., Burgio, L.D. et al. (1994). An operant approach to rehabilitation medicine: overcoming learned non-use by shaping. *J. Exp. Anal. Behav.*, **61**: 281–293.

Tecchio, F., Rossini, P.M., Pizzella, V., Cassetta, E. & Romani, G.L. (1997). Spatial properties and interhemispheric differences on the sensory hand cortical representation: a neuromagnetic study. *Brain Res.*, **29**: 100–108.

Tecchio, F., Pasqualetti, P., Pizzella, V., Romani, G. & Rossini, P.M. (2000). Morphology of somatosensory evoked fields: interhemispheric similarity as a parameter for physiological and pathological neural connectivity. *Neurosci. Lett.*, **287**: 203–206.

Timmerhuis, T.P., Hageman, G., Oosterloo, S.J. & Rozeboom, A.R. (1996). The prognostic value of cortical magnetic stimulation in acute middle cerebral artery infarction compared to other parameters. *Clin. Neurol. Neurosurg.* **98**: 231–236.

Traversa, R., Cicinelli, P., Bassi, A., Rossini, P.M. & Bernardi, G. (1997). Mapping of motor cortical reorganization afeter stroke. *Stroke*, **28**: 110–117.

Traversa, R., Cicinelli, P., Pasqualetti, P., Filippi, M.M. & Rossini, P.M. (1998). Follow-up of interhemispheric differences of motor evoked potentials from the 'affected' and 'unaffected' hemispheres in human stroke. *Brain Res.*, **803**: 1–8.

Traversa, R., Cicinelli, P., Oliveri, M. et al. (2000). Neurophysiological follow-up of motor output in stroke patients. *Clin. Neurophysiol.*, **111**: 1695–1703.

Triggs, W.J., Cros, D., Macdonell, R.A.L., Chiappa K.H., Fang, J. & Day, B.J. (1993). Cortical and spinal motor excitability during the transcranial magnetic stimulation silent period in humans. *Brain Res.*, **628**: 39–48.

Trompetto, C., Assini, A., Buccolieri, A., Marchese, R. & Abbruzzese, G. (2000). Motor recovery following stroke: a transcranial magnetic stimulation study. *Clin. Neurophysiol.*, **111**: 1860–1867.

Turton, A., Wroe, S., Trepte, N., Fraser, C. & Lemon, R.N. (1996). Contralateral and ipsilateral EMG responses to transcranial magnetic stimulation during recovery of arm and hand function after stroke. *Electroencephalogr. Clin. Neurophysiol.*, **101**: 316–328.

Twitchell, T.E. (1951). The restoration of motor function following hemiplegia in man. *Brain*, **74**: 443–480.

Vang, C., Dunbabin, D. & Kilpatrick, D. (1999). Correlation between functional and electrophysiological recovery in acute ischemic stroke. *Stroke*, **30**: 2126–2130.

Von Giesen, H-J., Roick, H. & Benecke, R. (1994). Inhibitory actions of motor cortex following unilateral brain lesions as studied by magnetic brain stimulation. *Exp. Brain Res.*, **99**: 84–96.

Wall, P.D. (1980). Mechanisms of plasticity of connection following damage in adult mammalian nervous system. In *Recovery of Function: Theoretical Consideration for Brain Injury Rehabilitation*, ed. P. Bach-y-Rita, pp. 91–106. Bern: Hans Huber.

Wall, P.D. & Egger, M.D. (1971). Formation of new connection in adult rat brains after partial deafferentation. *Nature*, **232**: 542–45.

Wassermann, E.M., Pascual-Leone, A. & Hallett, M. (1994). Cortical motor representation of the ipsilateral hand and arm. *Exp. Brain Res.*, **100**: 121–132.

Weiller, C. (1998). Imaging recovery from stroke. *Exp. Brain Res.*, **123**: 13–17.

Weiller, C. & Rijntjes, M. (1999). Learning, plasticity, and recovery in the central nervous system. *Exp. Brain Res.*, **128**: 134–138.

Weiller, C. & Chollet, F., Friston K.J., Wise, R.J.S. & Frackowiak, R.S.J. (1992). Functional reorganization of the brain in recovery from striatocapsular infarction in man. *Ann. Neurol.*, **31**: 463–472.

Wikström, H., Roine, R.O., Salonen, O. et al. (1997). Somatosensory evoked magnetic fields to median nerve stimulation: interhemispheric differences in a normal population. *Electroencephalogr. Clin. Neurophysiol.*, **104**: 480–487.

Wikström, H. Roine, R.O., Aronen, H.J. et al. (2000). Specific changes in somatosensory evoked magnetic fields during recovery from sensorimotor stroke. *Ann. Neurol.*, **47**: 353–360.

Witte, O.W. (1998). Lesion-induced plasticity as a potential mechanism for recovery and rehabilitative training. *Curr. Opin. Neurol.*, **11**: 655–662.

Wolf, S.L., Lecraw, D.E., Barton, L.A. & Jann, B.B. (1989). Forced use of hemiplegic upper extremities to reverse the effect of learned nonuse among chronic stroke and head-injured patients. *Exp. Neurol.*, **104**: 125–132.

Yousry, T.A., Schmid, U.D., Alkadhi. H. et al. (1997). Localisation of the motor hand area to a knob on the precentral gyrus: a new landmark. *Brain*, **120**: 141–157.

Ziemann, U., Lönnecker, S., Steinhoff, B.J. & Paulus, W. (1996). The effect of lorazepam on the motor cortical excitability in man. *Exp. Brain Res.*, **109**: 127–135.

Ziemann U., Ishii, K., Borgheresi, A. et al. (1999). Dissociation of the pathways mediating ipsilateral and contralateral motor-evoked potentials in human hand and arm muscles. *J. Physiol.*, **518**: 895–906.

8

Lesions of the periphery and spinal cord

Michael J. Angel,[1] Nicholas J. Davey,[2] Peter H. Ellaway[2] and Robert Chen[1]

[1]Toronto Western Hospital, Ontario, Canada
[2]Department of Sensorimotor Systems, Imperial College School of Medicine, Charing Cross Hospital, London, UK

Introduction

Functional recovery or compensation following nervous system injury may be facilitated by plasticity within the central nervous system. For example, activation of the visual cortex that occurs during Braille reading in the early blind (under 14 years of age) is of functional importance (Cohen et al., 1997) and there is convincing evidence that plasticity can play an adaptive role following deafferentation (Pascual-Leone & Torres, 1993). Whether this kind of functional reorganization occurs in the motor system is less clear.

In the motor system, the skilled use of our muscles requires the integrative actions of sensory feedback and descending motor commands, which result in appropriate activation of motoneurones through activation of spinal interneurons, i.e. sensorimotor integration (Baldissera et al., 1981). The corticospinal system, the vital component of volitional movement, controls spinal motoneuronal activity through interneuronally mediated pathways (Lundberg & Voorhoeve, 1962; Pierrot-Deseilligny, 1996; Alstermark et al., 1999), and through their direct monosynaptic contacts with spinal motoneurons (Jankowska et al., 1975). The alterations in the control of the corticospinal system have received the greatest attention in TMS studies of plasticity in humans.

The importance of tonic sensory input in regulating cortical excitability and cortical body part representation in the motor cortex was initially shown in animal studies wherein peripheral nerve injury triggers a massive reorganization in the rat (Sanes et al., 1990). It appears that the same holds true for the human cortex. TMS studies have shown dramatic changes in cortical map representation of muscles, and corticospinal excitability following transient deafferentation (Brasil-Neto et al., 1993), amputation (Chen et al., 1998a; Cohen et al., 1991a; Fuhr et al., 1992; Hall et al., 1990; Roricht et al., 1999; Schwenkreis et al., 2000, 2001), spinal cord injury (Levy et al., 1990a; Topka et al., 1991), immobilization (Liepert et al., 1995) and root avulsion (Mano et al., 1995). These changes can be rapid in onset, as demonstrated in transient ischemic deafferentation studies (Brasil-Neto et al., 1993) and can persist for up to 50 years following amputation (Roricht et al., 1999). Whether these changes are critical for restoring function or whether they are only an epiphenomenon of removing sensory feedback are as yet unknown. Furthermore, although much of the plasticity described thus far has been cortical in origin, other sites including spinal interneuronal systems, thalamus, cerebellum and other subcortical areas remain candidates for plastic changes following injury.

This chapter reviews plasticity of the CNS induced by lesions of the peripheral nerve and spinal cord as demonstrated by studies using TMS. Discussion will include known and postulated sites of plasticity, known and postulated transmitter systems that have permissive and modulatory roles in CNS plasticity, as well as possible functional significance.

Amputation

Amputation results in a marked decline in afferent feedback from peripheral nerves previously innervating the amputated body part. In addition to reducing input onto segmental and propriospinal interneurons in the cord, there is also a concomitant reduction of the tonic and phasic ascending sensory information to all supraspinal and cortical structures. Given the importance of sensorimotor integration at the cortical level, it is not surprising that amputation can lead to a pronounced change in the excitability of cortical circuitry. Here we discuss the extent and the mechanisms underlying plasticity that occurs after amputation and transient deafferentation using ischemic nerve block (INB). Although discussion will primarily relate to experiments using TMS, some references will be made to animal studies, which support or challenge findings from human experiments. Through the use of TMS, increased excitability of the corticospinal system can be inferred by (a) a decrease in motor threshold (usually defined as the strength of stimulation required to evoke a motor-evoked potential (MEP) of more than 50 μV, 50% of the time), (b) an increase in MEP amplitude, (c) an increase in the scalp area where MEPs can be evoked for a given muscle, (d) a decrease in intracortical inhibition, or an increase in intracortical facilitation using paired pulse TMS.

Single pulse TMS

Amputation may decrease MT and increase MEP amplitude

Hall et al. (1990) revealed that the motor cortex undergoes reorganization in congenital amputees. Using single pulse TMS, MEP amplitude in muscles proximal to the amputation following stimulation of the cortical representation of the stump musculature was shown to be larger compared to MEPs in homologous muscles in the intact limb. In addition, the motor threshold is reduced, and the area of scalp from which MEPs could be evoked contralateral to the amputated limb is enlarged compared to the corresponding scalp regions for the intact limb. Increased MEP amplitude in the muscles proximal to the amputated limb has also been shown in traumatic upper limb (Cohen et al., 1991a; Dettmers et al., 1999; Hall et al., 1990, Kew et al., 1994; Roricht et al., 1999, 2001) and lower limb amputees (Chen et al., 1998b; Fuhr et al., 1992; Hall et al., 1990).

In a study of lower limb amputees, the motor threshold (MT) was found to be significantly lower on the cortex, which controls muscles proximal to the amputation, indicating increased excitability of the pathway from cortex to spinal motoneurons (Chen et al., 1998a). To test the site of the changes induced by amputation, the differences in MT of TMS between the motor cortex contralateral to the amputation and the ipsilateral cortex, were compared to the MT evoked by transcranial electric stimulation (TES). To assess the contribution of alterations in 'spinal excitability', H-reflexes and activation of the motoneuron pool with spinal electrical stimulation (SES) were compared on the intact and amputated side. With TMS, which predominately activates the corticospinal neurones transsynaptically, the MT was lower on the cortex contralateral to the amputated limb. By contrast with TES, which activates corticospinal cells directly (Hallett, 2000; Rothwell, 1997), the MT was similar between the two sides. Furthermore, tests of 'spinal excitability' with SES showed no difference between the amputated and intact side. Thus, the site of plasticity predominately involved cortical neurons presynaptic to the corticospinal neurons, i.e. intracortical interneurons.

The effect of deafferentation on MT, however, has not been consistent in the literature. Decreases in MT have been recorded in lower limb amputees (Chen et al., 1998b) and upper limb amputees (Cohen et al., 1991a; Dettmers et al., 1999; Hall et al., 1990). By contrast, Roricht reported a decrease in MT following amputation of the forearm, but not following amputation of more proximal portions of the upper arm (Roricht et al., 1999). No changes in MT were reported in other studies examining upper limb amputees (Capaday et al., 2000; Kew et al., 1994; Schwenkreis et al., 2000). The reasons for the differences are not known. Possible factors include differences in stimulation parameters used or as yet undetermined patient factors such as degree of use of the amputated limb and time since amputation. Table 8.1 summarizes several indices of excitability of the corticospinal system affected by amputation.

Changes in cortical map size occur following amputation

The motor cortex is grossly organized somatotopically, with the representation of the face, hand, arm, and leg, moving laterally to medially. The expansion of the scalp area over which TMS can evoke MEP in muscles proximal to the amputated limb was a provocative finding. It has been suggested that the cortical representation of the stump had 'invaded' the cortical area that previously represented the amputated limb. Symmetrical map expansion of muscles proximal to the amputation can be due to increased cortical neuronal excitability, thereby making neurons more responsive to current spread from remote areas on the scalp, or recruitment of cortical neurons located in representation of the amputated limb through disinhibition or formation of new synapses (Ridding & Rothwell, 1997). A shift in the amplitude-weighted centre of gravity of the cortical maps was required to support the hypothesis of spatial shifts of cortical representations (Dettmers et al., 1999; Kew et al., 1994; Pascual-Leone et al., 1996; Schwenkreis et al., 2001).

Intracortical stimulation studies in animals following amputation confirmed that cortical neurons controlling stump musculature could be found within the cortical representation of the amputated limb. For example, amputation at the level of the elbow results in the ability to activate pyramidal tracts neurons within the hand region of the cortex that project to motoneurons of the stump musculature (Hu-Xin et al., 2000). Previously unresponsive pyramidal neurons corresponding to motoneurons of the stump

Table 8.1. Summary of studies on changes in corticospinal excitability following amputation, transient deafferentation and hand replant

Study	Subjects tested	MEP	MT	ICI	ICF
Cohen et al. (1991a)	Amp. UL ($n = 7$, AE 4, BE 1, E 1), congenitally absent hand 1	↑	↓	NA	NA
Dettmers et al. (1999)	Amp. UL ($n = 1$)	↑	↓	↓	↑
Capaday et al. (2000)	Amp. UL ($n = 6$, BE 3, AE 3)	NC	NC	NA	NA
Kew et al. (1994)	Amp. UL ($n = 6$, AE 1, BE 2, congenital BE 3)	↑	↓rarely	NA	NA
Roricht et al. (1999)	Amp. (UL, long term) ($n = 15$, BE 8, AE 7)	↑BE; ↓ AE	↓BE; ↑↓ AE	NA	NA
Schwenkreis et al. (2000)	Amp. UL ($n = 12$, AE 4, BE 8)	NC	NC	↓BE NC AE	NC ↑
Hall et al. (1990)	Amp. UL ($n = 4$, BE 1, AE 1, congenital BE 2)	↑; NC late amputee	↓; NC in late amputee	NA	NA
Fuhr et al. (1992)	Amp. LL ($n = 6$, BK)	↑	NA	NA	NA
Chen et al. (1998a)	Amp. LL ($n = 16$, AK 9, BK 7)	↑	↓	↓	↑NA
Brasil-Nato et al. (1993)	INB UL & LL ($n = 8$ BE 4, BK 6)	↑	NC	NA	NA
Ziemann et al.(1998)	INB with rTMS UL ($n = 6$, BE)	↑	NC	↓	↑
Roricht et al. (2001)	Hand replant ($n = 10$)	↑FDI; ↑ BB	NC	NA	NA

Key:

AE: above elbow, AK: above knee, Amp: amputation, BB: biceps brachii, BE: below elbow, BK: below knee, FDI: first dorsal interosseus, INB: ischemic nerve block, LL: lower limb, NA: not assessed, NC: no change, NS: not significant, rTMS: repetitive transcranial magnetic stimulation, UL: upper limb.

musculature were thus made excitable following limb amputation. Using TMS in humans, similar expansion of the cortical representation of muscles adjacent to an amputated limb has been demonstrated by shifts in the amplitude-weighted cortical map centre of gravity (CoG) towards the representation of the amputated body parts (Dettmers et al., 1999; Kew et al., 1994; Pascual-Leone et al., 1996; Schwenkreis et al., 2001). Expansion of cortical maps revealed by TMS correlate with fMRI evidence of increased blood flow in the motor cortex with activation of the muscle proximal to amputation (Dettmers et al., 1999; Kew et al., 1994).

Changes in cortical excitability have been shown to persist for more than 50 years (Roricht et al., 1999). The nature of increased excitability, however, was more variable than that observed in subjects with more recent amputation. For example, although most subjects with amputations at the forearm or elbow showed some indices of increased excitability, not all subjects showed typical changes in each of MEP amplitude, MT and CoG. It was suggested that this might reflect a 'decay of a previously more accentuated state of reorganization' (Roricht et al., 1999). Another significant finding in the study was a differential expression of plasticity depending on the location of the amputation. Increased cortical excitability was only seen in two out of seven subjects with proximal arm amputations, whereas seven of eight subjects with amputations at the level of the forearm had an increase in cortical excitability. Thus, sensorimotor control of proximal muscles (deltoid/trapezius muscles) may be different than those of more distal muscles.

To examine if amputation-induced increases in cortical excitability are reversible, patients with hand amputation were examined after their hands were surgically reattached. In this group, reversal of amputation-induced plasticity was not observed. Factors that may contribute to this include poor dexterity of the replanted hand, which would make fine skilled movements difficult. This may contribute to a persistence of use-dependent plasticity of motor cortex controlling muscles proximal to the amputation (Roricht et al., 2001). The reduced use of the replanted hand, coupled with an increase use of more proximal portions of the limb might influence the amount and pattern of ascending sensory feedback from the transplanted hand, thus making replanted hands resemble a 'partially deafferented' limb. A single subject fMRI study showed that, following hand amputation, the motor cortical areas activated by elbow flexion expanded towards the hand area (analogous to the CoG shift in TMS studies). After hand replantation, the areas activated by elbow flexion receded to the normal 'elbow area' (Giraux et al., 2001). Such a finding at least suggests that the amputation-induced cortical reorganization may be reversible.

Limitation of cortical maps measured by TMS

The seminal work by Sherrington revealed the variability in the somatotopic organization of the motor cortex (Leyton & Sherrington, 1917). His classic experiments on chimpanzees, gorillas and orang-utans demonstrated

pronounced overlap of adjacent body parts in the motor cortex. Even stimulation of the same point, albeit with large surface electrodes, often activated
different muscles. Jankowska's group employed the more refined technique
of intracortical stimulation, and intracellular recordings from spinal motoneurons, and showed that pyramidal cells with monosynaptic connections
to the same motoneuron may be separated by up to 20 mm (Jankowska et al.,
1975). Furthermore, pyramidal cells have since been shown to have multiple
axon collaterals that mediate both mono- and oligosynaptic recurrent excitation and inhibition of neighbouring corticospinal cells (Ghosh & Porter,
1988). These observations do not support a strict, within-limb somatotopic
organization of motor cortex (for review, see Schieber, 2001), and may provide the anatomical underpinnings of the amputation-induced changes in
cortical map. The term 'rapid reorganization' that occurs following deafferentation tacitly implies a rewiring of neuronal circuits. This may not be
the case, and it is conceivable that the excitability changes created by deafferentation reflect disinhibition of cortical connections, which are silent only
during certain behaviours, i.e. when subjects are quietly sitting during the
experiment. Care should be taken not to assume that tonically inhibited pools
of interneurons at rest are not active during certain motor tasks, and that
TMS-evoked maps obtained at rest reflect what goes on during behaviour.
During behaviours that incorporate multiple joints, like combined reaching
and grasp, there may be drastic changes in the organization of motor maps
(McKiernan et al., 1998). The subthreshold postsynaptic potentials in spinal
motoneurons are not detected in the MEPs evoked by TMS. Therefore, cortical motor maps only represent the most excitable motor pathways at rest, and
may underestimate the projections of pyramidal cells (cf. Jankowska et al.,
1975). However, TMS maps may also overestimate cortical excitability due
to current spread and the large distances between the coil and the underlying
cortex.

Persistence of function of deafferented cortex

The fate of the motor pathways from pyramidal cells of the amputated limb is
of particular interest. Because the muscles innervated by the target motoneurons of pyramidal cells have been removed, the methodological limitations
of TMS studies (and intracortical stimulation studies in animals) are clear. To
determine if cortical expansion of neighbouring muscles is 'at the expense'

of the motor cortex controlling a transiently deafferented limb, intraneural recordings of cortically evoked volleys in the median or ulnar nerve were obtained proximal to the cuff during transient ischemic nerve block of the hand. The observation that single pulse TMS in the presence of ischemic nerve block (INB) produced a significantly larger volley in the motor nerve, innervating the transiently denervated hand musculature, suggests there is a generalized increase in excitability of the corticospinal system (McNutly et al., 2002). A similar study has not yet been reported in amputees. If similar results occur in amputees, the cortical map expansion of neighbouring muscles that results from amputation is not at the spatial expense of the corticospinal system of the amputated limb. There are at present no TMS studies testing changes in the motor map corresponding to the amputated regions. Preserved transcallosal inhibition evoked by TMS within the cortical representation of the amputated limb supports the hypothesis that physiological connections of pyramidal cells corresponding to the lost limb are maintained (Roricht & Meyer, 2000). fMRI studies of imaginary finger tapping in a patient with a plegic hand following root avulsion revealed a larger activation of the sensorimotor cortical representation of the deafferented hand compared to the homologous cortex of the intact limb. Thus, function of cortical neurons controlling de-efferented muscles appears to be at least partially preserved.

Paired pulse TMS
Amputation results in decreased ICI and increased ICF

When a suprathreshold TMS test pulse is preceded by a subthreshold conditioning TMS pulse, the resulting MEP amplitude will vary depending on the condition-test interval (Kujirai et al., 1993). In the normal subjects, intracortical inhibition (ICI) occurs at interstimulus intervals (ISIs) between 1 and 5 ms, which produces a MEP that is smaller than test pulse alone. At ISI of 6–20 ms there is intracortical facilitation (ICF) with facilitation of the test MEP. Following amputation, there is a significant decrease in ICI in lower limb (Chen et al., 1998a)(Fig. 8.1), upper limb and forearm amputees (Dettmers et al., 1999; Schwenkreis et al., 2000). In proximal arm amputees there is an increase in ICF (Schwenkreis et al., 2000), and in lower limb amputees is also a non-significant increase in ICF (Chen et al., 1998a)(Fig. 8.1). Table 8.1 summarizes some of the excitability indices altered by amputation.

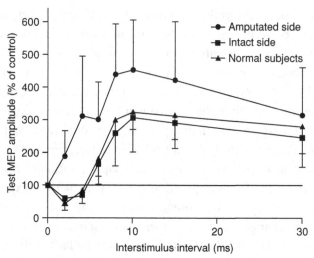

Fig. 8.1   Paired TMS study in lower limb amputees. MEPs were recorded from the quadriceps femoris muscle. Interstimulus interval (ISI) of 0 represents the MEP amplitude of the test pulse alone, which is defined as 100%. Each point represents an average of 11 subjects for the amputated side, seven subjects for the intact side, and seven normal subjects. On the intact side and in normal subjects, there was inhibition at ISIs of 2 and 4 ms and facilitation at ISIs of 6–30 ms. On the amputated side, there was more facilitation than on the intact side at all ISIs. Error bar indicates 1 standard error. (Adapted from Chen et al., 1998.)

Transient deafferentation studies reveal transmitters systems involved in cortical plasticity

Transient ischemic deafferentation (Bier's block or ischemic nerve block, INB) is a useful model of short-term plasticity in TMS studies (Brasil-Neto et al., 1993). Recently, this technique has been used to study the mechanisms, and the transmitters systems involved in the cortical plasticity that occurs following INB, and potentially after amputation. Animal studies have described powerful inhibition mediated by GABA releasing cortical interneurons, which, when blocked, resulted in cortical reorganization (Jacobs & Donoghue, 1991; for review see Sanes & Donoghue, 2000). Moreover, the network of cortical horizontal cells, which have synaptic actions on pyramidal cells, undergo plastic changes depending on the frequency of their input. The mechanism resembles that of long-term potentiation (LTP) and long-term depression (LTD) (Hess & Donoghue, 1994, 1996).

INB-induced cortical plasticity has been investigated in the presence of GABAergic agents and voltage-dependent ion channel blockers in order to disclose the possible components of deafferentation-induced plasticity (Ziemann et al., 1998; see also Chapter 6). A single dose of lorazepam (potentiates GABA$_A$ transmission) reduces MEP amplitude, and blocks the INB-induced decrease in ICI following single pulse TMS (Ziemann et al., 1998). A recent report on using ^{11}C-flumazenil binding in amputees has shown that GABA$_A$ receptors are up-regulated in the plastic motor cortex, perhaps as a compensatory mechanism for decreased activity of GABAergic interneurones (Capaday et al., 2000). Lamotrigine, which blocks voltage gated Na$^+$ and Ca^{2+} channels also decreases MEP size and blunts the INB plus TMS-induced increase in ICI (Ziemann et al., 1998). Activation of NMDA receptors also plays a role in deafferentation-induced plasticity. Dextromethorphan, a non-competitive NMDA antagonist, suppresses the INB plus rTMS-induced increase in ICI, but has no effect on the MEP amplitude (Ziemann et al., 1998). In summary, it is proposed that part of the increased cortical excitability following INB (and possibly amputation) is due to rapid removal of tonic GABA-mediated inhibition of cortical interneurons, thus disinhibiting corticospinal neurons. There may also be induction of NMDA-dependent LTP-like mechanisms, which through their network of horizontal connections provide increased excitatory drive to corticospinal neurons. The actions of voltage gated Na$^+$ and Ca^{2+} channels are non-specific, however, lamotrigine is believed to mediate its actions through inhibition of glutamate transmission (Leach et al., 1986). Change in LTD is also a candidate mechanism in corticospinal excitability modulation. Inhibition of LTD, via decreased metabotropic glutamate receptor activation and decreased L-type Ca^{2+} channel activation has been demonstrated following limb amputation in the anterior, but not posterior, cingulate cortex of rat (Wei et al., 1999). It is not known if changes in LTD occur in motor cortex following amputation.

Possible role of spinal cord plasticity

Thus far, discussion of plasticity in the CNS following amputation has been focused primarily in the cortex, with much less attention to changes in 'spinal excitability'. Special mention should be made, however, concerning the highly dynamic nature of spinal interneuronal excitability. The concept of functional (or behavioural-related) reorganization of spinal interneuronal systems has been borne out of recent in vivo cat experiments using fictive locomotion, which show that primary muscle spindle or tendon organ afferents can evoke inhibition of certain motoneurons at rest, and excitation of the same motoneurons during locomotion (Angel et al., 1996; Gossard et al., 1994; Guertin et al., 1995; McCrea et al., 1995; for review see McCrea, 2001. That is to say, the excitability of populations of spinal interneuronal systems profoundly changes during locomotion. Accordingly, the excitability of the interneuronal circuits at rest should not be rigidly extrapolated to those operational during behaviour. Finally, preliminary evidence suggests the spinal interneurons, which integrate the central pattern generator for locomotion with input from muscle and tendon afferents, undergo plasticity following partial dennervation of the limb (Whelan & Pearson, 1997). It is reasonable to hypothesize that similar interneuronal systems may be subserving the load-training enhancement of weight support and locomotion that is seen in spinal cord-injured patients (Barbeau et al., 1998; Dietz et al., 1998).

Spinal cord injury

It is becoming increasingly evident that spinal cord injury (SCI) results in changes in the organization of the CNS. Intuitively, it is to be expected that parts of the brain become redundant when muscles are paralysed as a result of SCI. The plasticity inherent in the brain results in functional changes to those potentially redundant areas such that they become redeployed in the control of musculature rostral to the level of the lesion. Another sign of plasticity in motor areas of the brain is the functional reorganization of corticospinal pathways following incomplete SCI that leaves some residual voluntary control of muscles. This is evident as changes in facilitatory and inhibitory cortical control of the surviving corticospinal neurons following partial severance of descending tracts. Finally, the spinal cord circuitry below the level of a lesion also shows adaptation to changed patterns of activity. Here, we review insights into the plastic reorganization of motor function that have been established using TMS of the motor cortex.

Before reviewing the consequences of SCI in terms of plasticity of CNS function, the direct impact of cord lesions on transmission in the corticospinal pathway needs assessment. In an early clinical assessment of the completeness of SCI, Gianutsos et al. (1987) demonstrated that motor-evoked potentials (MEPs) in response to TMS could be elicited from muscles over which a person had no voluntary control. Thus, the use of TMS demonstrated that a clinically complete lesion of the spinal cord, i.e. complete according to neurological examination, might contain axons that descend through the lesion and are capable of exciting motoneurons leading to muscle contraction.

Abnormally long latency and long duration MEPs in SCI may indicate prolonged corticospinal transmission to motoneurons, but might simply reflect peripheral motor nerve slowing. Central conduction delay between the motor cortex and the motoneuron pool can conveniently be assessed using a combination of TMS to measure total conduction delay and F-waves for peripheral motor nerve conduction time. Chang and Lien (1991) used this technique in subjects with neurologically incomplete injury to assess corticospinal conduction velocity in the region of the damaged spinal cord. The difference between the central delays to muscles above and below the lesion showed that the average conduction velocity through the damaged region was about half (32.1 m s^{-1}) the value for normal cord conduction (63.3 m s^{-1}). The method has proven to be an ideal diagnostic approach for subjects with coexisting entrapment neuropathy and spinal cord compression (Kaneko et al., 1996).

The presence and form of MEPs recorded below the level of a spinal cord lesion has mostly correlated well with the results of neurological and functional assessments (Ackermann et al., 1992; Davey et al., 1998; Dimitrijevic et al., 1992a). In the acute stages following SCI, the recovery (Tegenthoff, 1992) or early presence (Clarke et al., 1994) of MEPs preceded favourable clinical outcome in incomplete SCI subjects. In the case of spinal injury subjects with clinically complete lesions that appear to have residual connectivity but no voluntary control, so-called 'discomplete' subjects (Dimitrijevic et al., 1984), no MEP responses could be evoked below the lesion (Dimitrijevic et al., 1992a). Rather than indicate a limitation of TMS, a more probable explanation is that the surviving or recovered axons in the 'discomplete' subject are not corticospinal.

Another point to recognize before attributing any altered motor state in SCI to adaptation within the CNS, is that peripheral muscle atrophy through disuse may alter the characteristics of the MEP responses to TMS (Lissens &

Vanderstraeten, 1996). A reduced MEP amplitude may simply reflect a reduced muscle mass rather than a smaller corticospinal volley reaching the motoneurone pool; expressing the MEP amplitude as a percentage of the maximum M-wave response to peripheral motor nerve stimulation can help to avoid this problem.

Further information on the continuity of descending corticospinal connections to the motoneurone pool in SCI can be obtained by combining TMS with segmental reflex tests. Condition-test paradigms have revealed facilitation of H-reflexes by preceding TMS of the motor cortex. The facilitation reflects convergence of reflex and corticospinal pathways and has indicated preservation of corticospinal axons in some subjects who lack the ability to make a voluntary contraction of muscles (Hayes et al., 1992; Wolfe et al., 1996).

Cortical representation of muscles

The facility that TMS possesses to stimulate corticospinal neurones has been used extensively to map the motor cortex. Use of a figure-of-eight shaped stimulating coil, and due attention to its orientation over the scalp, can achieve more discrete stimulation of the brain than the conventional circular coil (Davey et al., 1994; Mills et al., 1992) and provide maps that are consistent to repeated observation. The majority of mapping studies in SCI have addressed the question of whether the motor cortical representation of muscles rostral to the site of a lesion changes after injury. Levy et al. (1990) showed an increased cortical field of the *biceps brachii* innervated above a SCI lesion. The field included an area normally associated with muscles that act on the digits, which were paralysed in their subjects. Subsequent studies in complete SCI (Cohen et al., 1991b; Topka et al., 1991) confirmed that the maps of cortical representation of muscles rostral to the cord lesion become enlarged. It was also shown that, for comparable intensities of TMS, a larger proportion of the motor pool was excited at a shorter latency than normal indicating that the excitability of the corticospinal system was enhanced. This was even the case for muscles of the abdominal wall (*rectus abdominis, external/internal obliques*), which normally have a relatively poor cortical representation and weak response to TMS (Topka et al., 1991). None of these studies actually distinguished whether the adaptation of the corticospinal pathway was occurring within the motor cortex or at the level of the spinal cord. This is because the response to TMS is affected by the excitability of both cortical cells and motoneurones. Cortical representation will appear larger for the same strength TMS if the threshold for excitation is lower simply due to increased excitability of the motoneurones. TMS is generally thought to excite pyramidal tract neurones presynaptically or at the level of the initial segment of the axon, whereas transcranial electrical stimulation (TES) excites corticospinal axons as they traverse white matter of the brain. Responses to TES are not influenced by changes in cortical excitability. Comparing the outcome of using the two techniques should distinguish between a cortical and spinal site of adaptation. To date, however, the only investigation of SCI using TES was simply for diagnostic purposes (Cheliout-Heraut et al., 1998). Other studies suggest that adaptation to the corticospinal pathway is likely to occur rostral to the motoneurones. Wolfe et al. (2001) found that 4-aminopyridine lowered threshold and latency, and increased the amplitude of MEP responses to TMS. The shortened latency suggests that the 4-aminopyridine may have improved conduction at the site of the lesion. However, compared with TMS, H-reflex and F-wave tests of excitability at the level of the motoneurones showed no changes in threshold or amplitude, suggesting that cortical excitability had altered. Caution should be exercised when comparing excitability to reflex stimuli and TMS, as the populations of motoneurones tested may not be the same (Morita et al., 1999). A study combining magnetic resonance spectroscopy and TMS has shown that metabolite changes indicating reorganization of synaptic connections or axonal sprouting are associated with weakened inhibition in the motor cortex of incomplete, well-recovered SCI subjects (Puri et al., 1998). In both studies such combinations of technique suggested that cortical reorganization had occurred.

It has been reported that an enlarged motor map for muscles rostral to the site of injury did not occur following incomplete SCI (Brouwer & Hopkins-Rosseel, 1997). This might indicate that partial preservation of sensory input is enough to retain normal cortical representation of muscles. However, evidence from Green et al. (1998) suggests that cortical adaptation does occur in incomplete injury. They employed EEG recording to measure changes in cortical representation directly as a component of the Bereitschaftspotential. They reported posteriorly shifted representation in complete SCI subjects but also in subjects with incomplete SCI.

The factors responsible for triggering the plastic changes in cortical function are unknown. Two plausible candidates are the withdrawal of sensory input and the effects of training. Temporary deafferentation by ischemic nerve block of the lower arm using a pressure cuff causes rapid (minutes) but reversible expansion of the cortical areas controlling more proximal muscles (Brasil-Neto et al., 1993). In SCI the cortical representation of muscles rostral to the site of a lesion has been examined (Streletz et al., 1995). The cortical map for musculature rostral to the lesion (*biceps brachii*) was already expanded 6 days postinjury, the earliest that examination took place. It is unlikely during such an acute stage of injury that the subjects would have experienced any training regime directed at the upper musculature. The short time lapse suggests therefore that the change may have been due to lasting effects of deafferentation. Even though the sensorimotor cortex is clearly deprived of sensory input following SCI, there is evidence that some representation is sustained. Cohen et al. (1991c) reported that TMS could elicit a tingling wave of sensation descending the leg in normal subjects but that in SCI the sensation was more definite.

The implications of cortical plasticity for SCI are not straightforward. Intuitively, there is benefit to be gained if potentially redundant areas of cortex are given over to the domain of unaffected muscles and result in enhanced control of those muscles. However, it is not clear whether such displacement of function can be reversed. This becomes an important issue if there is the potential for recovery from SCI. Recovery occurs in incomplete SCI, and the paralysis of muscles may only be temporary. Also, in the near future it is anticipated that surgical intervention will be employed to re-establish connectivity in the spinal cord and promote recovery. It would be important for appropriated cortical areas to be relinquished to allow functional recovery to accompany re-established connections. The evidence from experiments in which cortical adaptation occurred following temporary deafferentation by ischemic nerve block (Brasil-Neto et al., 1993) suggests that reorganization is reversible in the short term. However, such short-term adaptation is unlikely to involve sprouting and establishment of new synaptic connections. Until the potential for reversal of such new connections is known, caution should perhaps be exercised in directing occupational therapy at muscles above the lesion, and designed to compensate for movements affected by SCI, if there is the potential for recovery of function.

Corticospinal facilitation and recruitment

Excitability of the corticospinal system can be investigated by measuring the amount of facilitation of the MEP response to TMS that occurs with voluntary effort. The pattern of facilitation differs among muscle groups and appears to reflect the degree of corticospinal innervation (Taylor et al., 1997). In hand muscles of normal individuals, the facilitation reaches a maximum at 10% of a maximum voluntary contraction (MVC), whereas in leg muscles there is a more gradual increase in MEP amplitude with contraction strength. Following incomplete SCI, the pattern of facilitation of hand muscles (Fig. 8.2) continues beyond 10% MVC and appears more similar to that seen for leg muscles in normal subjects (Davey et al., 1999). An index of cortical excitability at rest can be provided by constructing recruitment curves of MEP amplitude with increasing strength of TMS. In incomplete SCI with good recovery, such recruitment curves for hand muscles are also less steep than normal (Davey et al., 1999). The fact that facilitation during voluntary contraction and recruitment for hand muscles in incomplete SCI show patterns of cortical excitability similar to those seen for normal leg muscles, could be interpreted simply as reflecting the reduced corticospinal innervation of motoneurones to hand muscles. Alternatively, since the SCI subjects were all long term, and would have experienced occupational therapy designed to improve hand function, the different patterns might reflect central adaptation of the corticospinal system.

Another sign of altered cortical excitability in incomplete SCI is the apparent increase in the late EMG burst seen after the silent period in response to TMS (Dimitrijevic et al., 1992b). Our own experience is that these longer latency responses can be evoked in the absence of voluntary effort and at a lower threshold than is needed to evoke a MEP following incomplete SCI (unpublished observation).

Cortical inhibitory circuitry

MEP responses to TMS in active muscle are followed by a silent period. Several mechanisms contribute to the silent period including cortical inhibitory circuits and reflex inhibition at a segmental level of the spinal cord (Chen et al., 1999). This makes it difficult to attribute any changes in the silent period to adaptation in the brain rather than the spinal cord. Application of TMS at a strength just subthreshold for eliciting a MEP can suppress the EMG activity

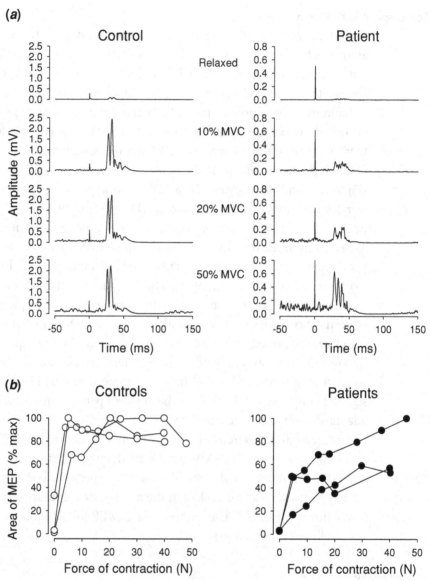

Fig. 8.2   Recruitment with increasing voluntary effort of MEP responses to TMS. (*a*) Averages
of rectified EMG of thenar muscles. Application of TMS at 10% above threshold in
the relaxed state, at different levels of voluntary contraction. The patient was well
recovered from incomplete spinal cord injury at C7 (ASIA grade D). (*b*) Size of the
MEP plotted against force of contraction for three control subjects and three well-
recovered SCI patients. The patients (all ASIA grade D) and subjects were selected
as having similar MVCs (range 80–111N). Note the less steep recruitment curves for
the SCI patients. (Adapted from Davey et al., 1999, with permission.)

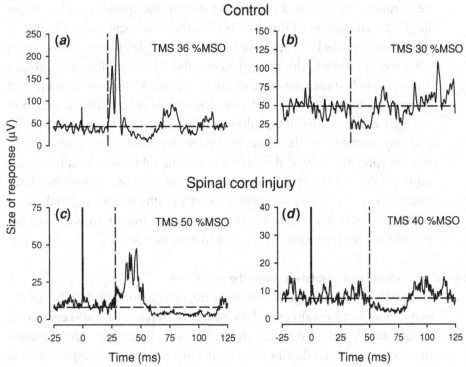

Fig. 8.3   Increased latency of MEPs and suppression of EMG to TMS in spinal cord injury. Averages of rectified EMG of thenar muscles and application of TMS during weak isometric voluntary contraction. Insets: strength of TMS in multiples of threshold for a MEP. (*a*), (*b*) Control subject. (*c*), (*d*) Well-recovered, incomplete spinal cord injury patient (C7, ASIA grade D). Horizontal dashed lines represent the mean level of voluntary EMG prior to TMS. The vertical dashed lines indicate latencies of MEPs (*a*), (*c*) and suppression of EMG (*b*), (*d*). Note the extra delays in the SCI patient and the particularly long latency of the inhibition.

associated with voluntary contraction. Davey et al. (1994) showed that such suppression can be attributed to activation of cortical inhibitory circuits. Figure 8.3 compares suppression of EMG in thenar muscles of a normal subject and a subject who has well-recovered sensorimotor function following incomplete SCI (Davey et al., 1998). In the SCI subject the MEP response to suprathreshold TMS is delayed compared with normal, as is the inhibition seen in response to TMS subthreshold for a MEP. However, the delay in onset of inhibition is considerably greater than for the MEP. The extra delay cannot be attributed to increased conduction time in the spinal cord, but rather implicates adaptation of the circuits that inhibit corticospinal output. The adaptation has also been observed in studies of single motor unit discharges (Smith et al., 2000a). This confirmed that the delayed inhibition is genuine and not simply due to masking within the gross EMG signal the inhibition of some motor units by the delayed excitation of others. The reduction in strength of cortical inhibition will presumably facilitate corticospinal output and may contribute to the recovery of voluntary actions. One problem with this interpretation is that the adaptation to the inhibitory circuitry occurs rapidly following SCI (possibly within days) whereas the recovery of motor function has a time course extending over months or a year (Smith et al., 2000b). Possibly, the down-regulation of cortical inhibition is a necessary prerequisite for the recovery processes to proceed.

Use-dependent plasticity and adaptation within the spinal cord

Long-term plastic changes in the brain are, in large part, likely to be use dependent, driven by regimes such as voluntary exercise (Pascual-Leone et al., 1995). For example, long-term improvements in hemiplegic hand function have been reported following constraint-induced exercise therapy and these are associated with adaptation of the corticospinal system assessed using transcranial stimulation (Liepert et al., 2000). Activity-dependent plasticity may occur within the spinal cord as well as the brain. Animal and human experiments show that afferent input can sensitize the spinal cord below a complete cord section (Wolpaw & Tennissen, 2001; Raineteau & Schwab, 2001). In human, the long-term effects of locomotor training in subjects with incomplete SCI improve weight support and stepping movements (Edgerton et al., 2001). Functional electrical stimulation has been commonly used to assist movement in cases of partial paralysis. It may also contribute to long-term adaptation within the CNS most evidently in locomotion when combined with weight support and locomotor training (Barbeau et al., 1998). The improvements are less evident and only temporary following complete SCI (Wirz et al., 2002). Evidently, recovery in incomplete SCI of automatic movements such as locomotion may involve plasticity of CNS function in either brain or spinal cord. Primates with incomplete SCI that spared ventral white matter do show locomotor patterns (Eidelberg et al., 1981). In this case the permissive descending tract may not have been corticospinal in origin, in which case its action would not have been revealed by TMS. This serves to remind us that the technique of TMS is limited in its application at present largely due to the testing of the crossed corticospinal pathway effecting voluntary movements.

Autonomic studies

Spinal cord injury results in impaired autonomic function and, potentially, the major complication of autonomic dysreflexia. TMS elicits a sympathetic skin response (SSR) but not below the level of a neurologically complete spinal cord lesion (Curt et al., 1996). In approximately 50% of subjects with incomplete lesions, SSRs could be evoked below the lesion level in the subjects who had not developed autonomic dysreflexia. Additionally, Cariga et al. (2002) have found that the spinal cord isolated below a complete lesion cannot support a SSR to lower limb nerve stimulation, even in cases with a cervical lesion well above the segmental output to the sympathetic chain. SSRs can thus be used to assess the integrity of autonomic spinal cord pathways and possibly to predict the likelihood of autonomic dysreflexia developing following a spinal cord injury.

Conclusions

Human TMS studies have made great advances in unveiling the nature and mechanisms of plasticity in the adult motor cortex following injury to the peripheral nervous system and spinal cord. By describing the plastic changes with TMS, insight has also been gained into the functional organization of the intact nervous system. In humans, TMS has shown that the selective activation of populations of corticospinal cells, as well as the amplitude and target of descending motor command, are under potent modulation from ascending sensory feedback. This cortical sensorimotor integration works both in parallel and in series with spinal interneuronal systems and undoubtedly helps humans perform accurate, smoothly executed movements. One must be cautious, however, extrapolating functional connectivity within the CNS from data obtained in the absence of motor behaviour.

Important initial findings that speak to the neurochemistry of plasticity include the important roles for GABAergic inhibition, NMDA transmission and voltage-gated ion channels. Although the preliminary description of plasticity in the cortex is well established via TMS, there is evidence of plasticity in subcortical and spinal systems. Due to its limitation of depth of penetration, TMS is not an effective tool at studying the extent of subcortical plasticity. Animal studies using intracortical stimulation and recording (e.g. Hu-Xin, 2000), as well as intracranial records obtained from surgical patients (Davis et al., 1998) will continue to be crucial complements to TMS. Ultimately, there is a need to develop therapeutic strategies that harness plasticity in ways that improve function in patients with nervous system lesions.

REFERENCES

Ackermann, H., Thomas, C., Guschlbauer, B. & Dichgans, J. (1992). Neurophysiological evaluation of sensorimotor functions of the leg: comparison of evoked potentials following electrical and mechanical stimulation, long latency muscle responses, and transcranial magnetic stimulation. *J. Neurophysiol.*, **239**: 218–222.

Alstermark, B., Isa, T., Ohki, Y. & Saito, Y. (1999). Disynaptic pyramidal excitation in forelimb motoneurons mediated via C(3)–C(4) propriospinal neurons in the *Macaca fuscata. J. Neurophysiol.*, **82**: 3580–3585.

Angel, M.J., Guertin, P., Jimenez, I. & McCrea, D.A. (1996). Group I afferents evoke disynaptic EPSPs in cat hindlimb motoneurones during fictive locomotion. *J. Physiol. (Lond.)*, **494**: 851–861.

Baldissera, F., Hultborn, H. & Illert, M. (1981). Integration in spinal neuronal systems. In *Handbook of Physiology – The Nervous System*, ed. J.M. Brookhart & V.B. Mountcastle, pp. 509–595. Bethesda: Williams and Wilkins.

Barbeau, H., Norman, K., Fung, J., Visintin, M. & Ladouceur, M. (1998). Does neurorehabilitation play a role in the recovery of walking in neurological populations? In *Neuronal Mechanisms for Generating Locomotor Activity*, ed. O. Kien, R.M. Harris-Warrick, L.M. Jordan, H. Hultborn & N. Kudo, *Ann. N.Y. Acad. Sci.*, **16**: 377–392.

Brasil-Neto, J., Valls-Sole, J., Pascual-Leone, A. et al. (1993). Rapid modulation of human cortical motor output following ischaemic nerve block. *Brain*, **116**, 511–525.

Brouwer, B. & Hopkins-Rosseel, D.H. (1997). Motor cortical mapping of proximal upper extremity muscles following spinal cord injury. *Spinal Cord*, **35**: 205–212.

Capaday, C., Richardson, M.P., Rothewll, J.C. & Brooks, D.J. (2000). Long-term changes of GABAergic function in the sensorimotor cortex of amputees: a combined magnetic stimulation and ^{11}C-flumazenil PET study. *Exp. Brain Res.*, **133**: 552–556.

Cariga, P., Cately, M., Mathias, C.J., Savic, G., Frankel, H.L. & Ellaway, P.H. (2002). Organisation of the sympathetic skin response in spinal cord injury. *J. Neurol. Neurosurg. Psychiatry*, **72**: 356–360.

Chang, C-W. & Lien, I-N. (1991). Estimate of motor conduction in human spinal cord: slowed conduction in spinal cord injury. *Muscle Nerve*, **14**: 990–996.

Cheliout-Heraut, F., Loubert, G., Masri-Zada, T., Aubrun, F. & Pasteyer, J. (1998). Evaluation of early motor and sensory evoked potentials in cervical spinal cord injury. *Neurophysiol. Clin.*, 39–55.

Chen, R., Corwell, B., Yaseen, Z., Hallett, M. & Cohen, L.G. (1998). Mechanisms of cortical reorganization in lower-limb amputees. *J. Neurosci.*, **18**: 3443–3450.

Chen, R., Lozano, A.M. & Ashby, P. (1999). Mechanism of the silent period following transcranial magnetic stimulation. Evidence from epidural recordings. *Exp. Brain Res.*, **128**: 539–542.

Clarke, C.E., Modarres-Sadeghi, H., Twomey, J.A. & Burt, A.A. (1994). Prognostic value of cortical magnetic stimulation in spinal cord injury. *Paraplegia*, **32**: 554–560.

Cohen, L.G., Bandinelli, S., Findley, T.W. & Hallet, M. (1991a). Motor reorganization after upper limb amputation in man: a study with focal magnetic stimulation. *Brain*, **114**: 615–627.

Cohen, L.G., Roth, B.J., Wassermann, E. et al. (1991b). Magnetic stimulation of the human cerebral cortex, an indicator of reorganization in motor pathways in certain pathological conditions. *J. Clin. Neurophysiol.*, **8**: 65.

Cohen, L.G., Topka, H., Cole, R.A. & Hallet, M. (1991c). Leg paresthesias induced by magnetic brain stimulation in subjects with thoracic spinal cord injury. *Neurology*, **41**: 1283–1288.

Cohen, L.G., Celnik, P., Pascual-Leone, A. et al. (1997). Functional relevance of cross-modal plasticity in the blind. *Nature*, **389**: 180–183.

Curt, A., Weinhardt, C. & Dietz, V. (1996). Significance of sympathetic skin responses in assessment of autonomic failure in subjects with spinal cord injury. *J. Auton. Nerv. Syst.*, **61**: 175–180.

Davey, N.J., Romaiguère, P., Maskill, D.W. & Ellaway, P.H. (1994). Suppression of voluntary motor activity revealed using transcranial magnetic stimulation of the motor cortex in man. *J. Physiol.*, **477**: 223–235.

Davey, N.J., Smith, H.C., Wells, E., Maskill, D.W., Ellaway, P.H. & Frankel, H.L. (1998). Responses of thenar muscles to transcranial magnetic stimulation of the motor cortex in patients with incomplete spinal cord injury. *J. Neurol. Neurosurg. Psychiatry*, **65**: 80–87.

Davey, N.J., Smith, H.C., Savic, G., Maskill, D.W., Ellaway, P.H. & Frankel, H.L. (1999). Comparison of input-output patterns in the corticospinal system of normal subjects and incomplete spinal cord injured patients. *Exp. Brain Res.*, **127**: 382–390.

Davis, K.D., Kiss, Z.H.T., Luo, L., Tasker, R.R., Lozano, A.M. & Dostrovsky, J.O. (1998). Phantom sensations generated by thalamic microstimulation. *Nature*, **391**: 385–387.

Dettmers, C., Liepert, J., Adler, T. et al. (1999). Abnormal motor cortex organization contralateral to early upper limb amputation in humans. *Neurosci. Lett.*, **263**: 41–44.

Dietz, V., Wirz, M., Curt, A. & Columbo, G. (1998). Locomotor pattern in paraplegic patients: training effects and recovery of spinal cord function. *Spinal Cord*, **36**: 380–390.

Dimitrijevic, M.R., Dimitrijevic, M.M., Faganel, J. & Sherwood, A.M. (1984). Suprasegmentally induced motor unit activity in paralyzed muscles of subjects with established spinal cord injury. *Ann. Neurol.*, **16**: 216–221.

Dimitrijevic, M.R., Hsu, C.Y. & McKay, W.B. (1992a). Neurophysiological assessment of spinal cord and head injury. *J. Neurotrauma*, **9**: 293–300.

Dimitrijevic, M.R., Kofler, M., McKay, W.B., Sherwood, A.M., Van der Linden, C. & Lissens, M.A. (1992b). Early and late lower limb motor evoked potentials elicited by transcranial magnetic motor cortex stimulation. *Electroencephalogr. Clin. Neurophysiol.*, **85**: 365–373.

Edgerton, V.R., Leon, R.D. & Harkema, S.J. (2001). Retraining the injured spinal cord. *J. Physiol.*, **533**: 15–22.

Eidelberg, E., Walden, J.G. & Nguyen, L.H. (1981). Locomotor control in macacque monkeys. *Brain*, **104**: 647–663.

Fuhr, P., Cohen, L.G., Dang, N. et al. (1992). Physiological analysis of motor reorganization following lower limb amputation. *Electroencephalogr. Clin. Neurophysiol.*, **85**: 53–60.

Ghosh, S. & Porter, R. (1988). Corticocortical synaptic influences on morphologically identified pyramidal neurones in the motor cortex of the monkey. *J. Physiol.*, **400**: 617–629.

Gianutsos, J., Eberstein, A., Ma, D., Holland, T. & Goodgold, J. (1987). A noninvasive technique to assess completeness of spinal cord lesions in humans. *Exp. Neurol.*, **98**: 34–40.

Giraux, P., Sirigu, A., Schneider, B. & Dubernard, J.M. (2001). Cortical reorganization in motor cortex after graft of both hands. *Nat. Neurosci.*, **4**: 691–692.

Gossard, J.P., Brownstone, R.M., Barajon, I. & Hultborn, H. (1994). Transmission in a locomotor-related group Ib pathway from hindlimb extensor muscles in the cat. *Exp. Brain Res.*, **98**: 213–228.

Green, J.B., Sora, E., Bialy, Y., Ricamato, A. & Thatcher, R.W. (1998). Cortical sensorimotor reorganization after spinal cord injury. *Neurology*, **50**: 1115–1121.

Guertin, P., Angel, M.J., Perreault, M-C. & McCrea, D.A. (1995). Ankle extensor group I afferents excite extensors throught the hindlimb during fictive locomotion in the cat. *J. Physiol.*, **487**: 197–209.

Hall, E.J., Flament, D., Fraser, C. & Lemon, R.N. (1990). Non-invasive brain stimulation reveals reorganised cortical outputs in amputees. *Neurosci. Lett.*, **116**: 379–386.

Hallett, M. (2000). Transcranial magnetic stimulation and the human brain. *Nature*, **406**: 147–150.

Hayes, K.C., Allatt, R.D., Wolfe, D.L., Kasai, T. & Hsieh, J. (1992). Reinforcement of subliminal flexion reflexes by transcranial magnetic stimulation of motor cortex in subjects with spinal cord injury. *Electroencephalogr. Clin. Neurophysiol.*, **85**: 102–109.

Hess, G. & Donoghue, J.P. (1994). Long-term potentiation of horizontal connections provides a mechanism to reorganize cortical maps. *J. Neurophysiol.*, **71**: 2543–2547.

Hess, G. & Donoghue, J.P. (1996). Long-term depression of horizontal connections in rat motor cortex. *Eur. J. Neurosci.*, **8**: 658–665.

Hu-Xin, Q., Stepniewaska, I. & Kaas J.H. (2000). Reorganization of primary motor cortex in adult macaque monkeys with long-standing amputations. *J. Neurophysiol.*, **84**: 2133–2147.

Jacobs, K. & Donoghue, J. (1991). Reshaping the cortical map by unmasking latent intracortical connections. *Science*, **251**: 944–947.

Jankowska, E., Padel, Y. & Tanaka, R. (1975). Projections of pyramidal tract cells to alpha-motoneurons innervating hindlimb muscles in the monkey. *J. Physiol.*, **249**: 637–667.

Kaneko, K., Kawai, S., Fuchigami, Y., Morita, H. & Ofuji, A. (1996). The effect of current direction induced by transcranial magnetic stimulation on the corticospinal excitability in human brain. *Electroencephalogr. Clin. Neurophysiol.*, **101**: 478–482.

Kew, J.J.M., Ridding, M.C., Rothwell, J.C. et al. (1994). Reorganization of cortical blood flow and transcranial magnetic stimulation maps in human subjects after upper limb amputation. *J. Neurophysiol.*, **72**: 2517–2524.

Kujirai, T., Caramia, M.D., Rothwell, J.C. et al. (1993). Corticocortical inhibition in human motor cortex. *J. Physiol.*, **471**: 501–519.

Leach, M.J., Marden, C.M. & Miller, A.A. (1986). Pharmacological studies on lamotrigine, a novel potential antiepileptic drug: II. Neurochemical studies on the mechanism of action. *Epilepsia*, **27**: 490–497.

Levy, W.J., Amassian, V.E., Traad, M. & Cadwell, J. (1990). Focal magnetic coil stimulation reveals motor cortical system reorganized in humans after traumatic quadriplegia. *Brain Res.*, **510**: 130–134.

Leyton, A.S.F. & Sherrington, C.S. (1917). Observations on the excitable cortex of the chimpanzee, orangutan, and gorilla. *Quart. J. Exp. Physiol.*, **11**: 135–222.

Liepert, J., Tegenthoff, M. & Malin, J.P. (1995). Changes of cortical motor area size during immobilization. *Electroencephalogr. Clin. Neurophysiol.*, **97**: 382–386.

Liepert, J., Bauder, H., Wolfgang, H.R., Miltner, W.H., Taub, E. & Weiller, C. (2000). Treatment-induced cortical reorganization after stroke in humans. *Stroke*, **31**: 1210–1216.

Lissens, M.A. & Vanderstraeten, G.G. (1996). Motor evoked potentials of the respiratory muscles in tetraplegic subjects. *Spinal Cord*, **34**: 673–678.

Lundberg, A. & Voorhoeve, P. (1962). Effects from the pyramidal tract on spinal reflex arcs. *Acta Physiol. Scand.*, **56**: 201–219.

McCrea, D.A. (2001). Spinal circuitry of sensorimotor control of locomotion. *J. Physiol.*, **533**: 41–50.

McCrea, D.A., Shefchyk, S.J., Stephens, M.J. & Pearson, K.G. (1995). Disynaptic group I excitation of synergist ankle extensor motorneurones during fictive locomotion in the cat. *J. Physiol.*, **487**: 527–539.

McKiernan, B.J., Maracario, J.K., Karrer, J.H. & Cheney, P.D. (1998). Corticomotoneural (CM) postspike effects on shoulder, elbow, wrist, digit, and intrinsic hand muscles during a reach and prehension task in the monkey. *J. Neurophysiol.*, **83**: 99–115.

McNutly, P.A., Macefield, V.G., Taylor, J.L. & Hallet, M. (2002). Cortically evoked neural volleys to the human hand are increased during ischemic block of the forearm. *J. Physiol.*, **538**: 279–288.

Mano, Y., Nakamuro, T., Tamura, R. et al. (1995). Central motor reorganization after anastomosis of the musculocutaneous and intercostal nerves following cervical root avulsion. *Ann. Neurol.*, **38**: 15–20.

Mills, K.R., Boniface, S.J. & Schubert, M. (1992). Magnetic brain stimulation with a double coil: the importance of coil orientation. *Electroencephalogr. Clin. Neurophysiol.*, **85**: 17–21.

Morita, H., Baumgarten, J., Petersen, N., Christensen, L.O. & Neilsen, J. (1999). Recruitment of extensor-carpi-radialis motor units by transcranial magnetic stimulation and radial-nerve stimulation in human subjects. *Exp. Brain Res.*, **128**: 557–562.

Pascual-Leone, A. & Torres, F. (1993). Plasticity of the sensorimotor cortex representation of the reading finger in Braille readers. *Brain*, **116**: 39–52.

Pascual-Leone, A., Dang, N., Cohen, L.G., Brasil-Neto, J.P., Cammarota, A. & Hallett, M. (1995). Modulation of muscle responses evoked by transcranial magnetic stimulation during acquisition of new fine motor-skills. *J. Neurophysiol.*, **74**: 1037–1045.

Pascual-Leone, A., Peris, M., Tormos, J.M., Pascual, A.P. & Catala, M.D. (1996). Reorganization of human cortical motor output maps following traumatic forearm amputation. *Neuroreport*, **7**: 2068–2070.

Pierrot-Deseilligny, E. (1996). Transmission of the cortical command for human voluntary movement through cervical propriospinal premotoneurons. *Progr. Neurobiol.*, **48**: 489–517.

Puri, B.K., Smith, H.C., Cox, I.J. et al. (1998). The human motor cortex following incomplete spinal cord injury: an investigation using proton magnetic resonance spectroscopy. *J. Neurol. Neurosurg. Psychiatry*, **65**: 748–754.

Raineteau, O. & Schwab, M.E. (2001). Plasticity of motor systems after incomplete spinal cord injury. *Nat. Rev. Neurosci.*, **2**: 263–273.

Ridding, M.C. & Rothwell, J.C. (1997). Stimulus/response curves as a method of measuring motor cortical excitability in man. *Electroencephalogr. Clin. Neurophysiol.*, **105**: 340–344.

Roricht, S. & Meyer, B-U. (2000). Residual function in motor cortex contralateral to amputated hand. *Neurology*, **54**: 984–987.

Roricht, S., Meyer, B.U., Niehaus, L. & Brandt, S.A. (1999). Long-term reorganization of motor cortex outputs after arm amputation. *Neurology*, **53**: 106–111.

Roricht, S., Machetanz, J., Irlbacher, K., Niehaus, L., Biemer, E. & Meyer, B.U. (2001). Reorganization of human motor cortex after hand replantation. *Ann. Neurol.*, **50**: 240–249.

Rothwell, J.C. (1997). Techniques and mechanisms of action of transcranial stimulation of the human motor cortex. *J. Neurosci. Methods*, **74**: 113–122.

Sanes, J.N. & Donoghue, J.P. (2000). Plasticity and primary motor cortex. *Annu. Rev. Neurosci.*, **23**: 393–415.

Sanes, J.N., Suner, S. & Donoghue, J.P. (1990). Dynamic organization of primary motor cortex output to target muscle in adult rats. I. Long-term patterns of reorganization following motor or mixed peripheral nerve lesion. *Exp. Brain Res.*, **79**: 479–491.

Schieber, M.H. (2001). Constraints on somatotropic organization in the primary motor cortex. *J. Neurophysiol.*, **86**: 2125–2143.

Schwenkreis, P., Witscher, K., Janssen, F. et al. (2000). Changes of cortical excitability in patients with upper limb amputation. *Neurosci. Lett.*, **293**: 143–146.

Schwenkreis, P., Witscher, K., Janssen, F. et al. (2001). Assessment of reorganization in the sensorimotor cortex after upper limb amputation. *Clin. Neurophysiol.*, **112**: 627–635.

Smith, H.C., Davey, N.J., Savic, G. et al. (2000a). Modulation of single motor unit discharges using magnetic stimulation of the motor cortex in incomplete spinal cord injury. *J. Neurol. Neurosurg. Psychiatry*, **68**: 516–520.

Smith, H.C., Savic, G., Frankel, H.L. et al. (2000b). Corticospinal function studied over time following incomplete spinal cord injury. *Spinal Cord*, **38**: 292–300.

Streletz, L.J., Belevich, J.K.S., Jones, S.M., Bhushan, A., Shah, S.H. & Herbison, G.J. (1995). Transcranial magnetic stimulation: cortical motor maps in acute spinal cord injury. *Brain Topography*, **7**: 245–250.

Taylor, J.L., Allen, G.M., Butler, J.E. & Gandevia, S.C. (1997). Effect of contraction strength on responses in biceps brachii and adductor pollicis to transcranial magnetic stimulation. *Exp. Res.*, **117**: 472–478.

Tegenthoff, M. (1992). Clinical applications of transcranial magnetic stimulation in acute spinal cord injury. In *Clinical Applications of Magnetic Transcranial Stimulation*, ed. M.A. Lissens, pp. 33–44. Leuven: Uitgeverij, Peters.

Topka, H., Cohen, L.G., Cole, R.A. & Hallet, M. (1991). Reorganization of corticospinal pathways following spinal cord injury. *Neurology*, **41**: 1276–1283.

Wei, F., Li, P. & Zhuo, M. (1999). Loss of synaptic depression in mammalian anterior cingulate cortex after amputation. *J. Neuorsci.*, **19**: 9346–9354.

Whelan, P.J. & Pearson, K.G. (1997). Plasticity in reflex pathways controlling stepping in the cat. *J. Neurophysiol.*, **78**: 1643–1650.

Wirz, M., Colombo, G. & Dietz, V. (2002). Long term effects of locomotor training in spinal humans. *J. Neurol. Neurosurg. Psychiatry*, **71**: 93–96.

Wolfe, D.L., Hayes, K.C., Potter, P.J. & Delaney, G.A. (1996). Conditioning lower limb H-reflexes by transcranial magnetic stimulation of motor cortex reveals preserved innervation in SCI subjects. *J. Neurotrauma*, **13**: 281–291.

Wolfe, D.L., Hayes, K.C., Hsieh, J.T. & Potter, P.J. (2001). Effects of 4-aminopyrridine on motor evoked potentials in patients with spinal cord injury: a double-blinded, placebo-controlled crossover trial. *J. Neurotrauma*, **18**: 757–771.

Wolpaw, J.R. & Tennissen, A.M. (2001). Activity-dependent spinal cord plasticity in health and disease. *Annu. Rev. Neurosci.*, **24**: 807–843.

Ziemann, U., Hallett, M. & Cohen, L. G. (1998). Mechanisms of deafferentation-induced plasticity in human motor cortex. *J. Neuroscience*, **18**: 7000–7007.

9

Functional relevance of cortical plasticity

Pablo A. Celnik[1] and Leonardo G. Cohen[2]

[1]Department of Physical Medicine and Rehabilitation, Johns Hopkins University, Baltimore, MD, USA
[2]Human Cortical Physiology Section, NINDS, NIH, Bethesda, MD, USA

Introduction

The human central nervous system (CNS) can change in response to new environmental challenges or lesions. While such changes are more pronounced in the developing brain, they are also present in adults. It has been a widely held belief that these alterations underlie behavioural modifications such as learning new skills or recovery of lost function after injuries. However, until recently there has been little evidence to support this assertion. The development of neuroimaging and neurophysiological techniques such as functional magnetic resonance imaging (fMRI), positron emission tomography (PET), event-related potentials, electroencephalography (EEG), magnetoencephalography (MEG) and transcranial magnetic stimulation (TMS), have demonstrated that neuroplastic modifications have functional implications.

TMS is a non-invasive technique that allows focal delivery of currents into the brain. It is possible to apply TMS to a specific cortical region and disrupt cortical activity there. Evaluation of the behavioural consequences of this disruption describes some of the functions of that part of the brain. TMS can therefore produce a 'virtual lesion' that lasts for milliseconds (Gerloff et al., 1997; Amassian et al., 1989). In the presence of brain reorganization, TMS could be applied to the reorganized cortical regions, while the subject performs a specific task. If TMS, by disrupting the activity of that part of the brain, results in altered performance, it could be inferred that the reorganized cortex plays an adaptive role. In this chapter, we will discuss experimental evidence leading to the identification of the functional role of neuroplasticity using TMS.

Technical considerations

TMS is a method used to deliver electrical currents to the brain, by inducing a large, rapidly changing, magnetic field. This magnetic field readily passes into the brain and elicits currents that flow in a plane parallel to the coil (Roth et al., 1991; Amassian et al., 1994; Maccabee et al., 1991a; Cohen et al., 1990). These currents depolarize the exposed neurons. Thus, two general types of effects can be observed with cortical stimulation. First, a response of the area stimulated that resembles normal function, such as a muscle twitch with stimulation over the motor cortex (Barker et al., 1985) or phosphenes with stimulation over the occipital cortex (Maccabee et al., 1991b). Second, disruptive effects on ongoing regional cortical activity (Fuhr et al., 1991; Ziemann et al., 1996). Thus, depending on the number and types of neurons stimulated, the disruption by one single stimulus can last up to 250 ms. However, when a train of TMS stimuli is used, it is possible to interrupt normal cortical activity for a more prolonged period of time (Gerloff et al., 1997; Pascual-Leone et al., 2000). Trains of stimuli (repetitive transcranial magnetic stimulation, rTMS) are now known to be more effective than single stimuli in inducing disruption of cortical activity (Luders et al., 1987; Henderson et al., 1979; Ojemann, 1983).

Functionally beneficial effects of plasticity

Plasticity in the blind

The idea that a cortical region in charge of processing visual information after visual input could be recruited to process information from a different sensory modality is relatively new (Pons, 1996; Kujala et al., 1995a, 1997). It has been reported that blind cats are more precise than sighted cats in localizing sound sources in space (Rauschecker, 1994). Similarly, blind humans may be able to perform auditory localization tasks better than sighted individuals (Muchnik et al., 1991). This behavioural enhancement of non-visual modalities in the blind is consistent with early neuroimaging studies showing increased occipital activation associated with performance of auditory or tactile tasks (Wanet-Defalque et al., 1988). It was also reported that the 'mismatch negativity', a cognitive evoked potential, has a more posterior scalp distribution in blind individuals than in sighted controls (Kujala et al., 1995b).

Similarly, MEG studies demonstrated that brain regions activated in association with performance of auditory discrimination tasks are located more posterior in the blind. Uhl et al. (1993) found increased activation in SPECT of inferior occipital regions in the blind relative to sighted controls, although these authors failed to find a task-dependent increase in occipital activity. All together, these findings suggested unmasking of non-visual processing modalities, auditory as well as somatosensory, in the visual cortex of blind individuals.

These studies in individuals who became blind at an early age indicated that the deafferented occipital areas of the brain remained active despite the lack of visual input. In a more recent study using PET, Sadato et al. demonstrated that the occipital cortex is one of the regions activated in a distributed network during Braille reading and tactile discrimination tasks in blind subjects, but not in sighted volunteers (Sadato et al., 1996). Even though an association between performing tactile discrimination tasks and activation of the occipital cortex was clearly demonstrated, the functional role of this occipital activation was still unclear. Could those metabolic modifications constitute a mere epiphenomenon unrelated to the task?

To address this question, TMS was used to disrupt different cortical areas while early blind individuals read Braille and embossed Roman letters. Results obtained in the blind group were later compared to those obtained from a group of sighted volunteers reading embossed Roman letters. Five subjects who became blind early in life and who were experienced Braille readers were studied while they read strings of 'grade I' non-contracted, non-word Braille letters. In addition, five sighted volunteers and four of the early blind subjects were studied while performing a tactile discrimination task requiring identification of the same embossed Roman letters. Subjects were asked to identify and read aloud letter-by-letter as fast and accurately as possible. Letters were presented with a specially designed device that shows five letters at a time and permits simultaneous triggering of the TMS train with the initiation of the sweeping motion to read Braille. Phonographic recordings of voice and EMG recording from hand muscles involved in the reading task were monitored. Overall accuracy in reading performance before TMS was around 95% in the different groups. In the blind, mid-occipital stimulation induced significantly more errors than the control condition (stimulation in the air). In addition, stimulation of occipital positions occasionally elicited

Table 9.1. Sample of subjective reports given by the early blind subjects when stimulation was applied over different scalp positions

Subject	Stimulated position	Comments
Subject 1	Mid-occipital	'When it gets near the end, I really know something is going on. I can't describe it.... The more you [stimulate] the more it builds. It's a collective thing.'
Subject 2	Parietal ipsilateral	'Where did that come from? Don't ask me. Where did I get that? The first two letters made perfect sense and after that it just fell apart. It felt like ... just bumps, random dots.'
Subject 3	Occipital contralateral	'I could feel the dots were there, but I couldn't interpret them.'
Subject 4	Parietal contralateral	'I couldn't do it. It read it completely wrong and I just couldn't go on. I read two letters and even they weren't right.'
Subject 5	Primary motor cortex contralateral	'I had trouble with the last one and I could feel my finger sort of moving up and down.'
	Occipital contralateral	'In the next to the last letter I was almost feeling a dot that wasn't there.'
	Mid-occipital	'I felt a phantom dot which wasn't there. Despite the fact I didn't get it wrong, it almost threw me off.'
	Parietal contralateral	'The fourth one felt like nothing in grade 1. It felt like a dot was missing, but it is really there.'

Note: Stimulation over both parietal and occipital areas induced misperception of the Braille letters. Whereas rTMS over the primary motor cortex induced reports consistent with induction of jerky movements similar to a tremor. These observations suggest that parietal and occipital areas under the coil (most likely Brodmann areas 17, 18, 19 and 7) are involved in active perceptual processing of somatosensory information during Braille reading in the early blind.

distorted somatosensory perceptions (Table 9.1). Blind subjects reported negative ('missing dots'), positive ('phantom dots'), and confusing sensations ('dots don't make sense'). Blind and sighted subjects performing the same task (reading embossed Roman letters) showed different effects with TMS. Mid-occipital stimulation induced more errors than control (stimulation in the air) in the blind, but not in sighted volunteers (Cohen et al., 1997), supporting the view that the occipital cortex is functionally active despite decades of visual deafferentation (Rushton, 1978) (Schmidt et al., 1996), and

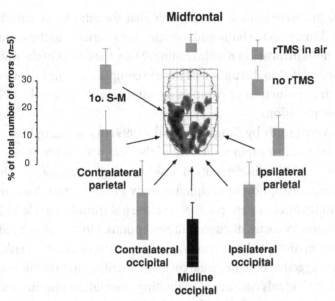

Fig. 9.1   The figure depicts the results of a PET study projected over the Taillarach map obtained from a blind subject while reading Braille letters. The bars represent the percentage of total number of errors incurred while subjects were reading Braille under transcranial magnetic stimulation in the different scalp positions. Mid-occipital position stimulation induced the largest number of Braille reading errors. When compared to control position (stimulation on the air), the blind group had significantly more errors than the control group. (Modified from Cohen et al., 1997.)

that it is actively engaged in meaningful processing of tactile information related to Braille reading and other tactile discrimination tasks (Fig. 9.1).

Since sensory processing for touch and vision seem to be segregated up to their arrival in primary reception areas (Brodmann areas 3, 1 and 2 for touch and 17 for vision), the first convergence of visual and somatosensory information in sighted mammals is thought to occur at cortical association sites, although a thalamic link between the two sensory modalities can not be excluded (Pons, 1996). It is possible that connections between visual and parietal association areas mediate transfer of somatosensory information to the occipital cortex in the blind. As such, what would be the role of the occipital cortex performing a tactile discrimination task? Since speech was unaffected by stimulation, and stimulation over parietal areas induced less errors than in the mid-occipital position, it can be concluded that input and output were spared. It is possible that the additional activation of the occipital cortex in the blind adds certain characteristics to the somatosensory perceptions involved in Braille reading. Thus, the effects of the mid-occipital TMS are related to disruption of a more complex discriminatory operation. Occasional induction of complex sensations with occipital TMS supports this interpretation.

In a recent study by Zangaladze et al. (1999) in normal sighted volunteers, TMS was used to explore the role of the occipital cortex during perform-ance of a tactile discrimination task (grating orientation). The authors found that disruption of occipital activity did not affect discrimination of different textures or perception of an electrical stimulus, while TMS over the somatosensory cortex disrupted all perceptions. On the other hand, occipital stimulation disrupted performance in the grating orientation task. Thus, the authors suggested that the visual cortex's contribution to tactile processing in sighted individuals consists of facilitating orientation discrimination, a task where visual imagery is heavily involved, but not other perceptions such as texture, detection of electrical stimulus or discrimination of a spacing task.

These results indicate that the occipital cortex contributes, to some extent, to tactile discriminatory functions in both sighted and blind individuals. It is conceivable that the magnitude of this contribution is larger in early blind individuals than in those who acquired blindness at a later age (Cohen et al., 1999). Additionally, the quality of that contribution appears to differ in sighted and blind individuals (Cohen et al., 1997). The finding that the oc-cipital cortex is a critical functioning component of the network involved in Braille reading supports the idea that perceptions are dynamically de-termined by the characteristics of the sensory inputs rather than by only the brain region that receives those inputs, at least in the case of early blind-ness (Pons, 1996; Rauschecker, 1995). These results indicate that cross-modal plasticity, as identified electrophysiologically or by neuroimaging techniques in human blind individuals, may play a functionally beneficial compensatory role.

A follow-up study was done on subjects who became blind after age 14 (late onset blind group, LOB). Eight subjects were studied using a combi-nation of H_2 ^{15}O PET and rTMS. The results in patients with late-onset blindness were compared with those obtained from subjects with early-onset blindness (Cohen et al., 1997). Except for small regions in the right inferior occipital gyrus and lingual gyrus, the occipital cortex was not activated in association with the tactile discrimination task in this late blind group. This finding was clearly in contrast to the activation of most of the visual cortex, including the primary visual regions in the congenitally blind (CB) and the early blind group (EOB). In addition, disruption of occipital activity by TMS did not affect the reading task in the LOB group. Therefore, the occipital cortex appears to play a fundamentally different role in LOB subjects compared to the other two groups. Taken together, neuroimaging and neurophysiological results provide evidence to support the concept of a window of opportunity for this form of functionally relevant cross-modal plasticity (Cohen et al., 1999). An interesting observation was a differential activation of occipital cortex in two subjects who became blind at ages 12 and 13 (in the EOB group) and the LOB group (including a subject blind at age 15), which suggests that the age boundary for the susceptible period of this form of cross-modal plasticity ranges between 13 and 15 years, close to that described for effectively treating strabismic amblyopia in humans (Epelbaum et al., 1993). The upper limit of the critical period for starting effective learning of a language is also considerably higher than previously estimated (Vargha-Khadem et al., 1997; Johnson, 1989). These findings are consistent with the hypothesis that puberty may mark a milestone in language acquisition (Lenneberg, 1969) and other plastic processes in the brain.

Auditory plasticity in the blind

Behavioural studies in cats determined that auditory localization skills in blind animals are superior to those in sighted animals (Rauschecker, 1994). Rauschecker et al. (1994) performing electrophysiological studies on visually deprived cats, found that neurons previously responsive to visual stimulation became activated by auditory or somatosensory stimulation (Korte, 1993). Behavioural studies in blind humans and near-sighted volunteers also reported better spatial localization skills when compared to sighted controls (Rice & Schusterman, 1965; Dufour Andre, 2000). In a behavioural and electrophysiological study by Roder et al. (1999) auditory localization in congenitally blind individuals was superior to sighted controls, but only when attending to sounds in the peripheral auditory space. Electrophysiological recordings suggested a compensatory reorganization of brain areas that may contribute to the improved spatial resolution for peripheral sound sources. Recently, Weeks et al. (2000) described cross-modal plastic changes between auditory and occipital cortical regions in blind individuals. They studied regional cerebral blood flow changes associated with performance of auditory localization tasks in congenitally blind subjects and in sighted controls. Sighted volunteers activated the primary auditory cortex with passive listening and the inferior parietal region with minimal bias to the right when they were asked to localize a sound in space. Congenitally blind subjects activated visual areas 18 and 19, and to a lesser degree the primary visual cortex (area 17) in addition to the inferior parietal cortex. This activation of the occipital cortex was positively correlated with activation of the parietal areas in the blind subjects but not in the sighted volunteers, implying that the visual cortex of the blind subjects is actively involved in the auditory spatial localization network (Weeks et al., 2000). However, the functional relevance of this activation of the occipital cortex in blind subjects has not been tested yet by TMS. But this may be possible in the near future, as one study has demonstrated recently the feasibility of testing auditory cortex function by slow-rate repetitive TMS (Lewald & Topper, 2002). In that study, rTMS produced a virtual lesion of the posterior parietal cortex outlasting the stimulation and resulting in a deterioration of sound localization relative to body coordinates.

Plasticity and dysphagia

This section briefly describes the correlation between cortical changes and clinical improvement of dysphagia as another example of functional beneficial plasticity. For a complete discussion on this topic, please refer to Chapter 11 of this book.

Swallowing function involves a complex sequence of motions leading to the transport of food and liquids from the mouth to the stomach while protecting the airway. When there is damage to the swallowing centres or their connections, as in stroke, dysphagia occurs. Almost one-third of stroke patients present with dysphagia (Gordon et al., 1987). However, most patients will recover within a few weeks (Barer, 1989). Recent studies demonstrated that the representation of oesophageal and pharyngeal muscles involved in swallowing function are bilaterally organized with some level of unilateral dominance

(Hamdy et al., 1996). This asymmetric hemispheric representation for swallowing could explain the occurrence of dysphagia in some strokes but not others. Hamdy et al., found that, in patients with dysphagia, TMS stimulation of the intact motor cortex elicited poorer motor responses than in patients without dysphagia, suggesting that in the dysphagic patients the dominant swallowing motor cortical representation was affected (Hamdy et al., 1997). In a different study, the same group performed serial swallowing evaluations, video-fluoroscopic barium swallowing, and motor mapping of the pharynx and thenar muscles. At presentation, 71% of the patients had signs of dysphagia. This percentage dropped to 46% at 1 month and 41% at 3 months. In the initial evaluation, pharyngeal motor maps in the intact hemisphere were smaller in dysphagic than in non-dysphagic patients, whereas maps in the affected hemisphere were similar. At 1 and 3 months pharyngeal motor maps increased only in patients who experienced substantial recovery. The authors concluded that recovery of dysphagia correlated with a representational change in the intact hemisphere (Hamdy et al., 1998), also suggesting that adaptation to a lesion in the swallowing representation may rely on the presence of an intact projection from the intact hemisphere that can develop increasing control over brainstem centres.

Functionally detrimental effects of plasticity

Extensive reorganizational changes in the somatosensory and motor cortices have been described after amputation. Studies in humans using magnetic source imaging demonstrated that the topographic representation of the face in the somatosensory cortex shifted an average of 1.5 cm toward the area that would normally receive input from the hand and fingers (Elbert et al., 1994). Kew et al. (1997) measured regional cerebral blood flow changes associated with vibrotactile stimulation (VS) of the pectoral region ipsilateral and contralateral to an amputated arm. VS ipsilateral to the stump activated a region of the contralateral S1 that extended ventrally to the trunk representation, extending into the hand representation. These results raised the hypothesis that the deafferented digit or hand/arm area had been activated by sensory input from the pectoral region.

In 1995, Flor et al. described a positive relationship between phantom limb pain and neuroplastic changes. Phantom limb pain after amputation is a condition characterized by sensations of pain in the missing limb. It is usually more common in the initial stages following amputations (Jensen & Rasmussen, 1995; Jensen et al., 1985), but in some cases, can be present for many years (Sunderland, 1978; Sherman, 1989). Using magnetic source imaging, Flor et al. studied subjects with different levels of phantom limb pain. They determined that the face representation in the somatosensory cortex experienced an almost fivefold larger medial shift for the subjects with phantom pain symptoms compared to the pain-free amputees. Additionally, the amount of phantom limb pain correlated with the amount of cortical reorganization. All other sensations, such as stump pain, non-painful stump and phantom sensations, presence of telescoping (the subjects experience a sensation where the phantom limb retracts towards, and often disappears in, the residual limb), or facial remapping (appearance of phantom sensations upon non-painful stimulation of the face) did not show this correlation. These findings raised the possibility that cortical reorganization may be related to a form of maladaptive plasticity.

To determine the functional role of this form of cortical reorganization, Birbaumer et al. (1997) anaesthetized subjects with phantom pain after amputation using a brachial plexus block. This intervention resulted in reduction of pain and reduction in the magnitude of plasticity. These findings were corroborated in a recent study on amputees where phantom pain reduction with the use of morphine was associated with diminished cortical reorganization (Huse et al., 2001).

In the motor domain, studies with TMS showed that stimulation over the sensorimotor cortex contralateral to the stump induced sensation of movement in the missing hand or fingers in patients with acquired amputation, but failed to do so in a patient with congenital absence of a limb. Furthermore, the cortical representations of muscles immediately proximal to the stump were larger than those of the homonymous muscles in the intact side (Cohen et al., 1991; Hall et al., 1990). These changes could reflect a true enlargement of the motor cortical representation or an increased excitability of a topographically unchanged motor representation. Later experiments demonstrated that these changes occur cortically (Chen et al., 1998; Fuhr et al., 1992; Roricht et al., 1999).

In a recent report, Karl et al. (2001) demonstrated that patients with phantom limb pain experienced more extensive motor reorganization than those without pain. The biceps representation of the amputated as compared to the intact side was more medial in all subjects, but only significantly different in the group with phantom limb pain. Optimal scalp positions for activation of the zigomaticus muscle with TMS was significantly different with a more medial representation in individuals with phantom limb pain relative to the non-pain group. Additionally, as in prior studies, the magnitude of motor cortex reorganization correlated well with the magnitude of phantom pain, the more intense pain the more medial was the optimal position of the zigomaticus representation.

Extensive information now exists showing marked cortical reorganization in the brain of adult amputees. Contrary to the past belief that neural plastic modifications have an adaptive and or preventive effect over phantom pain development (Katz, 1992; Ramachandran & Stewart, 1992a; Ramachandran et al., 1992b), cortical reorganizational changes in the case of the amputees appear to be associated with a significant functionally detrimental effect.

Conclusions

In summary, cortical and subcortical reorganization occur in both the immature and the mature CNS. The development of new non-invasive strategies allows an in-depth study of the functional role of these plastic changes. Understanding this role is important in designing strategies that could enhance plasticity when it plays a beneficial role and diminish it when it is deleterious.

REFERENCES

Amassian, V.E., Cracco, R.Q., Maccabee, P.J., Cracco, J.B., Rudell, A. & Eberle, L. (1989). Suppression of visual perception by magnetic coil stimulation of human occipital cortex. *Electroencephalogr. Clin. Neurophysiol.*, **74**: 458–462.

Amassian, V.E., Maccabee, P.J., Cracco, R.Q. et al. (1994). The polarity of the induced electric field influences magnetic coil inhibition of human visual cortex: implications for the site of excitation. *Electroencephalogr. Clin. Neurophysiol.*, **93**: 21–26.

Barer, D. (1989). The natural history and functional consequences of dysphagia after hemispheric stroke. *J. Neurol. Neurosurg. Psychiatry*, **52**: 236–241.

Barker, A.T., Jalinous, R. & Freeston, I. (1985). Non-invasive magnetic stimulation of human motor cortex. *Lancet*, 1106–1107.

Birbaumer, N., Lutzenberger, W., Montoya, P. et al. (1997). Effects of regional anesthesia on phantom limb pain are mirrored in changes in cortical reorganization. *J. Neurosci.*, **17**: 5503–5508.

Chen, R., Corwell, B., Yaseen, Z., Hallett, M. & Cohen, L. (1998). Mechanisms of cortical reorganization in lower-limb amputees. *J. Neurosci.*, **18**: 3443–3450.

Cohen, L.G., Roth, B.J., Nilsson, J. et al. (1990). Effects of coil design on delivery of focal magnetic stimulation. Technical considerations. *Electroencephalogr. Clin. Neurophysiol.*, **75**: 350–357.

Cohen, L., Bandinelli, S., Findley, T.W. & Hallett, M. (1991). Motor reorganization after upper limb amputation in man. A study with focal magnetic stimulation. *Brain*, **114**: 615–627.

Cohen, L.G., Celnik, P., Pascual-Leone, A. et al. (1997). Functional relevance of cross-modal plasticity in blind humans. *Nature*, **389**: 180–183.

Cohen, L.G., Weeks, R.A., Sadato, N., Celnik, P., Ishii, K. & Hallett, M. (1999). Period of susceptibility for cross-modal plasticity in the blind. *Ann. Neurol.*, **45**: 451–60.

Dufour, A. & Yannick, G. (2000). Improved auditory spatial sensitivity in near-sighted subjects. *Cogn. Brain Res.*, **10**: 159–165.

Elbert, T., Flor, H., Birbaumer, N. et al. (1994). Extensive reorganization of the somatosensory cortex in adult humans after nervous system injury. *Neuroreport*, **5**: 2593–2597.

Epelbaum, M., Milleret, C., Buisseret, P. & Dufier, J. (1993). The sensitive period for strabismic amblyopia in humans. *Ophthalmology*, **100**: 323–327.

Flor, H., Elbert, T., Knecht, S., Wienbruch, C., Pantev, C. & Larbig, W. (1995). Phantom limb pain as a perceptual correlate of massive cortical reorganization in upper extremity amputees. *Nature*, **375**: 482–484.

Fuhr, P., Agostino, R. & Hallett, M. (1991). Spinal motor neuron excitability during the silent period after cortical stimulation. *Electroencephalogr. Clin. Neurophysiol.*, **81**: 257–262.

Fuhr, P., Cohen. L.G., Dang, N. et al. (1992). Physiological analysis of motor reorganization following lower limb amputation. *Electroencephalogr. Clin. Neurophysiol.*, **85**: 53–60.

Gerloff, C., Corwell, B., Chen, R., Hallett, M. & Cohen, L. (1997). Stimulation over the human supplementary motor area interferes with the organization of future elements in complex motor sequences. *Brain*, **120**: 1587–1602.

Gordon, C., Langton-Hewer, R. & Wade, D.T. (1987). Dysphagia in acute stroke. *Br. Med. J.*, **295**: 411–414.

Hall, E.J., Flament, D., Fraser, C. & Lemon, R. (1990). Non-invasive brain stimulation reveals reorganized cortical outputs in amputees. *Neurosci. Lett.*, **116**: 379–386.

Hamdy, S., Aziz, Q., Rothwell, J.C. et al. (1996). The cortical topography of human swallowing musculature in health and disease. *Nat. Med.*, **2**: 1217–1224.

Hamdy, S., Aziz, Q., Rothwell, J.C. et al. (1997). Explaining oro-pharyngeal dysphagia after unilateral hemispheric stroke. *Lancet*, **350**: 686–692.

Hamdy, S., Aziz, Q., Rothwell, J.C. et al. (1998). Recovery of swallowing after dysphagic stroke relates to functional reorganization in the intact motor cortex. *Gastroenterology*, **115**: 1104–1112.

Henderson, D.C., Evans, J. R. & Dobelle, W. H. (1979). The relationship between stimulus parameters and phosphene threshold/brightness, during stimulation of human visual cortex. *Trans. Am. Soc. Artif. Intern. Organs.*, **25**: 367–371.

Huse, E., Larbig, W., Flor, H. & Birbaumer, N. (2001). The effect of opioids on phantom limb pain and cortical reorganization. *Pain*, **90**: 47–55.

Jensen, T.S. & Rasmussen, P. (1995). Phantom limb pain and related phenomena after amputation. *Textbook of Pain*, ed. P.D. Wall & R. Melzack, pp. 651–665. New York: Churchill Livingstone.

Jensen, T.S., Krebs, B., Nielsen, J. & Rasmussen, P. (1985). Immediate and long-term phantom limb pain in amputees: incidence, clinical characteristics and relationship to pre-amputation limb pain. *Pain*, **21**: 267–278.

Johnson, J.S. & Newport, E. (1989). Critical period effects in second language learning: the influence of maturational state on the acquisition of English as a second language. *Cogn. Psychol.*, **21**: 60–99.

Karl, A., Birbaumer, N., Lutzenberger, W., Cohen, L.G. & Flor, H. (2001). Reorganization of motor and somatosensory cortex in upper extremity amputees with phantom limb pain. *J. Neurosci.*, **21**: 3609–3618.

Katz, J. (1992). Psychophysiological contributions to phantom limbs. *Can. J. Psychiatry*, **37**: 282–298.

Kew, J.J., Halligan, P.W., Marshall, J.C. et al. (1997). Abnormal access of axial vibro-tactile input to deafferented somatosensory cortex in human upper limb amputees. *J. Neurophysiol.*, **77**: 2753–2764.

Korte, M. & Rauschecker, J. (1993). Auditory spatial tuning of cortical neurons is sharpened in cats with early blindness. *J. Neurophysiol.*, **70**: 1717–1721.

Kujala, T., Alho, K., Kekoni, J. et al. (1995a). Auditory and somatosensory event-related brain potentials in early blind humans. *Exp. Brain Res.*, **104**: 519–526.

Kujala, T., Huotilainen, M., Sinkkonen, J. et al. (1995b). Visual cortex activation in blind subjects during sound discrimination. *Neurosci. Lett.*, **183**: 143–146.

Kujala, T., Alho, K., Huotilainen, M. et al. (1997). Electrophysiological evidence for cross-modal plasticity in humans with early- and late-onset blindness. *Psychophysiology*, **34**: 213–216.

Lenneberg, E. (1969). On explaining language. *Science*, **9**: 635–643.

Lewald, J., Foltys, H. & Topper, R. (2002). Role of the posterior parietal cortex in spatial hearing. *J. Neurosci.*, **22**: RC207.

Luders, H., Lesser, R.P., Dinner, D.S. et al. (1987). Commentary: chronic intracranial recording and stimulation with subdural electrodes. In *Surgical Treatment of the Epilepsies*, ed. J. Engel, pp. 297–321. New York: Raven Press.

Maccabee, P.J., Amassian, V.E., Cracco, R.Q., Cracco, J.B., Eberle, L. & Rudell, A. (1991a). Stimulation of the human nervous system using the magnetic coil. *J. Clin. Neurophysiol.*, **8**: 38–55.

Maccabee, P.J., Amassian, V.E., Cracco, R.Q. et al. (1991b). Magnetic coil stimulation of human visual cortex: studies of perception. *Electroencephalogr. Clin. Neurophysiol. Suppl.*, **43**: 111–120.

Muchnik, C., Efrati, M., Nemeth, E., Malin, M. & Hildesheimer, M. (1991). Central auditory skills in blind and sighted subjects. *Scand. Audiol.*, **20**: 19–23.

Ojemann, G. (1983). Brain organization for language from the perspective of electrical stimulation mapping. *Behav. Brain Sci.*, **6**: 190–206.

Pascual-Leone, A., Walsh, V. & Rothwell, J. (2000). Transcranial magnetic stimulation in cognitive neuroscience – virtual lesion, chronometry, and functional connectivity. *Curr. Opin. Neurobiol.*, **10**: 232–237.

Pons, T. (1996). Novel sensations in the congenitally blind. *Nature*, **380**: 479–480.

Ramachandran, V.S., Rogers-Ramachandran, D. & Stewart, M. (1992a). Perceptual correlates of massive cortical reorganization. *Science*, **13**: 1159–1160.

Ramachandran, V.S., Stewart, M. & Rogers-Ramachandran, D. (1992b). Perceptual correlates of massive cortical reorganization. *Neuroreport*, **3**: 583–586.

Rauschecker, J.P. (1995). Compensatory plasticity and sensory substitution in the cerebral cortex. *Trends Neurosci.*, **18**: 36–43.

Rauschecker, J.P. & Kniepert, U. (1994). Enhanced precision of auditory localization behaviour in visually deprived cats. *Eur. J. Neurosci.*, **6**: 149–160.

Rice, C.E., Feinstein, S.H. & Schusterman, R. (1965). Echo-detection ability of the blind: size and distance factor. *J. Exp.*, **70**: 246–251.

Roder, B., Teder-Salejarvi, W., Sterr, A., Rosler, F., Hillyard, S.A. & Neville, H. (1999). Improved auditory spatial tuning in blind humans. *Nature*, **400**: 162–166.

Roricht, S., Meyer, B.U., Niehaus, L. & Brandt, S.A. (1999). Long-term reorganization of motor cortex outputs after arm amputation. *Neurology*, **53**: 106–111.

Roth, B.J., Saypol, J.M., Hallett, M. & Cohen, L. (1991). A theoretical calculation of the electric field induced in the cortex during magnetic stimulation. *Electroencephalogr. Clin. Neurophysiol.*, **81**: 47–56.

Rushton, D.N. & Brindley, G.S. (1978). Properties of cortical electrical phosphenes. In *Frontiers in Visual Science*, ed. S.S.J. Cool & E.L. Smith, pp. 574–593. New York: Springer-Verlag.

Sadato, N., Pascual-Leone, A., Grafman, J. et al. (1996). Activation of the primary visual cortex by Braille reading in blind subjects. *Nature*, **380**: 526–528.

Schmidt, E.M., Bak, M.J., Hambrecht, F.T., Kufta, C.V., ORourke, D.K. & Vallabhanath, P. (1996). Feasibility of a visual prosthesis for the blind based on intracortical micro-stimulation of the visual cortex. *Brain*, **119**: 507–522.

Sherman, R. (1989). Stump and phantom limb pain. *Neurol. Clin.*, **7**: 249–264.

Sunderland, S. (1978). *Nerves and Nerve Injuries*. Edinburgh: Churchill Livingstone.

Uhl, F., Franzen, P., Podreka, I., Steiner, M. & Deecke, L. (1993). Increased regional cerebral blood flow in inferior occipital cortex and cerebellum of early blind humans. *Neurosci. Lett.*, **19**: 162–164.

Vargha-Khadem, F., Carr, L.J., Isaacs, E., Brett, E., Adams, C. & Mishkin, M. (1997). Onset of speech after left hemispherectomy in a nine-year-old boy. *Brain*, **120**: 159–182.

Wanet-Defalque, M.C., Veraart, C., De Volder, A. et al. (1988). High metabolic activity in the visual cortex of early blind human subjects. *Brain Res.*, **19**: 369–373.

Weeks, R., Horwitz, B., Aziz-Sultan, A. et al. (2000). A positron emission tomographic study of auditory localization in the congenitally blind. *J. Neurosci.*, **20**: 2664–2672.

Zangaladze, A., Epstein, C.M., Grafton, S.T. & Sathian, K. (1999). Involvement of visual cortex in tactile discrimination of orientation. *Nature*, **401**: 587–590.

Ziemann, U., Lonnecker, S., Steinhoff, B.J. & Paulus, W. (1996). Effects of antiepileptic drugs on motor cortex excitability in humans: a transcranial magnetic stimulation study. *Ann. Neurol.*, **40**: 367–378.

10

Therapeutic uses of rTMS

Chip M. Epstein[1] and John C. Rothwell[2]

[1]Department of Neurology, Emoy Clinic, Atlanta, GA, USA
[2]Sobell Department, Institute of Neurology, London, UK

Introduction

The basic rationale for attempting to use rTMS as a therapeutic tool is that it is known to produce effects on cerebral cortex that outlast the stimulus. The assumption is that, in some cases, it may be possible to manipulate these long-term effects either to reverse the pathological processes responsible for the condition, or to change the excitability of remaining healthy systems so that they can compensate for the underlying disturbance. In this chapter we will consider the use of rTMS in psychiatric conditions and in movement disorders. However, before discussing clinical details, we consider the available data about the long-term effects of rTMS in healthy subjects from the standpoint of designing therapeutic trials on patients. In particular, we ask first whether rTMS can ever be targeted accurately enough at specific neural populations to achieve a therapeutic effect and, second, whether the effects it produces will last long enough to be used as a clinical treatment.

Effect on neural circuits, local

Most of our knowledge about the actions of rTMS comes from studies of the motor cortex, although a smaller number of investigations suggest that the basic principles may apply to visual (Boorojerdi et al., 2000) or frontal (Speer et al., 2000) cortex. As summarized in previous chapters, much of this work has described the effects of rTMS in terms of the excitability of the corticospinal output to single pulse TMS. Periods of low frequency (1 Hz) rTMS at intensities below, or around, resting motor threshold reduce the excitability of the corticospinal system, whereas frequencies above 5 Hz increase excitability, particularly if high intensities are used. These studies also suggest that the duration and depth of the after-effect increase with the number of stimuli given during rTMS (Maeda et al., 2000; Touge et al., 2001). No motor cortex studies in healthy subjects have demonstrated that rTMS can be used to affect specific neural circuits. However, Siebner et al. (1999b) did show that 5 Hz rTMS at 90% resting motor threshold could increase short interval corticocortical inhibition and lengthen the silent period in patients with dystonia without affecting motor threshold or the slope of the input–output function of MEP size vs. stimulus intensity. Munchau et al. (2002) gave rTMS over premotor cortex and showed that 1 Hz stimulation at 80% active motor threshold could modulate the time course of short latency paired pulse inhibition/facilitation at very specific intervals (ISI = 6 and 7 ms) without affecting motor threshold.

The conclusion from these initial studies must be that some measure of specificity may be produced by rTMS. Perhaps this can be increased in future studies by applying rTMS in conjunction with other inputs so that the effects are focused to particular circuits. In the sensorimotor cortex this could be done by pairing TMS with afferent stimulation or movement (for review see Boroojerdi et al., 2001). In other systems it may be possible to use TMS in conjunction with pharmacological inputs to strengthen/weaken particular neurotransmitter circuits. Work by Ziemann and others (for review see Boroojerdi et al., 2001) has shown that the effects of TMS can be modulated by a variety of drugs in therapeutic use.

Effects on neural circuits, distance

Ever since its first application, it has been clear that TMS may produce effects not only at the site of stimulation but also at distant connected sites. Thus, stimulation of motor cortex affects spinal motoneurones and muscle via at least two synaptic linkages. The same is true of central connections. For example, stimulation over one motor cortex affects the excitability of the contralateral motor areas via transcallosal connections (Ferbert et al., 1992; Siebner et al., 2000), stimulation over the frontal eye fields affects metabolic activity in parieto-occipital cortex (Paus et al., 1997), and stimulation over premotor cortex affects excitability of primary motor cortex (Gerschlager et al., 2001).

From a therapeutic viewpoint, the importance of these effects is that they may allow us to overcome one of the limitations of present stimulators, the ability to stimulate deep structures selectively without activating surface areas that overlie the point of interest. Since it is not possible to focus the magnetic field from a stimulator, any attempt to stimulate directly structures deep in the brain is contaminated by activation of all the structures superficial to that point. This means that any attempt to stimulate, for example, basal ganglia or amygdala in isolation is virtually impossible.

However, the data above suggest that it might be possible to target deep nuclei by activating inputs from superficial areas of cortex. A recent example of the success of this approach is a study by Strafella et al. (2001). They found that short bursts of 10 Hz motor threshold rTMS given for 30 min over frontal cortex reduced raclopride binding in the ipsilateral caudate nucleus compared with rTMS over occipital cortex. The effect lasted for up to 60 min after completion of rTMS. This would be compatible with the idea that rTMS of frontal cortex increased release of dopamine in the head of the caudate and this reduced the binding of raclopride to dopamine receptors. In effect, particular neural circuits in a deep structure had been influenced by stimulation at a superficial site.

Finally, it is worth noting that one of the characteristics of TMS is that its effects are proportional to the level of neuronal excitability at the time the stimulus is applied. This is why MEPs evoked in actively contracting muscles are larger than those evoked in muscles at rest. The same principle applies to central pathways, Ferbert et al. (1992) showed that the excitability of the transcallosal connections between motor cortices changed depending on whether subjects contracted one or both hands in a task. This opens up the possibility of increasing the specificity of targeting particular connections by giving rTMS at the same time as subjects perform a particular behavioural task.

Time course of rTMS effects

Perhaps the most problematic question about the therapeutic use of rTMS concerns the duration of its effect. In all studies on healthy subjects, effects have lasted only 30 min to 1 hour. This is too short to be of any practical benefit in disease, and has led several groups to use repeated (daily) administration of rTMS so that the effects might summate and last much longer. Workers using rTMS to treat depression routinely give treatments with rTMS every day for 2 weeks, and then report effects that last for days and weeks afterwards. Unfortunately, basic studies of repeated administration of rTMS are sorely lacking, and there is little to substantiate the claim that repeated administration of rTMS over several days may extend the duration of its after-effects. Only one study by Meada et al. (2000) has addressed the question. They found that the facilitatory effect of 20 Hz stimulation of motor cortex was increased when given to subjects on a second occasion up to 1 week after the first test. However, even though the *size* of the effect was larger, it was not clear whether or not the duration of the effect had changed. The latter is probably more important for therapeutic use. More work needs to be done on this very important practical point.

rTMS, lasting effects on behaviour vs. lasting effects on physiology

The majority of the studies that have investigated the mechanism of action of rTMS use physiological rather than behavioural outcome measures. Thus, work on the motor system has commonly used MEP threshold, MEP amplitude, paired pulse testing or silent period duration as a measure of rTMS effects. In the visual cortex, phosphene threshold has been measured, and in other areas, metabolic and EEG changes have also been described. However, relatively few studies have attempted to test whether any of these measures is of behavioural relevance. Most studies using motor cortex rTMS have failed to find any evidence for changes in task performance, despite changes in all of the measures above. In healthy subjects, Chen et al. (1997) found no effect on finger tapping speed, Muellbacher et al. (2001) found no effect on maximum force or acceleration, and Siebner et al. (1999b) found no effect on handwriting. Touge et al. (2001) showed that, although rTMS could affect the size of MEPs evoked at rest, it had no effect on the amplitude of MEPs evoked during voluntary contraction.

If rTMS is to be of therapeutic use, it will be essential to demonstrate behavioural benefits. It may be that the motor cortex is particularly resistant to behavioural changes, or that the tests that have been applied are too gross to detect changes in healthy individuals. Repetitive TMS of other areas has been reported to produce clearer behavioural changes, although the robustness of many of the findings is questionable. For example, Pascual-Leone et al. (1994) initially described quite a large effect of frontal rTMS on mood in healthy subjects. This was replicated, but only using much more sensitive measures by George et al. (1994), and also as an incidental finding by Greenberg et al. (1997) in a study of OCD (see below). However, three recent attempts to confirm the findings have failed (Hajak et al., 1998; Nedjat & Folkers, 1999; Mosiman et al., 2000). Kosslyn et al. (1999) reported a reduction in visual imagery after rTMS of occipital cortex

Finally it should be realized that the brains of neurological patients may react differently to rTMS than those of healthy volunteers. The data of Siebner et al. (1999b) using 5 Hz rTMS of motor cortex found effects on cortical inhibition and handwriting only in dystonic patients but not in healthy subjects. Similarly, single pulse TMS of SMA was reported to have effects on movement times in patients with Parkinson's disease but not in healthy subjects (Cunnington et al., 1996). The conclusion is that it may be easier to demonstrate behavioural effects of TMS in a damaged nervous system than in healthy individuals.

In summary, our understanding of the basic physiology of rTMS is still at a rudimentary stage and, at present, provides only hints at the possible specificity and duration of its after-effects on different areas of cortex. However, clinical studies that have been carried out suggest that some measure of success may be achieved, and this should provide further impetus to understand basic mechanisms.

Treatment of psychiatric disorders with rTMS

Attempts to treat psychiatric disorders with electromagnetism are far from new. In the first century AD, Roman physicians applied torpedo fish (electric rays) for a wide variety of conditions, including depression (Kellaway, 1946). Improved understanding of electricity in the mid-eighteenth century led rapidly to expanded medical applications. By 1840 a 'magneto-electric device', attributed to DuBois Raymond, was being used on patients with psychiatric disorders in Europe and North America. At the end of the nineteenth century, many physicians routinely employed electrotherapy machines and magnetism, usually from horseshoe magnets. In 1902 Pollacsek and Beer, in Vienna, patented an electromagnetic coil that was placed at the vertex of the skull for the treatment of 'depression and neuroses'. Such techniques eventually fell into obscurity as their lack of efficacy became clear. But, within several years of its discovery, non-focal transcranial magnetic stimulation (TMS) from circular coils was being delivered to patients with psychiatric disorders. These early efforts appear to have had their origin in hopeful expectation rather than in a detailed scientific model of brain function. A few years later, however, the treatment of psychiatric disorders with TMS had been transformed by neuroimaging studies and by improved understanding of TMS effects. This section reviews the present data in regard to mood disorders, schizophrenia, and obsessive–compulsive disorder.

Mood disorders

In 1994, George et al. reviewed the results of functional neuroimaging studies in depressed patients. PET scans had demonstrated that depressed patients show consistent focal decreases in cerebral metabolism in the prefrontal lobes, and treatment data indicated that prefrontal changes in regional cerebral blood flow predicted response to electroconvulsive therapy (Nobler et al., 1994). George and Wassermann proposed that stimulation of dorsolateral prefrontal cortex (DLPFC) might have antidepressant effects (George & Wasserman, 1994). Shortly afterwards, changes in mood were reported for both normal volunteers and depressed patients with rTMS over DLPFC. At present DLPFC represents by far the most common site of TMS treatment for depression. An extensive theoretical basis for this choice has been elaborated in the valence theory of mood.

The valence theory of mood regulation proposes that emotional state reflects a balance of neuronal activation in the left and right prefrontal regions. Relative overactivity on the left, or underactivity on the right, would produce positive mood states, including happiness. Relative underactivity on the left, or overactivity on the right, would produce negative emotions such as fear, sadness and depression. This dichotomy is also expressed in behavioural terms, the left dorsolateral prefrontal cortex (DLPFC) mediates approach to a rewarding stimulus, whereas the right DLPFC mediates withdrawal from an aversive stimulus. At least six different lines of evidence support this hemispheric asymmetry for the regulation of emotion and behaviour in the prefrontal lobes.

1. Clinical observations have correlated depression with lesions of the left hemisphere, while mania is more likely to follow injury to the right hemisphere (Robinson et al., 1984; Sackeim et al., 1982; Starkstein et al., 1987).

Mood changes are most common with lesions that involve the frontal pole rather than more posterior regions (Robinson et al., 1984). Among patients who have mainly unilateral Parkinson's disease, depression is significantly associated with greater left hemisphere involvement (Fleminger, 1991; Starkstein et al., 1990).

2. Positron emission tomography (PET) studies have implicated multiple brain areas in the regulation and expression of mood and emotion. Decreased regional cerebral blood flow (rCBF) in the anterior cingulate and left dorsolateral prefrontal cortex is especially correlated with depression (Baker et al., 1997; Baxter et al., 1989; Bench et al., 1995, Elliott et al., 1997; George et al., 1994; Martinot et al., 1990; Mayberg et al., 1997), and recovery to euthymia is accompanied by increases of rCBF in these same areas (Bench et al., 1995).

3. Quantitative EEG studies have repeatedly shown a relative or absolute increase in resting alpha activity over the left frontal region of depressed patients (Ahern & Schwartz, 1985; Davidson, 1992; Henriques & Davidson, 1990; Saletu et al., 1995; Tucker et al., 1981). Increased amplitude of alpha background, or 'synchronization', is considered a sign of reduced activation in the underlying cortex, thereby suggesting that cerebral underactivity in the left prefrontal region accompanies depression.

4. Assessments of mood during intracarotid amytal tests, which anaesthetize each cerebral hemisphere separately, indicate elation with right-sided anaesthesia and depression with left-sided injections (Christianson et al., 1993; Lee et al., 1990).

5. The antidepressant effects of vagus nerve stimulation appear to be mediated by the left vagus nerve, which connects ipsilaterally through the locus coeruleus and parabrachial nucleus to large areas of the forebrain. The latter include limbic regions thought to be involved in mood regulation and expression (Rush et al., 2000).

6. Finally, the effects of rTMS on mood support hemispheric asymmetry for regulation of emotion.

Interpreting the results of TMS on mood depends on knowledge about the differential effects of fast and slow stimulation frequencies (see Introduction). Assuming that stimulation-induced plasticity can modulate an imbalance of prefrontal activation in mood disorders, the valence theory would predict their alleviation by different types of TMS in specific areas. Depression might be improved by either fast left or slow right prefrontal TMS. Mania might be treated by either slow left or fast right TMS.

Published studies support three of these four possible combinations:

- Open and double-blind trials of fast rTMS over the left prefrontal cortex (Berman et al., 2000; Epstein et al., 1998; George et al., 1995, 1997, 2000; Pascual-Leone et al., 1996b) have demonstrated a significant fall in Hamilton depression scores among patients with both bipolar and unipolar depression. Benefit from fast rTMS has been observed after a single session (Szuba et al., 2001).
- Trials of slow TMS over the right DLPFC have also been shown to improve depression (Klein et al., 1999).
- Fast right rTMS had greater efficacy in alleviating symptoms of mania than fast left rTMS (Grisaru et al., 1998).
- In a comparison of fast and slow left prefrontal rTMS, better response to 20 Hz stimulation was associated with the degree of baseline hypometabolism, whereas response to 1 Hz rTMS tended to be associated with baseline hypermetabolism in that region (Kimbrell et al., 1999).

Thus the antidepressant effect of fast rTMS over the left DLPFC is consistent with therapeutic excitation of a relatively underactive left hemisphere in depression. The antimanic effect of fast rTMS over the right DLPFC is consistent with activation of an underactive right hemisphere in mania. The antidepressant effect of slow rTMS over the right DLPFC is consistent with inhibition of a relatively overactive right hemisphere in depression. Since the apparent benefit from TMS treatment of mood disorders persists for weeks or months, the cortical effects of multiple treatments may summate to produce much longer-lasting alterations in cortical excitability than those demonstrated with rTMS of the motor cortex. Long-term potentiation has been suggested as the neurophysiological basis of these changes, but has not yet been rigorously demonstrated.

Not all the arguments for the valence theory of mood are universally accepted. In particular, the incidence and lateralization of mood effects from cerebral lesions have remained controversial for more than 100 years, and many PET studies of depression have failed to show lateralized changes. Vagus nerve stimulation has not been tested on the right side sufficiently to determine whether its antidepressant effects are truly lateralized. The DLPFC has an important role in working memory processes, which show a different type of hemispheric lateralization and appear completely unrelated to the regulation of mood (Wagner et al., 1998). A few TMS studies with limited numbers of patients have failed to corroborate the results noted above. Furthermore, electroencephalographic and neuroimaging studies have demonstrated that TMS has effects at brain areas remote from the point of stimulation (Fox et al., 1997; Paus et al., 1997; Schutter et al., 2001) so that clinical changes may arise from unexpected sites.

A theory of lateralized mood regulation is not immediately compatible with the large number of studies that relate depression and mania to widely distributed systems of neurotransmitters. However, these vastly different models may be linked by animal studies and by the observation that strokes in the two hemispheres produce quite different long-term changes in S2 serotonin receptor binding (Mayberg et al., 1998). The degree of asymmetry showed a significant correlation with severity of depression scores. Thus the neurotransmitter systems linked to depression may express functionally important asymmetries under pathological conditions.

Animal studies of TMS are limited by physical difficulties in constructing very small magnetic coils (Cohen & Cuffin, 1991), because use of a coil much larger than the brain drastically reduces the efficiency of stimulation and prevents the focal application that is the distinguishing feature of most human research (Weissman et al., 1992). Many animal studies may therefore have inadvertently involved effects much smaller than those of a comparable magnetic field in humans. None the less, TMS in rats appears to produce changes in beta-adrenergic receptors and monoamines that are not duplicated by sham stimulation (Ben-Shachar et al., 1997; Fleischmann et al., 1996), and to alter gene expression in astroglia and in specific brain regions (Fujiki & Steward, 1997; Ji et al., 1998). Many, but not all, of these changes are similar to those produced by ECT.

An intriguing paradox is presented by several controlled studies of prefrontal TMS in normal volunteers, which showed acute effects on mood (George et al., 1996; Martin et al., 1997; Pascual-Leone et al., 1996a) but in an unexpected direction. For the normal subjects, who were tested shortly after stimulation, left-sided TMS tended to decrease happiness, and right-sided TMS to decrease sadness. These immediate effects are diametrically opposite to those reported with depressed patients. At present, any explanation for this dissociation is entirely speculative. One possibility is that in normal individuals, homeostatic mechanisms resist any acute perturbations of the neuronal activity that regulates mood, and these mechanisms transiently overcompensate in the brief time frame of the acute studies. A model for such effects could be the prolonged hyperpolarization that follows epileptic seizures.

Schizophrenia

Schizophrenia is characterized by both negative and positive symptoms. Among the most flagrant of the latter are auditory hallucinations. The experience of auditory hallucinations has been correlated on neuroimaging with increased activity in the primary auditory cortex of the middle and superior temporal gyri, along with speech areas in the left temporal-parietal region (d'Alfonso et al., in press). Based on the hypothesis that reduction of the neuronal activity in these regions might alleviate auditory hallucinations, several studies have involved low-frequency rTMS to left temporal–parietal and auditory cortex. Hoffman et al. (1999) reported improvement in hallucination severity among three of three patients in an open label study and subsequently in eight of 12 hallucinating patients in a sham-controlled study of slow rTMS to the left temporal–parietal region (Hoffman et al., 2000). D'Alfonso et al. (in press) applied TMS at 1 Hz and 80% of motor threshold to the region of the left auditory cortex for a total of ten daily sessions in eight treatment-resistant schizophrenic patients. Auditory hallucinations improved significantly, but did not remit completely in any of their patients.

Obsessive–compulsive disorder (OCD)

OCD is characterized by recurrent thoughts, feelings, or images that compel repetitive behaviours. These phenomena are not experienced as pleasant. Recent models of OCD postulate abnormal activity in cortico-striatal-pallido-thalamic (CSPT) circuits, which include orbitofrontal cortex and DLPFC. Regional cerebral blood flow studies (Rauch et al., 1994) and surgical lesions (Lippitz et al., 1999) suggest a critical role for the right hemisphere. Using 20 Hz rTMS at 80% of motor threshold to treat a group of 12 OCD patients, Greenberg et al. (1997) found a significant reduction of compulsive urges with right lateral prefrontal stimulation. This effect lasted at least 8 hours. However, there was no significant change after left prefrontal or parieto-occipital stimulation. Interpreting these results in more detail is complicated by the apparent existence of separate ventral and dorsal CSPT pathways, with potentially opposite effects on OCD symptoms. Fast right rTMS produced brief immediate mood elevations in these non-depressed patients, just as it has in normal volunteers.

Treatment of movement disorders with rTMS

Most of the published studies on rTMS in patients with movement disorders have focused on the motor cortex, with the simple rationale that it might be useful to try to increase motor cortical excitability in patients with hypokinetic disorders, whereas it might be appropriate to decrease excitability in hyperkinetic disorders. As we shall see below, the logic of this approach is not entirely clear. Other groups have targeted frontal areas of cortex. Given that this is now known to produce changes in levels of dopamine in the basal ganglia (Strafella et al., 2001), there may now be a *post-hoc* justification for the method, although it is fair to say that this was not clear at the time the studies were performed.

Parkinson's disease

Pascual-Leone et al. (1994) were the first to suggest that 5 Hz rTMS of motor cortex at 90% resting threshold could improve performance in the grooved pegboard test in patients with Parkinson's disease, particularly if they were in the OFF state after overnight withdrawal of l-DOPA. The stimuli were applied during performance of the test, and given the intensity used it is surprising that no overt movements were evoked during active movement. When the experiment was repeated by Ghabra et al. (1999), overt movements were clear, and these interfered with task performance in many of the patients. Decreasing the stimulus intensity prevented this from happening but did not improve performance in the task. Tergau et al. (1999) also applied rTMS (500 stimuli at 90% resting threshold to motor cortex) at 1, 5, 10 and 20 Hz, and again reported no change in performance on a walking task nor on a simple reaction time task. In contrast to these negative results, Siebner et al. (1999) gave patients 2250 stimuli at 90% resting threshold and 5 Hz and reported an improvement in performance of an arm pointing task. Patients' movements became faster and smoother without loss of accuracy. A sham stimulation session where the coil was applied at 45 degrees to the mid frontal cortex had no effect on task performance.

There are several problems with all these studies. First, the main logic of the intervention is to try to increase motor cortical excitability in order to compensate in some way for bradykinetic movement commands. However, studies with single pulse TMS have suggested that, in the resting state, the slope of the input–output curve relating stimulus intensity to MEP amplitude is steeper in patients than in healthy subjects (Valls-Sole et al., 1994). If anything, this suggests a basal hyper- rather than hypo-excitability of motor cortex in Parkinson's disease. In any case, rTMS at 5 Hz is not thought to be the most effective way of increasing cortical excitability. Maeda et al. (2000) found that, in most healthy subjects, 5 Hz stimulation failed to produce any change in cortical excitability; only 10 or 20 Hz reliably increased excitability.

The second problem in such studies, especially those that give positive results, is lack of good control data. Reducing the stimulus intensity by tilting the coil away from the scalp, or even removing it from the head, gives patients a clear sign that the sham treatment is not as strong as the real treatment. Given the marked and persistent improvements that can be observed after placebo treatments, it is vital to control for patient expectation as well as possible.

The studies on motor cortex above have used only a single application of rTMS. Two other groups have employed repeated treatment designs after stimulation of frontal areas of cortex in order to increase the overall efficacy of treatment. Both Mally and Stone (1999a, b) and Shimamoto et al. (2001) have employed a variety of stimulus rates, intensities and number of stimuli given through a round coil. They have reported substantial improvements in clinical scores that last weeks or months after the end of treatment. However, further control trials are needed to remove possible contaminating placebo effects.

Dystonia and Gilles de la Tourette's syndrome

There is some evidence for increased excitability of motor cortex in both these conditions. In dystonia, the slope of the input–output relation between stimulus intensity and MEP amplitude is steeper than normal, as is the relation between level of background contraction and MEP amplitude. In both dystonia and Tourette's syndrome, paired pulse tests reveal reduced short latency intracortical inhibition. On this basis, two groups have tried to reduce motor cortex excitability by using low frequency rTMS.

Siebner et al. (1999) gave 1800 stimuli at 90% resting threshold and 1 Hz to motor cortex and found that this increased levels of intracortical inhibition in patients, increased the duration of the silent period and improved handwriting for up to 30 min. There was no effect on any of these parameters in healthy controls. Karp et al. (1997) reported a similar improvement in tics after 1 Hz stimulation of motor cortex in patients with Tourette's syndrome.

REFERENCES

Ahern, G.L. & Schwartz, G.E. (1985). Differential lateralization for positive and negative emotion in the human brain, EEG spectral analysis. *Neuropsychologia*, **23**: 745–755.

Baker, S.C., Frith, C.D. & Dolan, R.J. (1997). The interaction between mood and cognitive function studied with PET. *Psychol. Med.*, **27**: 565–578.

Baxter, L.R.J., Schwartz, J.M., Phelps, M.E. et al. (1989). Reduction of prefrontal cortex glucose metabolism common to three types of depression. *Arch. Gen. Psychiatry*, **46**: 243–250.

Ben-Shachar, D., Belmaker, R.H., Grisaru, N. & Klein, E. (1997). Transcranial magnetic stimulation induces alterations in brain monoamines. *J. Neural. Transmiss.*, **104**: 191–197.

Bench, C.J., Friston, K.J., Brown, R.G., Scott, L.C., Frackowiak, R.S. & Dolan, R.J. (1994). The anatomy of melancholia – focal abnormalities of cerebral blood flow in major depression. *Psychol. Med.*, **22**: 607–615.

Bench, C.J., Frackowiak, R.S. & Dolan, R.J. (1995). Changes in regional cerebral blood flow on recovery from depression. *Psychol. Med.*, **25**: 247–261.

Berman, R.M., Narasimhan, M., Sanacora, G. et al. (2000). A randomized clinical trial of repetitive transcranial magnetic stimulation in the treatment of major depression. *Biol. Psychiatry*, **47**: 332–337.

Boroojerdi, B., Prager, A., Muellbacher, W. & Cohen, L.G. (2000). Reduction of human visual cortex excitability using 1 Hz transcranial magnetic stimulation. *Neurology*, **54**: 1529–1531.

Boroojerdi, B., Ziemann, U., Chen, R., Butefisch, C.M. & Cohen, L.G. (2001). Mechanisms underlying motor cortex plasticity. *Muscle Nerve*, **24**: 602–613.

Chen, R., Classen, J., Gerloff, C. et al. (1997). Depression of motor cortex excitability by low-frequency transcranial magnetic stimulation. *Neurology*, **48**: 1398–1403.

Christianson, S.A., Saisa, J., Garvill, J. & Silfvenius, H. (1993). Hemisphere inactivation and mood-state changes. *Brain Cogni.*, **23**: 127–144.

Cohen, D. & Cuffin, B.N. (1991). Developing a more focal magnetic stimulator. Part I, Some basic principles. *J. Clin. Neurophysiol.*, **8**: 102–111.

Cunnington, R., Iansek, R., Thickbroom, G.W. et al. (1996). Effect of magnetic stimulation over the supplementary motor area on movements in Parkinson's disease. *Brain*, **119**: 815–822.

d'Alfonso, A.A.L., Aleman, A., Kessels, R.P.C. et al. (2002). Transcranial magnetic stimulation of left auditory cortex in patients with schizophrenia, effects on hallucinations and neurocognition. *J. Neuropsych. Clin. Neurosci.* (in press).

Davidson, R.J. (1992). Anterior cerebral asymmetry and the nature of emotion. *Brain Cogn.*, **20**: 125–151.

Elliott, R., Baker, S.C., Rogers, R.D. et al. (1997). Prefrontal dysfunction in depressed patients performing a complex planning task, a study using positron emission tomography. *Psychol. Med.*, **27**: 931–942.

Epstein, C., Figiel, G.S., McDonald, W.M., Amazon-Leece, J. & Figiel, L. (1998). Rapid-rate transcranial magnetic stimulation in young and middle-aged refractory depressed patients. *Psychiat. Ann.*, **28**: 36–39.

Ferbert, A., Priori, A., Rothwell, J.C., Day, B.L., Colebatch, J.G. & Marsden, C.D. (1992). Interhemispheric inhibition of the human motor cortex. *J. Physiol.*, **453**, 525–546.

Fleischmann, A., Sternheim, A., Etgen, A.M., Li, C., Grisaru, N. & Belmaker, R.H. (1996). Transcranial magnetic stimulation downregulates beta-adrenoreceptors in rat cortex. *J. Neural. Transmiss.*, **103**: 1361–1366.

Fleminger, S. (1991). Left-sided Parkinson's disease is associated with greater anxiety and depression. *Psychol. Med.*, **21**: 629–638.

Fox, P., Ingham, R., George, M.S. et al. (1997). Imaging human intra-cerebral connectivity by PET during TMS. *Neuroreport*, **8**: 2787–2891.

Fujiki, M. & Steward, O. (1997). High frequency transcranial magnetic stimulation mimics the effects of ECS in upregulating astroglial gene expression in the murine CNS. *Mol. Brain Res.*, **44**: 301–308.

George, M.S. & Wasserman, E.M. (1994). Rapid-rate transcranial magnetic stimulation and ECT. *Convuls. Ther.*, **10**: 251–254.

George, M.S., Ketter, T.A. & Post, R.M. (1994). Prefrontal cortex dysfunction in clinical depression. *Depression*, **2**: 59–72.

George, M.S., Wassermann, E.M., Williams, W.A. et al. (1995). Daily repetitive transcranial magnetic stimulation (rTMS) improves mood in depression. *Neuroreport*, **6**: 1853–1856.

George, M.S., Wassermann, E.M., Williams, W.A. et al. (1996). Changes in mood and hormone levels after rapid-rate transcranial magnetic stimulation (rTMS) of the prefrontal cortex. *J. Neuropsych. Clin. Neurosci.*, **8**: 172–180.

George, M.S., Wassermann, E.M., Kimbrell, T.A. et al. (1997). Mood improvement following daily left prefrontal repetitive transcranial magnetic stimulation in patients with depression, a placebo-controlled crossover trial. *Am. J. Psychiatry*, **154**: 1752–1756.

George, M.S., Nahas, Z., Molloy, M. et al. (2000). A controlled trial of daily left prefrontal cortex TMS for treating depression. *Biol. Psychiatry*, **48**: 962–970.

Gerschlager, W., Siebner, H.R. & Rothwell, J.C. (2001). Decreased corticospinal excitability after subthreshold 1 Hz rTMS over lateral premotor cortex. *Neurology*, **57**: 449–455.

Ghabra, M.B., Hallett, M. & Wassermann, E.M. (1999). Simultaneous repetitive transcranial magnetic stimulation does not speed fine movement in PD. *Neurology*, **52**: 768–770.

Greenberg, B.D., George, M.S., Martin, J.D. et al. (1997). Effect of prefrontal repetitive transcranial magnetic stimulation in obsessive-compulsive disorder, a preliminary study. *Am. J. Psychiatry*, **154**, 867–869.

Grisaru, N., Chudakov, B., Yaroslavsky, Y. & Belmaker, R.H. (1998). Transcranial magnetic stimulation in mania, a controlled study. *Am. J. Psychiatry*, **155**: 1608–1610.

Hajak, G., Cohrs, S., Tergau, F. et al. (1998). Sleep and rTMS. *Electroencephal. Clin. Neurophysiol.*, **107**: 92.

Henriques, J.B. & Davidson, R.J. (1990). Regional brain electrical asymmetries discriminate between previously depressed and healthy control subjects. *J. Abnormal Psychol.*, **99**: 22–31.

Hoffman, R.E., Boutros, N.N., Berman, R.M. et al. (1999). Transcranial magnetic stimulation of left temporo-parietal cortex in three patients reporting hallucinated 'voices'. *Biol. Psychiatry*, **46**: 130–132.

Hoffman, R.E., Boutros, N.N, Hu, S., Berman, R.M., Krystal, J.H. & Charney, D.S. (2000). Transcranial magnetic stimulation and auditory hallucinations in schizophrenia. *Lancet*, 355.

Ji, R.R., Schlaepfer, T.E., Aizenman, C.D. et al. (1998). Repetitive transcranial magnetic stimulation activates specific regions in rat brain. *Proc. Natl Acad. Sci., USA*, **95**: 15635–15640.

Karp, B.I., Wassermann, E.M., Porter, S. & Hallett, M. (1997). Transcranial magnetic stimulation acutely decreases motor tics. *Neurology*, **48**: A397.

Kellaway, P. (1946). The part played by electric fish in the early history of bioelectricity and electrotherapy. *Bull. Hist. Med.*, **20**: 112–137.

Kimbrell, T.A., Little, J.T., Dunn, R.T. et al. (1999). Frequency dependence of antidepressant response to left prefrontal repetitive transcranial magnetic stimulation (rTMS) as a function of baseline cerebral glucose metabolism. *Biol. Psychiatry*, **46**: 1603–1613.

Klein, E., Kreinen, I., Chistyakov, A. et al. (1999). Therapeutic efficacy of right prefrontal slow repetitive transcranial magnetic stimulation in major depression. A double blind controlled study. *Arch. Gen. Psychiatry*, **56**: 315–320.

Kosslyn, S.M., Pascual-Leone, A., Felician, O. et al. (1999). The role of area 17 in visual imagery, convergent evidence from PET and rTMS. *Science*, **284**: 167–170.

Lee, G.P., Loring, D.W., Meader, K.J. & Brooks, B.B. (1990). Hemispheric specialization for emotional expression, a reexamination of results from intracarotid administration of sodium amobarbital. *Brain Cogn.*, **12**, 267–280.

Lippitz, B.E., Mindus, P., Meyerson, B.A., Kihlstrom, L. & Lindquist, C. (1999). Lesion topography and outcome after thermocapsulotomy or gamma knife capsulotomy for obsessive-compulsive disorder, relevance of the right hemisphere. *Neurosurgery*, **44**: 452–458.

Maeda, F., Keenan, J.P., Tormos, J.M., Topka, H. & Pascual-Leone, A. (2000). Interindividual variability of the modulatory effects of repetitive transcranial magnetic stimulation on cortical excitability. *Exp. Brain Res.*, **133**: 425–430.

Mally, J. & Stone, T.W. (1999a). Improvement in parkinsonian symptoms after repetitive transcranial magnetic stimulation. *J. Neurol. Sci.*, **162**, 179–184.

Mally, J. & Stone, T.W. (1999b). Therapeutic and 'dose dependent' effect of repetitive microelectroshock induced by transcranial magnetic stimulation in Parkinson's disease. *J. Neurosci. Res.*, **57**: 935–940.

Martin, J.D., George, M.S., Greenberg, B.D. et al. (1997). Mood effects of prefrontal repetitive high-frequency TMS in healthy volunteers. *CNS Spectrums*, **2**: 53–68.

Martinot, J.L., Hardy, P., Feline, A. et al. (1990). Left prefrontal glucose hypometabolism in the depressed state, a confirmation. *Am. J. Psychiatry*, **147**: 1313–1317.

Mayberg, H.S., Brannan, S.K., Mahurin, R.K. et al. (1997). Cingulate function in depression, a potential predictor of treatment response. *Neuroreport*, **8**: 1057–1061.

Mayberg, H.S., Robinson, R.G., Wong, D.F. et al. (1998). PET imaging of cortical S2 serotonin receptors after stroke, lateralized changes and relationship to depression. *Am. J. Psychiatry*, **145**: 937–943.

Mossiman, U.P., Toscji, N., Kresse, A.E., Post, A. & Keck, M.E. (2000). Effects of repetitive transcranial magnetic stimulation of left prefrontal cortex in healthy volunteers. *Psychiat. Res.*, **94**: 251–256.

Muellbacher, W., Ziemann, U., Boroojerdi, B. & Hallett, M. (2001). Effect of low frequency TMS on motor excitability and basic motor behaviour. *Clin. Neurophysiol.*, **111**: 1002–1007.

Munchau, A., Bloem, B., Irlbacjer, K., Trimble, M. & Rothwell, J.C. (2002). Functional connectivity of human motor and premotor cortex explored with transcranial magnetic stimulation. *J. Neurosci.*, **22**: 554–561.

Nedjat, S. & Folkers, H.W. (1999). Induction of a reversible state of hypomania by rapid rate transcranial stimulation over the left prefrontal lobe. *J. ECT*, **15**: 166–168.

Nobler, M.S., Sackeim, H.A., Prohovnik, I. et al. (1994). Regional cerebral blood flow in mood disorders. III. Treatment and clinical response. *Arch. Gen. Psychiatry*, **51**: 884–897.

Pascual-Leone, A., Valls-Sole, J., Brasil-Neto, J.P. cammarota, A., Grafman, J. & Hallett, M. (1994). Akinesia in Parkinson's disease. II. Shortening of choice reaction time and movement time with subthreshold repetitive transcranial motor cortex stimulation. *Neurology*, **44**: 892–898.

Pascual-Leone, A., Catala, M.D. & Pascual-Leone, A. (1996a). Lateralized effect of rapid-rate transcranial magnetic stimulation of the prefrontal cortex on mood. *Neurology*, **46**: 499–502.

Pascual-Leone, A., Rubio, B., Pallard, F. & Catalan, M.D. (1996b). Rapid-rate transcranial magnetic stimulation of left dorsolateral prefrontal cortex in drug-resistant depression. *Lancet*, **348**: 233–237.

Paus, T. Jech, R., Thompson, C.J., Comeau, R., Peters, T. & Evans, A.C. (1997). Transcranial magnetic stimulation during positron emission tomography, a new method for studying connectivity of the human cerebral cortex. *J. Neurosci.*, **17**: 3178–3184.

Rauch, S.L., Jenike, M.A., Alpert, N.M. et al. (1994). Regional cerebral blood flow measured during symptom provocation in obsessive-compulsive disorder using oxygen 15-labeled carbon dioxide and positron emission tomography. *Arch. Gen. Psychiatry*, **51**: 62–70.

Robinson, R.G., Kubos, K.L., Starr, L.B., Rao, K. & Price, T.R. (1984). Mood disorders in stroke patients. Importance of location of lesion. *Brain*, **107**: 81–93.

Rush, A.J., George, M.S., Sackeim, H.A. et al. (2000). Vagus nerve stimulation (VNS) for treatment-resistant depressions, a multicenter study. *Biol. Psychiatry*, **47**: 276–286.

Sackeim, H.A., Greenberg, M.S., Weiman, A.L., Gur, R.C., Hungerbuhler, J.P. & Geschwind, N. (1982). Hemispheric asymmetry in the expression of positive and negative emotions. Neurologic evidence. *Arch. Neurol.*, **39**: 210–218.

Saletu, B., Brandstatter, N., Metka, M. et al. (1995). Double-blind, placebo-controlled, hormonal, syndromal and EEG mapping studies with transdermal oestradiol therapy in menopausal depression. *Psychopharmacology*, **122**, 321–329.

Schutter, D.J.L.G., van Honk, J., d'Alfonso, A.L., Postma, A. & de Haan, E.H.F. (2001). Effects of slow rTMS at the right dorsolateral prefrontal cortex on EEG asymmetry and mood. *Neuroreport*, **12**: 445–447.

Shimamoto, H., Takasaki, K., Shigemori, M., Imaizumi, T., Ayabe, M. & Shoji, H. (2001). Therapeutic effect and mechanism of repetitive transcranial magnetic stimulation in Parkinson's disease. *J. Neurol.*, **248**: III 48–52.

Siebner, H.R., Mentschel, C., Auer, C. & Conrad, B. (1999a). Repetitive transcranial magnetic stimulation has a beneficial effect on bradykinesia in Parkinson's disease. *Neuroreport*, **10**: 589–594.

Siebner, H.R., Tormos, J.M., Ceballos-Baumann, A.O. et al. (1999b). Low frequency repetitive transcranial magnetic stimulation of the motor cortex in writers' cramp. *Neurology*, **52**: 529–537.

Siebner, H.R., Peller, M., Willoch, F. et al. (2000). Lasting cortical activation after repetitive TMS of the motor cortex, a glucose metabolic study. *Neurology*, **22**: 956–962.

Speer, A.M., Willis, M.W., Herscovitch, P. et al. (2000). Intensity-dependent rCBF changes during 1 Hz rTMS over the left primary motor and prefrontal cortices. *Biol. Psychiatry*, **47**: 105S.

Starkstein, S.E., Robinson, R.G. & Price, T.R. (1987). Comparison of cortical and subcortical lesions in the production of poststroke mood disorders. *Brain*, **110**: 1045–1059.

Starkstein, S.E., Preziosi, T.J., Bolduc, P.L. & Robinson, R.G. (1990). Depression in Parkinson's disease. *J. Nerv. Ment. Dis.*, **178**: 27–31.

Strafella, A.P., Paus, T., Barrett, J. & Dagher, A. (2001). Transcranial magnetic stimulation of the human prefrontal cortex induces dopamine release in the caudate nucleus. *J. Neurosci.*, **21**: RC157.

Szuba, M.P., O'Reardon, J.P., Rai, A.S. et al. (2001). Acute mood and thyroid stimulating hormone effects of transcranial magnetic stimulation in major depression. *Biol. Psychiatry*, **50**: 22–27.

Tergau, F., Wassermann, E.M., Paulus, W. & Ziemann, U. (1999). Lack of clinical improvement in patients with Parkinson's disease after low and high frequency repetitive transcranial magnetic stimulation. *Electroencephalgr. Clin. Neurophysiol.*, **51** (suppl.): 281–288.

Touge, T., Gerschlager, W., Brown, P. & Rothwell, J.C. (2001). Are the after-effects of low-frequency rTMS on motor cortex excitability due to changes in the efficacy of cortical synapses? *Clin. Neurophysiol.*, **112**: 2138.

Tucker, D.M., Stenslie, C.E., Roth, R.S. & Shearer, S.L. (1981). Right frontal lobe activation and right hemisphere performance. Decrement during a depressed mood. *Arch. Gen. Psychiatry*, **38**: 169–174.

Valls-Sole, J., Pascual-Leone, A., Brasil-Neto, J.P., Cammorat, A., McShane, L. & Hallett, M. (1994). Abnormal facilitation of the response to transcranial magnetic stimulation in patients with Parkinson's disease. *Neurology*, **44**: 735–741.

Wagner, A.D., Poldrack, R.A., Eldridge, L.L., Desmond, J.E., Glover, G.H. & Gabrieli, J.D. (1998). Material-specific lateralization of prefrontal activation during episodic encoding and retrieval. *Neuroreport*, **9**: 3711–3717.

Wassermann, E.M. (1998). Risk and safety of repetitive transcranial magnetic stimulation, report and suggested guidelines from the International Workshop on the Safety of Repetitive Transcranial Magnetic Stimulation, June 5–7, 1996. *Electroencephalogr. Clin. Neurophysiol.*, **108**: 1–16.

Weissman J.D., Epstein C.M. & Davey K.R. (1992). Magnetic brain stimulation and brain size, relevance to animal studies. *Electroencephalogr. Clin. Neurophysiol.*, **85**: 215–219.

Ziemann, U., Paulus, W. & Rothenburger, A. (1997). Decreased motor inhibition in Tourette's disorder, evidence from transcranial magnetic stimulation. *Am. J. Psychiatry*, **154**: 1277–1284.

11

Rehabilitation

David Gow,[1] Chris Fraser[2] and Shaheen Hamdy[1]

[1]Department of GI Sciences and Medicine, University of Manchester, Hope Hospital, Eccles Old Road, Salford M6 8HD, UK
[2]Department of Medicine, Royal Bolton Hospital Farnworth, Bolton BL4 OJR, UK

Introduction

Neurological rehabilitation can be defined as the institution of therapy to maximize the degree of recovery within a given individual following a neurological insult. It has been suggested that neurological rehabilitation is based around the phenomenon of neuronal plasticity which is thought to play a crucial role in recovery from neurological injury and in particular stroke. For the design and implementation of effective rehabilitative strategies it is essential to consider three components: (i) an understanding of the nature of the initial insult, (ii) an understanding of the manner in which recovery may occur and (iii) an objective measure of the result of therapeutic interventions employed.

Each of these components can be addressed in part with transcranial magnetic stimulation and the area of recovery from disability following stroke has received most attention. In particular, TMS has been used to investigate motor reorganization following stroke, which has led to a greater understanding of the potential recovery patterns that occur. TMS may also have a role in the induction of plasticity itself and has potential to become a rehabilitative tool in recovery from neurological injury.

In this chapter we will review how TMS has been utilized in the study of spontaneous recovery, explore the role of TMS in quantifying rehabilitation and examine how TMS has been applied to studies aimed at influencing the recovery process with therapeutic intervention.

Mechanisms of recovery from unilateral hemispheric stroke

Unilateral hemispheric stroke (UHS) has many advantages as a model for investigating recovery from neurological injury. First, it is a common disorder leading to a large potential target group. Second, the nature of the insult is radiologically and clinically definable. Lastly, it allows the unique opportunity for the study of the pattern of recovery associated with damage to anatomically discrete areas of the brain. To comprehensively review recovery following UHS, we will consider the evidence for contralateral limb and midline structure dysfunction separately.

TMS and contralateral limb recovery
Insight from non-TMS studies

In contrast to the focal investigation of the motor cortex and its immediate connections that TMS allows, other brain imaging modalities have the advantage of being able to investigate the whole cerebral matrix. We will review the data from functional neuroimaging concentrating on positron emission tomography and functional magnetic resonance imaging, two techniques that are particularly suited to concurrently assessing multiple cerebral domains.

Positron emission tomography (PET)

Much of the poststroke PET work comes from studies conducted by the MRC cyclotron unit in London. In the early 1990s this group presented a collection of three papers, which examined cerebral activation during movements of the affected hand following recovery from UHS. They initially showed in addition to activation of the affected hemisphere (AH) consistent coactivation of the unaffected hemisphere (UH) with voluntary activity of the affected hand in comparison to the unaffected hand (Chollet et al., 1991). Further studies compared the activation seen with movement of the recovered hand with control populations of normal individuals (Weiller et al., 1992, 1993). The areas activated in these studies were numerous and varied and included UH cerebellum, premotor cortex, primary sensorimotor cortex and, bilaterally, the anterior inferior parietal lobe in addition to supplementary motor area (SMA). These findings have, in part, been further validated by other PET workers, e.g. Seitz et al. (1998) and Nelles et al. (1999a,b).

It is worth noting that the findings of Weiller et al. (1993) were possibly contaminated by the presence of mirror movements. It should, however, be remembered that the presence of mirror movements is, to some degree, related to the task that is performed but, where present, they raise doubt over the validity of observed activation in the UH. This has led to a 'chicken and egg' scenario, as to whether the mirror movements were a cause of the UH activation seen during affected limb movements or a reflection of the ipsilateral contribution to recovery (Weiller et al., 1993). The latter point is of interest as the observed mirror movements may reflect a degree of motor outflow operating within a system where the normal interhemispheric inhibitory balance has been altered. Nevertheless, activation observed within the UH must be considered more secure if mirror movements are not present. Our understanding of this area has been furthered to some degree with functional magnetic resonance imaging (fMRI) as will be described below.

Functional magnetic resonance imaging (fMRI)

In considering fMRI protocols in this section we will essentially be focusing on the technique of blood oxygen level dependent imaging (BOLD). Using this technique Cramer et al. (1997) showed similar findings to the PET work in terms of degree and areas of activation seen with movements of the recovered hand. However, only one in ten of the subjects displayed mirror movements in this paper and, as the population in question had an excellent functional outcome, this suggested that the ipsilateral activity may be a constituent of recovery rather than a consequence of mirror activation (Cramer et al., 1997). Further fMRI evidence presented by Cao et al. (1998) showed UH activation in the sensorimotor cortex during sequential finger movements in a group of patients with moderate–good recovery from hemiparetic stroke.

The conclusion from the available functional imaging data is that bilateral hemispheric recruitment takes place following UHS with multiple cerebral regions playing a role in recovered affected limb movement. It is perhaps reasonable at this point to discuss the area of recovery from poststroke aphasia in which activation of the UH has also been observed. The initial PET studies carried out in both Wernicke's and Broca's aphasia found an increased degree of right hemisphere activation in affected individuals compared to controls during language tasks (Weiller et al., 1995; Buckner et al., 1996). These papers suggested a role for the UH in recovery from poststroke aphasia. This work is contradicted to some degree by the PET study of Heiss et al. (1999) and the fMRI study of Rosen et al. (2000), which, although showing consistent activation of the right hemisphere, noted that recovery was, however, greatest in the group with residual perilesional activity in the AH. Overall, the aphasia work reveals increased UH activation during language tasks compared to controls, but seems to suggest that it is the degree of residual activity within the damaged left hemisphere, which mitigates recovery.

Insight from TMS studies

TMS has been used to predict functional recovery following UHS with agreement across the literature that, in the acute poststroke phase, the inability to elicit motor evoked potentials (MEPs) following focal stimulation of the affected hemisphere (AH) correlates with a poor functional outcome. Conversely, the persistence of contralateral MEPs in this time window, regardless of the clinical grade of the patients deficit, is a good marker of favourable outcome (Rapisarda et al., 1996; Trompelto et al., 2000; D'Olhaberriague et al., 1997). In addition, the latencies of responses elicited in the acute phase are prolonged and shorten in line with recovery (Heald et al., 1993; Turton et al., 1996).

However, with the available data from functional imaging suggesting a contribution of both the UH and AH in recovery from UHS, TMS has been utilized to study the potential contribution of the magnetically accessible motor projections of both the AH and UH during the acute (<48 hours) and chronic (18 months) poststroke phases.

Ipsilateral pathways

Before we examine data from TMS studies, it is important to briefly describe the physiology of the ipsilateral motor projections that are known to exist in health. These pathways are more pronounced in youth and become progressively more difficult to demonstrate after the age of 10 years old, the degradation being thought to be mediated by increasing transcallosal inhibition from the contralateral hemisphere (Muller et al., 1997). Ipsilateral MEPs (iMEPs) can be variably elicited by TMS in upper limbs of normal adults with tonic contraction of the target muscle (Wassermann et al., 1991; Carr et al., 1994). They are more readily elicitable from proximal rather than from distal muscles (Carr et al., 1994). If present, the representation tends to be separate from the optimal site for producing contralateral MEPs, the threshold tends to be higher and the amplitude smaller with longer latency (Wassermann et al., 1994).

Given this evidence of a persistence of an ipsilateral motor projection into adulthood and the data from studies in posthemispherectomy children where a surprising degree of motor function was retained following the procedure, the potential contribution of this tract to motor recovery following UHS was of interest to the neuroscience community (Carr et al., 1993).

TMS investigation of the unaffected hemisphere following UHS

The potential role of the UH was first investigated in detail by Turton et al. (1996), who studied the contralateral and ipsilateral EMG responses to TMS of four upper limb muscles in 21 UHS patients and related these to functional outcome. The initial assessments took place within 5 weeks and were then performed at regular intervals for the next 12 months. The patients were grouped at 6 weeks following ictus depending on whether they were able (group A, $n = 8$) or unable (group B, $n = 13$) to perform a standardized peg test. These groups were then considered to represent good and poor functional outcome, respectively.

In line with the published work the authors highlighted the poor functional outcome associated with initial absence of contralateral MEPs (cMEPs) and, in addition, the initial prolonged latencies of cMEPs where present, which shortened in line with clinical improvement (Rapisarda et al., 1996; Trompelto et al., 2000; D'Olhaberriague et al., 1997; Heald et al., 1993).

The protocol for eliciting iMEPs was as follows: the generated iMEPs were only considered 'secure' if they were elicitable at thresholds as low or lower than the threshold for cMEPs. This methodology was based in part on reducing the likelihood of current spread to the opposite hemisphere resulting in a measurable MEP. However, should the threshold for obtaining a cMEP from the damaged hemisphere be higher in the poor functional outcome group than the favourable outcome group, then the likelihood of obtaining iMEPs in the former group would be increased as a function of threshold of stimulation. Indeed in health, iMEPs are normally only elicitable at thresholds above that for the equivalent contralateral muscles (Wassermann et al., 1994).

However, accepting this caveat, more iMEPs were elicited from the UH in the poor outcome group than in the favourable outcome group. The authors concluded that ipsilateral projections do exist but they do not play a beneficial role in functional outcome. This area was further studied by

Netz et al. (1997), who compared 15 UHS patients with 15 normal control subjects. The assessments took place in the chronic phase poststroke (mean time postictus, 18 +/− 21 months).

The patients were again subdivided into poor and good functional outcome groups ($n = 10$ and 5, respectively). There was a significant difference in the proportion of individuals with iMEPs in the poor outcome group (iMEPs were identified in all ten patients) when compared to the good outcome group (iMEPs present in one out of five patients) and normal individuals (iMEPs present in two out of 12). In the poor outcome group the iMEPs were elicitable at lower thresholds than in the other groups, but always significantly higher than the threshold for cMEPs from the UH. The iMEPs also had a longer latency than the equivalent cMEP. This again added further evidence to the suggestion that the presence of iMEPs following UHS was not associated with a favourable functional outcome.

Caramia and colleagues used a bimodal approach utilizing TMS and transcranial Doppler (TCD) to assess ipsilateral activation following UHS (Caramia et al., 2000). They studied 14 patients with TMS at 48 hours and with TMS+TCD at 6 months. They chose an anterior site outside M1 (likely SMA/prefrontal cortex) for generation of iMEPS and, although absent at 48 hours, they were present (during relaxation) in all recovered hands at 6 months postictus. TCD, which measured ipsilateral middle cerebral artery mean flow velocity, was also elevated during ipsilateral recovered hand movement compared to patient's normal hand. The authors concluded first that ipsilateral activation occurs during recovery from UHS, second, that areas outside ipsilateral M1 may be recruited and, third, that it takes some time for this neuromatrix to be established. It is, however, not clear how the observed changes correlated with individual functional outcome in this study.

Conclusions from TMS studies in peripheral limb model

Taken together, both the TMS and functional imaging data support the contention that both AH and UH mechanisms contribute to the recovery process. Whether the UH mechanisms play a favourable role in the functional recovery has yet to be established. Anecdotal evidence exists with the observations of Miller Fisher, who observed dramatic deterioration of two patients who, whilst recovering from pure motor stroke, then suffered a further contralateral pure motor stroke. Following injury to the initially unaffected hemisphere reparalysis of the original partially recovered hemiparesis resulted thus implying a major functional role for the UH in recovery (Fisher, 1992). The ipsilateral pathway may importantly originate from outside M1. The characterization of potential pathways utilized when iMEPs are demonstrated has recently been revisited by Ziemann and colleagues. Using TMS, they have concluded that the ipsilateral responses are probably mediated via an ipsilateral cortico-reticular or cortico-propriospinal projection. Also, they present a patient with complete agenesis of the corpus callosum, who had large ipsilateral responses again suggesting the contribution of opposite hemisphere inhibitory mechanisms mediated via the callosum on the suppression in health of these ipsilateral projections (Ziemann et al., 1999). The functional significance of these projections in terms of recovery is, however, still not established. One potential reason why the TMS data do not concur entirely with the neuroimaging data is that, although with fMRI and PET large bihemispheric networks of activation have been noted, it is by no means certain that all these areas will be accessible with TMS. This may be due to excessive threshold for activation, anatomical localization outside of M1 or because they are polysynaptic neural networks and in this setting TMS may be an inadequate investigative tool. Perhaps future studies with rTMS to disrupt targeted areas of UH temporarily may reveal the functional relevance of UH compensatory mechanisms.

TMS and midline muscle recovery

Central representation of midline structure

To understand how midline motor function recovers following UHS, it is essential to understand how the central organization of these midline structures differs from that of peripheral limbs. TMS has been instrumental in the investigation of cortical control of midline structures and has advanced understanding beyond that gained from the classic direct cortical stimulation experiments of Penfield (1937) and subsequent investigators (Woolsey et al., 1979). Weighed against the obvious advantage of excellent spatial resolution, the major limitation of these highly focal direct stimulation studies is that they were exclusively unilateral investigations that failed to provide detailed information about symmetry. The direct stimulation experiments did, however, reveal a degree of inter-individual variability in the cortical representation of midline muscles, which may have occurred as a consequence of interhemispheric asymmetry. In its role as a surrogate for direct cortical stimulation, what TMS lacks in spatial accuracy is balanced by the advantage of being non-invasive, reproducible and having the capacity for bihemispheric stimulation.

TMS has been used to examine the cortical representation of various midline structures including orofacial and swallowing musculature (Hamdy et al., 1996; Urban et al., 1997; Muellbacher et al., 1998). TMS investigation of the cortico-lingual pathway has revealed that in health both contralateral and ipsilateral MEPs (recorded via a fitted mouthpiece with in-built recording electrodes) can be generated with unilateral hemispheric stimulation.

The resultant iMEPs were of smaller amplitude and longer latency than the cMEPs, therefore mirroring the peripheral limb data to some extent. There was, however, no difference in the amplitude or latency of the contralateral responses generated via stimulation of each hemisphere. As no formal mapping was performed, it was therefore not possible to demonstrate whether asymmetrical cortical representations of lingual muscles with similar excitability thresholds were present or not (Muellbacher et al., 1999).

With respect to the swallowing musculature the cortical representation of the following muscles: right and left mylohyoid, pharynx and oesophagus (the latter recorded via an indwelling catheter with in-built recording electrodes) were mapped on both hemispheres by Hamdy et al. (1996). The representational area of the four muscles was subsequently compared to subject handedness. The results revealed that the swallowing muscles were arranged somatotopically with the oral muscles (mylohyoid) laterally and the swallowing muscles (pharynx and oesophagus) medially. The representations for all muscles were asymmetric and this asymmetry was also unrelated to handedness. Discordance was also demonstrated in a pair of monozygotic twins, suggesting that genetic factors have little influence on the development of this midline representational asymmetry.

Mechanism of deficit following UHS

Given this bilateral cortical innervation, the crucial question remains: why should a functional deficit ensue following UHS and moreover does the apparent asymmetry play a role in the observed clinical phenotypes? The mechanism for dysphagia following UHS was explored by Hamdy et al., who examined the corticopharyngeal projections in a large number of pure unilateral stroke patients (Hamdy et al., 1997). Half of the studied patients were dysphagic and half not. They reasoned that, if there were a functional asymmetry of swallowing cortical representation, damage to the 'dominant' hemisphere would result in dysphagia. The results showed that TMS of the damaged hemisphere produced little or no response in either group of patients, and that stimulation of the undamaged hemisphere tended to evoke much larger responses in the non-dysphagic than in the dysphagic subjects. Thus the size of the remaining cortical projection to the swallowing muscles may determine the presence or absence of dysphagia.

Mechanism of recovery following UHS in the midline model

TMS has been used to investigate recovery from lingual and swallowing dysfunction following UHS (Muellbacher et al., 1998, 1999). We will initially consider the swallowing data. Given that dysphagia following stroke is usually a transient phenomenon, and that most patients recover within weeks of ictus, it follows that the swallowing system must have a significant capacity for functional recovery (Barer, 1989). It is of particular interest how this recovery is achieved within an asymmetrically bilaterally represented system. Hamdy et al. recruited 28 patients with UHS in whom videofluoroscopic evaluation of swallowing and TMS mapping of pharyngeal and thenar motor representations were performed at 1 week, 1 month and 3 months postictus (Hamdy et al., 1998).

The patients were grouped into dysphagic (71%) and non-dysphagic by the baseline videofluoroscopic data. The magnitude of the pharyngeal motor representations on both the AH and UH were then correlated with the presence or absence of dysphagia at each time-point. Non-dysphagic and persistently dysphagic patients showed little change in either hemisphere at 1 and 3 months compared with presentation, but dysphagic patients who recovered had an increased pharyngeal representation in the UH at 1 and 3 months without change in the affected hemisphere (Fig. 11.1, see colour plate at www.cambridge.org/9780521114462).

This work therefore indicated that recovery from dysphagia following UHS relates to expansion of the pharyngeal representation within the UH, which suggests a role for the UH in recovery from midline structure dysfunction following UHS. This compares with functional imaging in the peripheral model showing consistent activation of the UH following tasks of the recovered hand; however, this was not replicated in the peripheral

TMS work (Turton et al., 1996; Netz et al., 1997). It is worth noting, however, that the optimal scalp position for obtaining a pharyngeal MEP is a number of centimetres anterior to that of the hand. This is of relevance as functional imaging has consistently demonstrated activation of premotor and supplementary motor areas within the UH, Caramia et al. noted the presence of iMEPS in six recovered stroke patients when stimulating an anterior (premotor or supplementary motor) area (Caramia et al., 2000). It may be that the pharyngeal responses noted after recovery from dysphagia are generated from these magnetically accessible anterior secondary motor cortical areas.

Muellbacher et al. (1999) investigated the role of the UH in the motor recovery from unilateral lingual paralysis following hemispheric stroke. Six patients were examined with TMS in the symptomatic phase of lingual paralysis and again after complete recovery. The cortical motor output patterns were compared to 40 control subjects. In most healthy subjects there was a degree of asymmetry, but stimulation of either hemisphere invariably evoked both cMEPs and iMEPs. At baseline in the patient population, stimulation of the UH evoked similar responses to that of the healthy controls but stimulation of the AH failed to evoke any responses. After recovery, only one patient showed evidence of normal bilateral evoked responses from the AH, leaving five patients who recovered function without restoration of the cortico-lingual output from the damaged hemisphere. Therefore, it is suggested that recovery took place in the majority due to the effective utilization of the uncrossed ipsilateral pathways.

TMS demonstrates in these two studies evidence of beneficial changes occurring within the UH resulting in recovery from midline muscle dysfunction following UHS. As mentioned TMS has not been able to demonstrate such clear evidence in the peripheral muscles but, as previously stated, it may be that the relevant structures involved in reorganization may not be magnetically accessible or may not have been explored in these studies (Turton et al., 1996; Netz et al., 1997).

TMS evaluation of physical rehabilitative approaches

Physical rehabilitative therapy is administered almost universally following neuronal injury. This is particularly true of stroke where the capacity for 'plasticity' has been extensively documented, and the therapists involved are focused on exploiting this potential for repair. TMS has been used to assess the efficacy of various physical therapeutic strategies following unilateral hemispheric stroke, which we will proceed to review (Liepert et al., 2000; Traversa et al., 1997) (see also Chapter 7).

Evidence for the potential efficacy of physical therapy from animal work

As a background to the TMS work in rehabilitation, we will initially consider the data pertaining to potential mechanisms and induction of functional recovery from animal stroke models. In adult monkeys following limited lesioning of the hand area of M1, the comparative effects of spontaneous (without postlesion behavioural training) and encouraged (constraint+repetitive training paradigm) recovery have been studied (Nudo et al., 1996; Nudo & Milliken, 1996; Nudo, 1997). This body of work utilized the technique of intracortical microstimulation (ICMS) to map the hand area of M1, where a limited (30% of total area) lesion was subsequently made.

In the monkeys who were allowed to recover spontaneously a contraction of the remaining undamaged hand area of M1 was observed at 4 months postlesion. However, in the group which received constraint therapy plus repetitive training postinjury, a net gain of 10% of the hand area was observed when ICMS studies were performed following restoration of manual skills to normal levels (Fig. 11.2). It was noted that unimpaired limb constraint alone did not help preserve the hand cortical representation and therefore it is concluded that the physical therapy of repetitive task training was the driving force behind the observed reorganization. For an excellent review on this area of work, see Nudo and Plautz (2001).

The available evidence from animal studies suggested a role for physical therapy in driving reorganization following cortical injury and provided the impetus for TMS investigations of human subjects undergoing neurorehabilitation programmes.

TMS evidence for the reorganizational potential of current neurorehabilitation techniques

TMS has been used to investigate the neuronal correlates underlying the documented improvements that occur with physical therapy. Traversa et al. (1997) mapped the motor cortical output to the affected abductor digiti

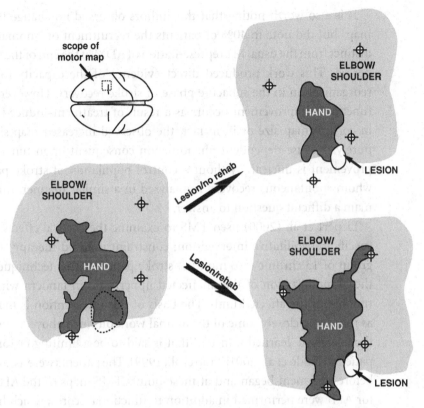

Fig. 11.2   Summary of functional remodelling of the hand representation in the primary motor cortex after a stroke-like injury. Data were derived from hundreds of microelectrode penetrations using microstimulation techniques to determine evoked movements in anaesthetized monkeys. These studies, and others like them, demonstrate that the uninjured tissue adjacent to a cortical injury undergoes functional reorganization that can be modulated by postinjury behavioural training. (Reproduced with kind permission, Nudo, 1997.)

minimi (ADM) pre- and post-8 to 10 weeks of Bobath rehabilitation in 15 subacute stroke patients (Bobath, 1970). In addition to the TMS measures, Canadian stroke scales and Barthel disability scales were also performed (Cote et al., 1986; Mahoney & Barthel, 1965). The authors observed an initial decrease in the cortical map of the AH ADM compared to the UH and healthy control maps followed by a significant expansion after the period of neurorehabilitation, which correlated with an improvement in Canadian stroke and Barthel disability scores.

It is also worth noting that the authors observed no change in the UH maps but did note in 40% of patients the recruitment of 'anomalous sites' distinct from the usual M1 representation of ADM at the end of the treatment period. This work produced direct evidence of the capacity for cortical reorganization in the subacute phase of stroke recovery. However, whether functional improvement occurs as a result of treatment-induced increases in cortical map size or if, in fact, the observed increased map size relates purely to a use-dependent phenomenon consequent upon functional improvement is unclear. Without a control population of stroke patients in whom spontaneous recovery is analysed in a similar manner, this will remain a difficult question to answer.

Liepert et al. (2000) used TMS to examine the cortical effects of a very specific rehabilitative intervention: constraint induced therapy (CIT) in a group of 13 chronic (>6 months) stroke patients. This technique involves the immobilization of the unaffected upper limb in tandem with intense training of the affected limb. The basis of this intervention is that, as well as mirroring closely some of the animal work outlined above, it also tackles the perceived 'learned non-use' that is said to be a limiting factor in these patients (Nudo et al., 2001; Taub et al., 1999). The patients were assessed twice before treatment began and at these points TMS maps of the AH and UH for APB were performed in addition to functional scores, which had a bias towards movements which are encountered in day-to-day tasks. This served as a strict baseline to the post-therapy measurements which were performed at +1 day, +4 weeks and +6 months postintervention which consisted of CIT for 12 days. At baseline there were 40% fewer 'active' areas in the AH vs. UH, a ratio which was essentially reversed at 1 day post-therapy. This effect persisted at 4 weeks but at this stage, although the increased reactivity of the AH persisted, the numbers of active sites in the UH increased. By 6 months in the eight patients who were studied, the map increase in the AH was still present but, by this time, the activity between the two hemispheres was essentially equal. These results were also mirrored by the functional scores.

Various explanations for the cortical changes are possible. The authors suggested that the CIT may produce long-lasting changes in the cortical inhibitory network or perhaps the enhancement of synaptic strength within pre-existing synaptic connections. Given that the unaffected limb was immobilized during the intervention period, it may be that the initial changes are related to a use-dependent mechanism, i.e. a negative influence on UH map size and that this persists in the AH due to increased utilization of the paretic limb following the period of training, i.e. a positive influence on AH map size. However, given the short length of the intervention, it is unlikely that the results were contaminated by natural spontaneous recovery, especially given the chronic nature of the patients studied. It is still difficult to tease out from the rehabilitation literature a plasticity-inducing manoeuvre with resultant demonstrable changes in cortical physiology, which unequivocally results in a consequent functional benefit.

The relationship between beneficial manipulation of neuronal plasticity following recovery and functional improvement that TMS has shown great potential both in helping to elucidate normal patterns of recovery, thus identifying potential therapeutic targets and, in addition, allowing an objective measure of these interventions to be performed. It is essential that this link continues to be objectively explored if we are going to be able to obtain the rehabilitative 'holy grail', which is the institution of evidence-based therapy programmes with accurate neuroscientific foundations to maximize an individual's functional status following neurological insults.

Sensory-induced plasticity

Modulation of sensory input may also play a central role in sensorimotor cortical plasticity and consequently in neurorehabilitation. Much of the evidence that changes in sensory input can alter the excitability of motor cortex (cross-system plasticity), comes from the observation, both in animals and humans, that reduction in sensory feedback from a body site, by denervation, prolonged positional stasis, or ischemic nerve block can induce changes in motor representation (Donoghue et al., 1990; Sanes et al., 1992; Brasil-Neto et al., 1993; Ridding & Rothwell, 1997; Cohen et al., 1993). In human studies, however, there has been little to suggest that the effects outlast the manipulation. Nonetheless, it has recently been shown that, although motor maps may show little long-lasting change, there is a residual increase in their sensitivity to other inputs, which may last for up to 1 hour (Ziemann et al., 1998). Given this effect, Hamdy et al. (1998) wondered whether modifications of the technique might allow changes in sensory input to drive long-term changes in human motor cortex organization. Evidence for such an effect would have clear relevance for the rehabilitation of motor disabled patients after CNS injury.

In this study, a 10 minutes' train of electrical stimuli was applied to the pharynx of healthy subjects at a just perceived intensity using a pair of intraluminal electrodes. Motor cortex projections to pharynx were measured before and after this conditioning input using TMS. The authors found that, following the pharyngeal input, cortico-pharyngeal evoked responses were increased for 30 minutes after pharyngeal stimulation, without changes in brainstem reflexes, or in responses evoked to transcranial electrical stimulation. The implication was that short-term (sensory) stimuli could induce longer-term changes in motor cortical excitability, providing evidence for a driven 'cross-system' effect to increased input. More recent work has suggested that the direction of these changes in swallowing motor cortex is highly dependent on the stimulus frequency, intensity and duration used. Fraser et al. (1999) showed that, whilst medium to low frequency stimulation (≤ 10 Hz) was excitatory, high frequency pharyngeal stimulation (> 10 Hz) resulted in long-lasting cortical inhibition and a reduction in the pharyngeal motor map. In addition, the stronger the stimulation the more pronounced the effect; however, 20 minutes of stimulation appeared no better than 10 minutes. Since this initial description in the pharynx, other workers have demonstrated that stimulation of muscle afferents in the hand can also produce analogous effects, albeit with longer trains of stimulation (Ridding et al., 2001).

Sensory-induced plasticity and changes in function

Whilst evidence from the swallowing model in healthy subjects appears to show a clear effect of sensory stimulation on motor cortex organization, the critical question remains: can sensory induced plasticity alter function, as a prelude to formulating stimulation therapies to promote functional recovery after injury? In another study by Fraser et al. (2001) functional magnetic resonance imaging was used to demonstrate that those patterns of pharyngeal input associated with enhanced motor cortical excitability, could alter the recruitment pattern of cortical activations associated with the task of swallowing. The group was able to show that pharyngeal stimulation resulted in functionally stronger, bilateral, cortical (sensorimotor) activation in areas related to swallowing (Fig. 11.3, see colour plate at www.cambridge.org/9780521114462).

Despite this finding, there has been no direct demonstration in the human that any form of plasticity-inducing stimuli produces a measurable improvement in function after cerebral injury. Of relevance, however, the effects of pharyngeal stimulation on swallowing have recently been investigated in acute dysphagic stroke patients (Fraser et al., 2001). The application of 10 minutes of 5 Hz of pharyngeal electrical stimulation at 75% of the intensity maximally tolerated by the patient was used. The stimulation resulted in a long-term (60 minutes) increase in swallowing cortico-bulbar excitability predominantly within the undamaged, but not the damaged, hemisphere (Fig. 11.4, see colour plate at www.cambridge.org/9780521114462). Critically, this was strongly associated with an improvement in swallowing using videofluoroscopy, the standard marker of swallowing performance during the same time frame (Fraser et al., 2001). The exciting implication from these results is that sensory input to the human adult brain can be programmed to promote beneficial changes in plasticity that result in an improvement of function after cerebral injury. Whilst the more long-term (days to weeks) effects of this approach still need to be established, the observations hold great promise for future neurorehabilitative strategies.

Repetitive transcranial magnetic stimulation (rTMS) of the swallowing motor cortex

Properties of rTMS relevant to rehabilitation

Repetitive transcranial magnetic stimulation is a non-invasive method capable of producing long-lasting alterations in cortical properties. The accepted maxim is that fast rate stimulation (5 Hz and above) increases cortical excitability, which is thought to be mediated by saturation of intracortical inhibitory mechanisms (Pascual-Leone et al., 1993, 1994; Berardelli et al., 1998). In contrast slow frequency (1 Hz) reduces cortical excitability by enhancing inhibitory tone, which is quantifiable by single pulse TMS, in particular by measurement of cortical silent periods, and paired pulse techniques (Berardelli et al., 1999; Chen et al., 1997; Wassermann et al., 1996; Wu et al., 2000). The duration and magnitude of any resulting alteration in cortical properties are related to the exact frequency, length and intensity of the stimulation. In addition, properties intrinsic to the model under consideration are likely to exert influence over the final observed effects.

Although alterations in cortical inhibitory tone following fast and slow rTMS have been extensively documented by neurophysiological methods, the exact cortical cellular mechanism by which rTMS produces these observed effects is as yet unknown. Potential candidates include: alteration in neurotransmitter levels, gene induction, manipulation of neurotrophic factors and the much-vaunted induction of synaptic plasticity (Ben-Shachar et al., 1997, 1999; Hausmann et al., 2000; Keck et al., 2000; Muller et al., 2000). The latter is the most commonly cited explanation for the 'plastic' changes noted in human rTMS experiments and, although pharmacological manipulation has suggested a role for NMDA receptors, which are required for long-term potentiation of synapses in this process, given the lack of corroborative animal models some doubt has been cast on this assertion (Ziemann et al., 1998; Wassermann & Lisanby, 2001).

Features of the pharyngeal model relevant to rehabilitation

The human swallowing motor cortex is an interesting model in which to investigate potential neuroplasticity inducing interventions for a number of different reasons. First, its bilateral asymmetrical cortical representation provides an interesting contrast from the lateralized organization of peripheral limbs and, second, the clinical model of recovery from dysphagia following UHS strongly implicates the UH, which may be a valuable target for therapeutic intervention. Following from the observed effects of afferent stimulation of the pharynx, which produced long-lasting changes in the excitability of the swallowing motor cortex in health and following dysphagic stroke, the latter importantly associated with documented functional benefit, it became intriguing as to whether such changes could be produced by more direct methods of cortical stimulation.

rTMS of pharyngeal motor cortex

Given the possibility of inducing lasting cortical change and the premise that swallowing recovery from dysphagic stroke relates to cortical reorganization in the UH, we sought to evaluate rTMS as a potential tool for influencing this process. We proceeded to examine the effects of limited trains of fast rate rTMS (5 Hz) on the dominant swallowing motor cortex. In assessing the 'dose' of rTMS to be administered, we chose 5 Hz frequency, which was optimal for up-regulating cortical excitability following afferent stimulation.

We used an intensity of 80% of the pharyngeal motor threshold capped at 120% of the contralateral APB. The frequency and intensity factors were allied to a total of 100 pulses (given in two 5 second 50 pulse trains with an intertrain interval of 1 minute). The basis of this 'recipe' formulation is of relevance as one of the limiting factors in potential therapeutic rTMS research has often been the utilization of arbitrary 'dosing' schedules.

Given the possible underlying mechanism of how rTMS might induce change in the motor cortex, we decided to look at changes in excitability as measured by single pulse TMS over a period of 2 hours post-intervention. In nine healthy individuals the effect of active 5 Hz rTMS to the dominant pharyngeal motor cortex was compared with a sham procedure, which utilized an anterior coil tilt. Active stimulation resulted in a significant increase in cortical excitability lasting for more than 1 hour poststimulation (Fig. 11.5). This effect was not seen with the sham. The time frame of this effect is of great interest. As the increase in excitability is not evident immediately, it is unlikely that this enhancement is explained simply by LTP. The magnitude of this effect is not as great as that produced by pharyngeal electrical stimulation, which is probably related to the fact that the sensory projection provides a more directed input to M1 than rTMS at the scalp. Although the rTMS data are only available in healthy subjects, there is sufficient promise to proceed to

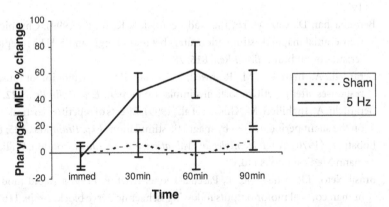

Fig. 11.5   A comparison of the change in TMS-evoked pharyngeal MEP size before and after 5 Hz rTMS or sham stimulation. Mean percentage change from baseline is plotted (error bars=SEM) for a group of nine healthy individuals. (Unpublished data.)

investigate the effect in dysphagic stroke patients. There may be a role for combining rTMS with sensory stimulation to optimize the 'up-regulation' of the pharyngeal motor representation in dysphagic subjects.

Conclusions

We can see that TMS has been a valuable tool in rehabilitation research. It has been used successfully to provide individual prognostic information following neuronal injury thus allowing accurate treatment and resource planning. It has also been able to demonstrate biological features of recovery including neuroplastic reorganization following injury. In helping to quantify therapeutic interventions and providing measurable surrogate markers for recovery, it will further the quest for providing directed neurorehabilitative therapy with demonstrable beneficial biological effects. Lastly TMS may also have potential as a therapeutic entity in its own right.

REFERENCES

Barer, D.H. (1989). The natural history and functional consequences of dysphagia after hemispheric stroke. *J. Neurol. Neurosurg. Psychiatry*, **52**: 236–241.

Ben-Shachar, D., Belmaker, R.H., Grisaru, N. & Klein, E. (1997). Transcranial magnetic stimulation induces alterations in brain monoamines. *J. Neural. Transm.*, **104**: 191–197.

Ben-Shachar, D., Gazawi, H., Riboyad-Levin, J. & Klein, E. (1999). Chronic repetitive transcranial magnetic stimulation alters beta-adrenergic and 5-HT2 receptor characteristics in rat brain. *Brain Res.*, **816**: 78–83.

Berardelli, A., Inghilleri, M., Rothwell, J.C. et al. (1998). Facilitation of muscle evoked responses after repetitive cortical stimulation in man. *Exp. Brain Res.*, **122**: 79–84.

Berardelli, A., Inghilleri, M., Gilio, F. et al. (1999). Effects of repetitive cortical stimulation on the silent period evoked by magnetic stimulation. *Exp. Brain Res.*, **125**: 82–86.

Bobath, B. (1970). *Adult Hemiplegia: Evaluation and Treatment*. London: William Heinemann Medical Books Ltd.

Brasil-Neto, J.P., Valls-Sole, J., Pascual-Leone, A. et al. (1993). Rapid modulation of human cortical motor outputs following ischaemic nerve block. *Brain*, **116**: 511–525.

Buckner, R.L., Corbetta, M., Schatz, J., Raichle, M.E. & Petersen, S.E. (1996). Preserved speech abilities and compensation following prefrontal damage. *Proc. Natl Acad. Sci., USA*, **93**: 1249–1253.

Cao, Y., D'Olhaberriague, L., Vikingstad, E.M., Levine, S.R. & Welch, K.M. (1998). Pilot study of functional MRI to assess cerebral activation of motor function after poststroke hemiparesis. *Stroke*, **29**: 112–122.

Caramia, M.D., Palmieri, M.G., Giacomini, P., Iani, C., Dally, L. & Silvestrini, M. (2000). Ipsilateral activation of the unaffected motor cortex in patients with hemiparetic stroke. *Clin. Neurophysiol.*, **111**: 1990–1996.

Carr, L.J., Harrison, L.M., Evans, A.L. & Stephens, J.A. (1993). Patterns of central motor reorganization in hemiplegic cerebral palsy. *Brain*, **116**: 1223–1247.

Carr, L.J., Harrison, L.M. & Stephens, J.A. (1994). Evidence for bilateral innervation of certain homologous motoneurone pools in man. *J. Physiol.*, **475**: 217–227.

Chen, R., Classen, J., Gerloff, C. et al. (1997). Depression of motor cortex excitability by low-frequency transcranial magnetic stimulation. *Neurology*, **48**: 1398–1403.

Chollet, F., DiPiero, V., Wise, R.J., Brooks, D. J., Dolan, R.J. & Frackowiak, R.S. (1991). The functional anatomy of motor recovery after stroke in humans: a study with positron emission tomography. *Ann. Neurol.*, **29**: 63–71.

Cohen, L.G., Brasil-Neto, J.P., Pascual-Leone, A. & Hallett, M. (1993). Plasticity of cortical motor output organization following deafferentation, cerebral lesions, and skill acquisition. *Adv. Neurol.*, **63**: 187–200.

Cote, R., Hachinski, V.C., Shurvell, B.L., Norris, J.W. & Wolfson, C. (1986). The Canadian Neurological Scale: a preliminary study in acute stroke. *Stroke*, **17**: 731–737.

Cramer, S.C., Nelles, G., Benson, R.R. et al. (1997). A functional MRI study of subjects recovered from hemiparetic stroke. *Stroke*, **28**: 2518–2527.

D'Olhaberriague, L., Espadaler Gamissans, J.M., Marrugat, J. Valls, A., Oliveras Ley, C. & Seoane, J.L. (1997). Transcranial magnetic stimulation as a prognostic tool in stroke. *J. Neurol. Sci.*, **147**: 73–80.

Donoghue, J.P., Suner, S. & Sanes, J.N. (1990). Dynamic organization of primary motor cortex output to target muscles in adult rats. II. Rapid reorganization following motor nerve lesions. *Exp. Brain Res.*, **79**: 492–503.

Fisher, C.M. (1992). Concerning the mechanism of recovery in stroke hemiplegia. *Can. J. Neurol. Sci.*, **19**: 57–63.

Fraser, C., Hamdy, S., Rothwell, J.C. & Thompson, D.G. (1999). Sensory-induced reorganisation of human swallowing motor cortex displays differential frequency dependent patterns. *NeuroImage*, **9**: A507.

Fraser, C., Hobday, D., Power, M. et al. (2001a). A functional study of sensory dependent brain reorganisation during swallowing. *Gastroenterology*, **120**: A713.

Fraser, C., Power, M., Hamdy, S. et al. (2001b). Driving plasticity in adult human motor cortex improves functional performance after cerebral injury. *Clin. Neurophysiol.*, **112**: S86.

Hamdy, S., Aziz, Q., Rothwell, J.C. et al. (1996). The cortical topography of human swallowing musculature in health and disease. *Nat. Med.*, **2**: 1217–1224.

Hamdy, S., Aziz, Q., Rothwell, J.C. et al. (1997). Explaining oropharyngeal dysphagia after unilateral hemispheric stroke. *Lancet*, 350: 686–692.

Hamdy, S., Aziz, Q., Rothwell, J.C. et al. (1998a). Recovery of swallowing after dysphagic stroke relates to functional reorganization in the intact motor cortex. *Gastroenterology*, 115: 1104–1112.

Hamdy, S., Rothwell, J.C., Aziz, Q., Singh, K.D. & Thompson, D.G. (1998b). Long-term reorganization of human motor cortex driven by short-term sensory stimulation. *Nat. Neurosci.*, 1: 64–68.

Hausmann, A., Weis, C., Marksteiner, J., Hinterhuber, H. & Humpel, C. (2000). Chronic repetitive transcranial magnetic stimulation enhances c-fos in the parietal cortex and hippocampus. *Brain Res. Mol. Brain Res.*, 76: 355–362.

Heald, A., Bates, D., Cartlidge, N.E., French, J.M. & Miller, S. (1993). Longitudinal study of central motor conduction time following stroke. 2. Central motor conduction measured within 72 h after stroke as a predictor of functional outcome at 12 months. *Brain*, 116: 1371–1385.

Heiss, W.D., Kessler, J., Thiel, A., Ghaemi, M. & Karbe, H. (1999). Differential capacity of left and right hemispheric areas for compensation of poststroke aphasia. *Ann. Neurol.*, 45: 430–438.

Keck, M.E., Sillaber, I., Ebner, K. et al. (2000). Acute transcranial magnetic stimulation of frontal brain regions selectively modulates the release of vasopressin, biogenic amines and amino acids in the rat brain. *Eur. J. Neurosci.*, 12: 3713–3720.

Liepert, J., Bauder, H., Wolfgang, H.R., Miltner, W.H., Taub, E. & Weiller, C. (2000). Treatment-induced cortical reorganization after stroke in humans. *Stroke*, 31: 1210–1216.

Mahoney, F. & Barthel, D. (1965). Functional evaluation: the Barthel index. *MD State Med. J.*, 14: 61–85.

Muellbacher, W., Artner, C. & Mamoli, B. (1998). Motor evoked potentials in unilateral lingual paralysis after monohemispheric ischaemia. *J. Neurol. Neurosurg. Psychiatry*, 65: 755–761.

Muellbacher, W., Artner, C. & Mamoli, B. (1999). The role of the intact hemisphere in recovery of midline muscles after recent monohemispheric stroke. *J. Neurol.*, 246: 250–256.

Muller, K., Kass Iliyya, F. & Reitz, M. (1997). Ontogeny of ipsilateral corticospinal projections: a developmental study with transcranial magnetic stimulation. *Ann. Neurol.*, 42: 705–711.

Muller, M.B., Toschi, N., Kresse, A.E., Post, A. & Keck, M.E. (2000). Long-term repetitive transcranial magnetic stimulation increases expression of brain derived neurotrophic factor and cholecystokinin mRNA, but not neuropeptide tyrosine mRNA in specific areas of rat brain. *Neuropsychopharmacology*, 23: 205–215.

Nelles, G., Spiekermann, G., Jueptner, M. et al. (1999). Reorganization of sensory and motor systems in hemiplegic stroke patients. A positron emission tomography study. *Stroke*, **30**: 1510–1516.

Netz, J., Lammers, T. & Homberg, V. (1997). Reorganization of motor output in the non-affected hemisphere after stroke. *Brain*, **120**: 1579–1586.

Nudo, R.J. (1997). Remodeling of cortical motor representations after stroke: implications for recovery from brain damage. *Mol. Psychiatry*, **2**: 188–191.

Nudo, R.J. & Milliken G.W. (1996). Reorganization of movement representations in primary motor cortex following focal ischemic infarcts in adult squirrel monkeys. *J. Neurophysiol.*, **75**: 2144–2149.

Nudo, R.J., Wise, B.M., SiFuentes, F. & Milliken, G.W. (1996). Neural substrates for the effects of rehabilitative training on motor recovery after ischemic infarct. *Science*, **272**: 1791–1794.

Nudo, R.J., Plautz, E.J. & Frost S.B. (2001). Role of adaptive plasticity in recovery of function after damage to motor cortex. *Muscle Nerve*, **24**: 1000–1019.

Pascual Leone, A., Houser, C.M., Reese, K. et al. (1993). Safety of rapid-rate transcranial magnetic stimulation in normal volunteers. *Electroencephalogr. Clin. Neurophysiol.*, **89**: 120–130.

Pascual Leone, A., Valls Sole, J., Wassermann, E.M. & Hallett, M. (1994). Responses to rapid-rate transcranial magnetic stimulation of the human motor cortex. *Brain*, **117**: 847–858.

Penfield, W. B.E. (1937). Somatic motor and sensory representation in the cerebral cortex in man as studied by electrical stimulation. *Brain*, **60**: 389–443.

Rapisarda, G., Bastings, E., de Noordhout, A.M., Pennisi, G. & Delwaide, P.J. (1996). Can motor recovery in stroke patients be predicted by early transcranial magnetic stimulation? *Stroke*, **27**: 2191–2196.

Ridding, M.C. & Rothwell, J.C. (1997). Stimulus/response curves as a method of measuring motor cortical excitability in man. *Electroencephalogr. Clin. Neurophysiol.*, **105**: 340–344.

Ridding, M.C., McKay, D.R., Thompson, P.D. & Miles, T.S. (2001). Changes in corticomotor representations induced by prolonged peripheral nerve stimulation in humans. *Clin. Neurophysiol.*, **112**: 1461–1469.

Rosen, H.J., Petersen, S.E., Linenweber, M.R. et al. (2000). Neural correlates of recovery from aphasia after damage to left inferior frontal cortex. *Neurology*, **55**: 1883–1894.

Sanes, J.N., Wang, J. & Donoghue, J.P. (1992). Immediate and delayed changes of rat motor cortical output representation with new forelimb configurations. *Cereb. Cortex*, **2**: 141–152.

Seitz, R.J., Hoflich, P., Binkofski, F., Tellmann, L., Herzog, H. & Freund, H.J. (1998). Role of the premotor cortex in recovery from middle cerebral artery infarction. *Arch. Neurol.*, **55**: 1081–1088.

Taub, E., Uswatte, G. & Pidikiti, R. (1999). Constraint-induced movement therapy: a new family of techniques with broad application to physical rehabilitation – a clinical review. *J. Rehabil. Res. Dev.*, **36**: 237–251.

Traversa, R., Cicinelli, P., Bassi, A., Rossini, P.M. & Bernardi, G. (1997). Mapping of motor cortical reorganization after stroke. A brain stimulation study with focal magnetic pulses. *Stroke*, **28**: 110–117.

Trompetto, C., Assini, A., Buccolieri, A., Marchese, R. & Abbruzzese, G. (2000). Motor recovery following stroke: a transcranial magnetic stimulation study. *Clin. Neurophysiol.*, **111**: 1860–1867.

Turton, A., Wroe, S., Trepte, N., Fraser, C. & Lemon, R.N. (1996). Contralateral and ipsilateral EMG responses to transcranial magnetic stimulation during recovery of arm and hand function after stroke. *Electroencephalogr. Clin. Neurophysiol.*, **101**: 316–328.

Urban, P.P., Hopf, H.C., Fleischer, S., Zorowka, P.G. & Muller Forell, W. (1997). Impaired cortico-bulbar tract function in dysarthria due to hemispheric stroke. Functional testing using transcranial magnetic stimulation. *Brain*, **120**: 1077–1084.

Wassermann, E.M. & Lisanby, S.H. (2001). Therapeutic application of repetitive transcranial magnetic stimulation: a review. *Clin. Neurophysiol.*, **112**: 1367–1377.

Wassermann, E.M., Fuhr, P., Cohen, L.G. & Hallett, M. (1991). Effects of transcranial magnetic stimulation on ipsilateral muscles. *Neurology*, **41**: 1795–1799.

Wassermann, E.M., Pascual Leone, A. & Hallett, M. (1994). Cortical motor representation of the ipsilateral hand and arm. *Exp. Brain Res.*, **100**: 121–132.

Wassermann, E.M., Grafman, J., Berry, C. et al. (1996). Use and safety of a new repetitive transcranial magnetic stimulator. *Electroencephalogr. Clin. Neurophysiol.*, **101**: 412–417.

Weiller, C., Chollet, F., Friston, K.J., Wise, R.J. & Frackowiak, R.S. (1992). Functional reorganization of the brain in recovery from striatocapsular infarction in man. *Ann. Neurol.*, **31**: 463–472.

Weiller, C., Ramsay, S.C., Wise, R.J., Friston, K.J. & Frackowiak, R.S. (1993). Individual patterns of functional reorganization in the human cerebral cortex after capsular infarction. *Ann. Neurol.*, **33**: 181–189.

Weiller, C., Isensee, C., Rijntjes, M. et al. (1995). Recovery from Wernicke's aphasia: a positron emission tomographic study. *Ann. Neurol.*, **37**: 723–732.

Woolsey, C.N., Erickson, T.C. & Gilson, W.E. (1979). Localization in somatic sensory and motor areas of human cerebral cortex as determined by direct recording of evoked potentials and electrical stimulation. *J. Neurosurg.*, **51**: 476–506.

Wu, T., Sommer, M., Tergau, F. & Paulus, W. (2000). Lasting influence of repetitive transcranial magnetic stimulation on intracortical excitability in human subjects. *Neurosci. Lett.*, **287**: 37–40.

Ziemann, U., Corwell, B. & Cohen, L.G. (1998a). Modulation of plasticity in human motor cortex after forearm ischemic nerve block. *J. Neurosci.*, **18**: 1115–1123.

Ziemann, U., Hallett, M. & Cohen, L.G. (1998b). Mechanisms of deafferentation-induced plasticity in human motor cortex. *J. Neurosci.*, **18**: 7000–7007.

Ziemann, U., Ishii, K., Borgheresi, A. et al. (1999). Dissociation of the pathways mediating ipsilateral and contralateral motor-evoked potentials in human hand and arm muscles. *J. Physiol.*, **518**: 895–906.

12

New questions

Mark Hallett, Eric M. Wassermann and Leonardo G. Cohen

NINDS, NIH, Bethesda, MD, USA

The future is ever a misted landscape, no man foreknows it, but at cyclical turns
There is a change felt in the rhythm of events

> ROBINSON JEFFERS
> Prescription of Painful Ends (l. 3–4). Oxford Book of American Verse, The. F.O. Matthiessen, ed. (1950) Oxford University Press.

The 1990s have witnessed a dramatic burst of knowledge about plasticity. Understanding the importance of plasticity and mechanisms of plasticity and the use of transcranial magnetic stimulation (TMS) as a tool to study human biology have developed at about the same time. It is clear from this book that contributions from TMS studies to plasticity have been enormous. What are the prospects for the future? It is impossible to know exactly what will happen. Simple extrapolations from what is happening now are relatively obvious, and to some extent have been noted in the earlier chapters. There may be new discoveries that will change directions.

It is clear that TMS will not be the only tool to study plasticity, many different techniques will play a role in both basic science and human investigations. For human studies, neuroimaging is very powerful, and EEG and MEG will likely play a greater role to improve time resolution. TMS will likely continue to be used to study the physiology of plasticity, but the bigger growth area may well be in the use of TMS to influence plasticity. Such uses may well expand to therapeutics. These are the topics that we will consider in some more detail.

Use of TMS to explore plasticity

TMS can be used to map the cortex and assess its excitability. Knowing how much capability there is for change in these features is to assess plasticity itself. Knowing how much difference there has been after an intervention is to assess the result of a plastic change. From a practical point of view, we assess plasticity by making interventions and looking at the resultant change. One of the major goals of future work will be to relate human results to basic science findings, and it is likely that TMS will be useful in this regard.

Mapping different regions of the cortex has been done by recording responses as a function of moving the magnetic coil over the surface of the scalp. This should give information as to where relevant neurons are, and what their 'excitability' is. Most frequently this has been done in the motor system recording motor evoked potential (MEP) amplitudes. It has been pointed out that mapping can be confounded by changes in excitability (Ridding & Rothwell, 1997). If the excitability of a region is increased, then the map size apparently expands. This is because a stimulus actually outside the region may spread sufficient current to the active region to make it appear that it is included in the active region. There are no established ways to separate this confound, and it would be valuable to do so. We note that there are similar problems in neuroimaging; an increased magnitude of response in a fixed region may appear as a larger region. Whether a voxel is activated in neuroimaging still remains a statistical issue.

The accuracy of mapping seems very good, but the resolution could use improvement. The figure-of-eight coil was a big improvement over the circular coil, but there have not been substantial improvements since then. Other coil shapes, such as the four-leaf coil (Roth et al., 1994), or smaller size coils might be possible with further technical advances.

There is now the capability of visualizing in real time the location of a mapping coil on an individual's brain using a previously obtained MRI scan. This can aid mapping, particularly in the non-motor areas, and is likely to be used more in the future.

Another future addition to mapping comes from the anatomical fact that not all neurons are similarly oriented. Maps are usually constructed with the current flowing in the same direction, but different sets of neurons may be activated with current flows in different directions. Thus the map may differ with each orientation of the coil. This is clearly a time-consuming problem, since mapping with the coil in one direction is already a long procedure.

Excitability of the cortex is clearly not a single nor simple measure. There are many aspects, including:

1. the net level of polarization of the membranes of the output neurons. They can be firing at slow or fast rates or not firing at all. The absence of firing is not a fully defined state because the cells could be close to their firing level or profoundly inhibited.
2. efficacy of excitatory synapses. This is a function of the number of synapses and their strength. This aspect is rather independent of the level of neuronal polarization, and should be kept separately in mind.
3. efficacy of inhibitory synapses. Again, this is a function of synaptic number and strength. There appear already to be many types of inhibition functioning within the cortex.

The measures that are in common use at present include motor threshold, MEP size (or, in more complete investigations, MEP recruitment curve giving MEP size as a function of stimulus intensity), and paired-pulse studies for (short interval) intracortical inhibition (ICI) and intracortical facilitation (ICF). We need to learn more about all of these measures to be better able to relate any results to basic mechanisms. The least well understood is MEP size/recruitment. Moreover, while ICI and ICF are often thought of as separate phenomena, distinct in time, it is likely that there are both excitatory and inhibitory events occuring during both time intervals. This may be one of the reasons that ICI seems so non-specific in assessment of different neurologic disorders.

A number of types of inhibition are already established. Short interval intracortical inhibition thought to be mediated largely by $GABA_A$ receptor mechanisms, long interval intracortical inhibition thought to be mediated largely by $GABA_B$ receptor mechanisms, cutaneous inhibition thought to be mediated by cholinergic mechanisms, the silent period thought to be similar to long interval intracortical inhibition, and transcallosal inhibition. It is clear that there is also inhibition of inhibition (Sanger et al., 2001). Other types may well be established. It will be critical to know more about inhibitory mechanisms, not only because changes in inhibition are one facet of plasticity, but also because reductions of inhibition seem to play a role in facilitating plastic changes.

Use of TMS to influence brain excitability

TMS has been used to modify the excitability of the cerebral cortex. Application of 1 Hz TMS to the motor cortex for a short period of time, for example, is capable of eliciting measurable decreases in cortical excitability and/or depression of function (Wassermann et al., 1996; Chen et al., 1997; Boroojerdi et al., 2000). There is also evidence that these effects may generalize to other areas including the visual (Kosslyn et al., 1999; Boroojerdi et al., 2000), parietal (Hilgetag et al., 2001) and prefrontal (Speer et al., 2000) cortices. While the mechanisms underlying this are not understood, given the similarity of this paradigm with those used to elicit long-term depression in vitro, it has been commonly thought that they may involve changes in synaptic plasticity (Chen et al., 1997).

High-frequency rTMS (above 5 Hz or so) applied to the motor cortex (Pascual-Leone et al., 1993, 1994b) can saturate the inhibitory capacity of the cortical network and produce increasing excitability as indicated by the spread of evoked activity from low threshold (hand) to higher threshold (shoulder) muscles and spontaneous jerks persisting after the end of the stimulating train. This increased excitability can also last for minutes (Pascual-Leone et al., 1993, 1994b). Milder increases in MEP amplitude were also described immediately after brief trains of 5 Hz rTMS (Berardelli et al., 1998). Such increases, while desirable in certain situations, may lead to complications like seizures and require careful monitoring, expert supervision, and careful following of safety guidelines, as well as proper institutional monitoring by IRBs and (in the USA) FDA.

The future of TMS as a tool for neurophysiology and therapeutic intervention depends largely on better understanding its effects. While the mechanism of the MEP has been worked out fairly well, the lasting effects of rTMS, which may have the greatest potential for scientific and clinical impact, are not well understood. Progress in this area will require advances in three overlapping pursuits: exploring the nature of the functional changes produced by rTMS, efforts to make them stronger and longer lasting, and the development of animal models to help with the first two.

While tempting and potentially informative analogies have been drawn from these phenomena to long-term potentiation (LTP) and long-term depression (LTD), it is clear that the effects observed after rTMS do not involve long-term changes in synaptic efficacy. The excitatory changes mentioned above are, when produced with subconvulsive combinations of frequency and intensity of stimulation, transient, lasting minutes at the longest. The inhibitory phenomenon, when produced with 10–15 min of 1 Hz stimulation, persists for perhaps an order of magnitude longer, but we have not observed any changes lasting more than 2 hours. Therefore, while these phenomena might represent precursors of LTD and LTP, they may result in less durable changes. Certain manipulations, for instance reversible deafferentation of the studied limb segment (Ziemann et al., 1998a,b), may alter conditions in the cortex such that TMS can produce longer-lasting facilitatory changes. Furthermore, this form of stimulation-induced plasticity shares many features, such as threshold for induction, input specificity and dependence on NMDA receptor activation with the basic features of LTP, suggesting that rTMS-induced plasticity and LTP are mediated by the same mechanisms.

Human experimentation aimed at characterizing these changes might profitably concentrate on some of the following issues: first, simple experiments could be done to determine the location of the change, at least in the motor, and possibly the visual cortex. This task has been started for 1 Hz motor cortex depression. Touge and coworkers (Touge et al., 2001) demonstrated that the depression was not apparent during a mild voluntary contraction of the target muscle. This is good evidence against a change in the strength of any set of synapses in the path of the stimulus from the horizontal cortical axons to the muscle since such a change would be measurable as greater MEP excitability at any level of drive or inhibition of the cortical or spinal motoneurons. Siebner et al. (1999b) showed that 1 Hz rTMS increased stimulus-evoked intracortical inhibition, suggesting the involvement of cortical GABAergic interneurons. Similar studies should be done on the facilitatory effect of high-frequency stimulation. Work in this area has begun. For instance, Wu et al. (2000) found facilitatory changes in the motor cortex using the paired-pulse paradigm after treatment with 5 and 15 Hz rTMS. The pharmacology of these effects might also be worth exploring. For instance, the facilitation following high-frequency rTMS could involve a purely presynaptic effect, such as the accumulation of Ca^{2+} that produces post-tetanic potentiation. On the other hand, it could also involve a synaptic change as a precursor to LTP. It is possible to identify post-tetanic potentiation. Samii et al. (1998) used phenytoin, a blocker of post-tetanic potentiation, but not LTP, to show that postexercise facilitation was not due to post-tetanic potentiation.

A central feature of LTP is its dependence on converging and temporally related inputs. This implies that facilitation of MEPs by high-frequency rTMS should be easier to produce or longer lasting when TMS is applied in combination with afferent stimulation from another source. LTP has been demonstrated in the motor cortex of animals with simultaneous stimulation of the somatosensory cortex and the ventrolateral thalamus (Iriki et al., 1991). While thalamic stimulation is not practical in humans, this type of experiment has been done with a combination of rTMS and somatosensory stimulation (Stefan et al., 2000). Combining rTMS with specific sensory inputs might be useful for enhancing various types of training or even for extinguishing undesirable associations as in anxiety spectrum disorders or addictions.

Certain features also distinguish LTD. One is that it is considerably easier to induce after priming stimulation with brief exposure to stimulation that activates N-methyl-D-aspartate receptors, e.g. high-frequency stimulation even below the threshold required to induce LTP (Abraham & Tate, 1997; Abraham et al., 2001). Experiments in this area may help both to clarify the basis of the rTMS depressant effect and to help to make a reasonable candidate therapy in disorders such as epilepsy.

Finally, if the effects of TMS are to be fully understood and optimized, animal models will have to be developed. So far, a number of studies have looked at corticospinal activation, i.e. the physiological basis of the MEP, in primates and other animals. Many others have examined the biochemical and transcriptional effects of exposure to TMS in rodents (Wassermann & Lisanby, 2001). These studies have used coils of various sizes, all of which have been too large to reproduce the conditions of human TMS and very likely produce currents that pervade the entire brain and activate neurons in regions that lie too deep to reach in humans with conventional equipment. The resulting data have served mainly to confuse among clinicians. Recent studies using specially designed stimulating coils (Keck et al., 2000) have begun to approach a realistic model, but an easier and more certain approach may be to use focal electrical stimulation. For instance, an appropriate rat model for the putative effects of rTMS treatment in depression might involve electrical stimulation of the frontal cortex and assays of neurotransmitters or gene transcription in the diencephalon and limbic areas.

Use of TMS to influence plasticity

The recognition that neuroplasticity can be functionally beneficial (Cohen et al., 1997), but also may be unrelated to function or even potentially maladaptive (Ramachandran et al., 1992; Yang et al., 1994; Flor et al., 1995, 1998; Birbaumer et al., 1997), raises a new question: Is it possible to up-regulate plasticity when it is beneficial and down-regulate it when it is mal-adaptive (Pons, 1998)? Stimulation delivered to a body part can predictably increase the excitability of its cortical representation (Hamdy et al., 1998) and, when applied to the paretic hand of stroke patients, enhance motor performance (Conforto et al., 2002). TMS could modulate cortical plasticity in a way similar to the modulation of cortical excitability described above. Some recent studies appear to support this contention. For example, acute deafferentation induced by ischemic nerve block leads to a rapid facilitation of cortical motor outputs to muscles immediately above the deafferentation level, that can be modulated by application of TMS. The deafferentation-induced plastic changes can be up-regulated by direct stimulation of the 'plastic' cortex and, probably through inhibitory projections, down-regulated by stimulation of the opposite cortex (Ziemann et al., 1998a). Similarly, motor training results in use-dependent plasticity in the human motor cortex that may contribute to the beneficial effects of preperformance practice in musicians and athletes and be the first step in skill acquisition (Classen et al., 1998). This form of plasticity, influenced by GABA-related disinhibi-tion of intracortical networks and NMDA and muscarinic receptor activation (Butefisch et al., 2000, 2002; Sawaki et al., 2002), can be enhanced by applica-tion of TMS to the plastic cortex during the training process (Bütefisch et al., 1999).

Applications to therapeutics

The idea that TMS can influence cortical excitability and plasticity itself has already been extended to therapeutics. This is a very active area of invest-igation. No therapeutic effect is very dramatic at this time, but it is fair to say that the best locus for stimulation and the optimal pattern of number of pulses, frequency and intensity have not been determined. It can be noted in this regard that rapid rTMS, if delivered at just threshold intensity, may actually reduce cortical excitability (Modugno et al., 2001).

In some circumstances, a reasonable goal would be to increase cortical excitability. The observation that TMS, delivered in just the right way, can speed up the RT in patients with Parkinson's disease, led to the idea that rTMS might be able to be used for therapy (Pascual-Leone et al., 1994a). It is already clear that continuous deep brain stimulation (DBS) of the pallidum or subthalamic nucleus can be useful for ameliorating symptoms in patients with Parkinson's disease. In an initial rTMS trial using the Purdue pegboard, this seemed to be the case (Pascual-Leone et al., 1994a), but the finding was not reproduced (Ghabra et al., 1999). On the other hand, other studies have suggested an improvement in pointing performance after rTMS (Siebner et al., 1999a) and an improvement on the UPDRS (Siebner et al., 2000). TMS repeated over long periods of time may be beneficial (Shimamoto et al., 1999), and this suggests that multiple applications may lead to a longer-term plasticity.

Depression is characterized by cortical hypometabolism and is known to respond to ECT. Can rTMS treatments increase cortical excitability and improve mood? Early observations indicated that high rate rTMS applied to the left dorsolateral prefrontal cortex may improve depression giving hope that this might replace electroconvulsive shock treatment (ECT) (George et al., 1995; Triggs et al., 1999). These results are holding up in controlled trials (George et al., 2000). A recent review that found seven controlled trials and five suitable for a meta-analysis suggested that there is a statistically valid antidepressive effect (McNamara et al., 2001). Another review is more cautious (Wassermann & Lisanby, 2001). Like ECT, multiple treatments are used and are apparently necessary implying a long-term influence of the TMS. Additionally, there is some attention to the idea that rTMS may have value in mania (Yaroslavsky et al., 1999).

The idea that cortical activity could be depressed by 1 Hz rTMS has attracted clinical interest in the area of epilepsy (Tergau et al., 1999). Another early application has been schizophrenic auditory hallucinosis (Hoffman et al., 2000). Low rate rTMS delivered to the right dorsolateral prefrontal cortex may also be helpful in depression (Klein et al., 1999) suggesting a ying–yang effect on mood from right and left frontal cortices. Again, all of these applications have required multiple applications suggesting that repeated rTMS eventually leads to a longer-lasting cortical change.

A logical rationale was developed for why low-frequency rTMS might be useful in dystonia. Physiological findings in dystonia reveal an decrease in intracortical inhibition. Since rTMS delivered over the primary motor cortex at 1 Hz can induce an increase in inhibition, it was proposed that it might ameliorate the deficit. A study showed a normalization of the intracortical inhibition and some modest improvement in performance (Siebner et al., 1999b), but only a single therapeutic session was employed.

In therapeutics, a long-term effect will be needed if there is going to be any value, if we are going to stick with external magnets. The rTMS studies could potentially point the way for continuous stimulation therapy like DBS. On the other hand, long-term effects do seem possible given the TMS effect on plasticity. In addition to optimizing number of pulses, frequency and intensity, as noted above, it might also be valuable to explore varying patterns of stimulation with variations in rhythm of pulses and intensities. There have already been some attempts at this using rTMS with series of paired stimuli. (Sommer et al., 2001).

Conclusion

Our succinct conclusion and recommendation comes from Sophocles:

These things are in the future; we needs must do what lies at hand.

SOPHOCLES. *Antigone, l. 1334*

REFERENCES

Abraham, W.C. & Tate, W.P. (1997). Metaplasticity: a new vista across the field of synaptic plasticity. *Prog. Neurobiol.,* **52**: 303–323.

Abraham, W.C., Mason-Parker, S.E., Bear, M.F., Webb, S. & Tate, W.P. (2001). Heterosynaptic metaplasticity in the hippocampus in vivo: a BCM-like modifiable threshold for LTP. *Proc. Natl Acad. Sci., USA,* **98**: 10924–10929.

Berardelli, A., Inghilleri, M., Rothwell, J.C. et al. (1998). Facilitation of muscle evoked responses after repetitive cortical stimulation in man. *Exp. Brain Res.,* **122**: 79–84.

Birbaumer, N., Lutzenberger, W., Montoya, P. et al. (1997). Effects of regional anesthesia on phantom limb pain are mirrored in changes in cortical reorganization. *J. Neurosci.,* **17**: 5503–5508.

Boroojerdi, B., Bushara, K.O., Corwell, B. et al. (2000). Enhanced excitability of the human visual cortex induced by short-term light deprivation. *Cereb. Cortex,* **10**: 529–534.

Bütefisch, C.M., Khurana, V., Davis, B., Kopylev, L. & Cohen, L.G. (1999). Modulation of use-dependent plasticity in human motor cortex. *Soc. Neurosci. Abstr.*, **25**: 384.

Bütefisch, C.M., Davis, B.C., Wise, S.P. et al. (2000). Mechanisms of use-dependent plasticity in the human motor cortex. *Proc. Natl Acad. Sci., USA*, **97**: 3661–3665.

Bütefisch, C.M., Davis, B.C., Sawaki, L. et al. (2002). Modulation of use-dependent plasticity by D-amphetamine. *Ann. Neurol.*, **51**: 59–68.

Chen, R., Classen, J., Gerloff, C. et al. (1997). Depression of motor cortex excitability by low-frequency transcranial magnetic stimulation. *Neurology*, **48**: 1398–1403.

Classen, J., Liepert, J., Wise, S.P., Hallett, M. & Cohen, L.G. (1998). Rapid plasticity of human cortical movement representation induced by practice. *J. Neurophysiol.*, **79**: 1117–1123.

Cohen, L.G., Celnik, P., Pascual-Leone, A. et al. (1997). Functional relevance of cross-modal plasticity in blind humans. *Nature*, **389**: 180–183.

Conforto, A.B., Kaelin-Lang, A. & Cohen, L.G. (2002). Increase in hand muscle strength of stroke patients after somatosensory stimulation. *Ann. Neurol.*, **51**: 122–125.

Flor, H., Elbert, T., Knecht, S. et al. (1995). Phantom-limb pain as a perceptual correlate of cortical reorganization following arm amputation. *Nature*, **375**: 482–484.

Flor, H., Elbert, T., Muhlnickel, W., Pantev, C., Wienbruch, C. & Taub, E. (1998). Cortical reorganization and phantom phenomena in congenital and traumatic upper-extremity amputees. *Exp. Brain Res.*, **119**: 205–212.

George, M.S., Wassermann, E.M., Williams, W.A. et al. (1995). Daily repetitive transcranial magnetic stimulation (rTMS) improves mood in depression. *Neuroreport*, **6**: 1853–1856.

George, M.S., Nahas, Z., Molloy, M. et al. (2000). A controlled trial of daily left prefrontal cortex TMS for treating depression. *Biol. Psychiatry*, **48**: 962–970.

Ghabra, M.B., Hallett, M. & Wassermann, E.M. (1999). Simultaneous repetitive transcranial magnetic stimulation does not speed fine movement in PD. *Neurology*, **52**: 768–770.

Hamdy, S., Rothwell, J.C., Aziz, Q., Singh, K.D. & Thompson, D.G. (1998). Long-term reorganization of human motor cortex driven by short-term sensory stimulation. *Nat. Neurosci.*, **1**: 64–68.

Hilgetag, C.C., Theoret, H. & Pascual-Leone, A. (2001). Enhanced visual spatial attention ipsilateral to rTMS-induced 'virtual lesions' of human parietal cortex. *Nat. Neurosci.*, **4**: 953–957.

Hoffman, R.E., Boutros, N.N., Hu, S., Berman, R.M., Krystal, J.H. & Charney, D.S. (2000). Transcranial magnetic stimulation and auditory hallucinations in schizophrenia. *Lancet*, **355**: 1073–1075.

Iriki, A., Pavlides, C., Keller, A. & Asanuma, H. (1991). Long-term potentiation of thalamic input to the motor cortex induced by coactivation of thalamocortical and corticocortical afferents. *J. Neurophysiol.*, **65**: 1435–1441.

Keck, M.E., Sillaber, I., Ebner, K. et al. (2000). Acute transcranial magnetic stimulation of frontal brain regions selectively modulates the release of vasopressin, biogenic amines and amino acids in the rat brain. *Eur. J. Neurosci.*, **12**: 3713–3720.

Klein, E., Kreinin, I., Chistyakov, A. et al. (1999). Therapeutic efficacy of right prefrontal slow repetitive transcranial magnetic stimulation in major depression: a double-blind controlled study. *Arch. Gen. Psychiatry*, **56**: 315–320.

Kosslyn, S.M., Pascual-Leone, A., Felician, O. et al. (1999). The role of area 17 in visual imagery: convergent evidence from PET and rTMS. *Science*, **284**: 167–170.

McNamara, B., Ray, J.L., Arthurs, J. & Boniface, S. (2001). Transcranial magnetic stimulation for depression and other psychiatric disorders. *Psychol. Med.*, **31**: 1141–1146.

Modugno, N., Nakamura, Y., MacKinnon, C.D. et al. (2001). Motor cortex excitability following short trains of repetitive magnetic stimuli. *Exp. Brain Res.*, **140**: 453–459.

Pascual-Leone, A., Houser, C.M., Reese, K. et al. (1993). Safety of rapid-rate transcranial magnetic stimulation in normal volunteers. *Electroencephalogr. Clin. Neurophysiol.*, **89**: 120–130.

Pascual-Leone, A., Valls-Solé, J., Brasil-Neto, J., Cammarota, A., Grafman, J. & Hallett, M. (1994a). Akinesia in Parkinson's Disease. II. Effects of subthreshold repetitive transcranial motor cortex stimulation. *Neurology*, **44**: 892–898.

Pascual-Leone, A., Valls-Solé, J., Wassermann, E.M. & Hallett, M. (1994b). Responses to rapid-rate transcranial magnetic stimulation of the human motor cortex. *Brain*, **117**: 847–858.

Pons, T.P. (1998). Reorganizing the brain. *Nat. Med.*, **4**: 561–562.

Ramachandran, V.S., Stewart, M. & Rogers-Ramachandran, D.C. (1992). Perceptual correlates of massive cortical reorganization. *Neuroreport*, **3**: 583–586.

Ridding, M.C. & Rothwell, J.C. (1997). Stimulus/response curves as a method of measuring motor cortical excitability in man. *Electroencephalogr. Clin. Neurophysiol.*, **105**: 340–344.

Roth, B.J., Maccabee, P.J., Eberle, L.P. et al. (1994). In vitro evaluation of a 4-leaf coil design for magnetic stimulation of peripheral nerve. *Electroencephalogr. Clin. Neurophysiol.*, **93**: 68–74.

Samii, A., Chen, R., Wassermann, E.M. & Hallett, M. (1998). Phenytoin does not influence postexercise facilitation of motor evoked potentials. *Neurology*, **50**: 291–293.

Sanger, T.D., Garg, R.R. & Chen, R. (2001). Interactions between two different inhibitory systems in the human motor cortex. *J. Physiol.*, **530**: 307–317.

Sawaki, L., Boroojerdi, B., Kaelin-Lang, A. et al. (2002). Cholinergic influences on use-dependent plasticity. *J. Neurophysiol.*, **87**: 166–171.

Shimamoto, H., Morimitsu, H., Sugita, S., Nakahara, K. & Shigemori, M. (1999). Therapeutic effect of repetitive transcranial magnetic stimulation in Parkinson's disease. *Rinsho Shinkeigaku*, **39**: 1264–1267.

Siebner, H.R., Mentschel, C., Auer, C. & Conrad, B. (1999a). Repetitive transcranial magnetic stimulation has a beneficial effect on bradykinesia in Parkinson's disease. *Neuroreport*, 10: 589–594.

Siebner, H.R., Tormos, J.M., Ceballos-Baumann, A.O. et al. (1999b). Low-frequency repetitive transcranial magnetic stimulation of the motor cortex in writer's cramp. *Neurology*, 52: 529–537.

Siebner, H.R., Rossmeier, C., Mentschel, C., Peinemann, A. & Conrad, B. (2000). Short-term motor improvement after sub-threshold 5-Hz repetitive transcranial magnetic stimulation of the primary motor hand area in Parkinson's disease. *J. Neurol. Sci.*, 178: 91–94.

Sommer, M., Tergau, F., Wischer, S. & Paulus, W. (2001). Paired-pulse repetitive transcranial magnetic stimulation of the human motor cortex. *Exp. Brain Res.*, 139: 465–472.

Speer, A.M., Kimbrell, T.A., Wassermann, E.M. et al. (2000). Opposite effects of high and low frequency rTMS on regional brain activity in depressed patients. *Biol. Psychiatry*, 48: 1133–1141.

Stefan, K., Kunesch, E., Cohen, L.G., Benecke, R. & Classen, J. (2000). Induction of plasticity in the human motor cortex by paired associative stimulation. *Brain*, 123: 572–584.

Tergau, F., Naumann, U., Paulus, W. & Steinhoff, B.J. (1999). Low-frequency repetitive transcranial magnetic stimulation improves intractable epilepsy. *Lancet*, 353: 2209.

Touge, T., Gerschlager, W., Brown, P. & Rothwell, J.C. (2001). Are the after-effects of low-frequency rTMS on motor cortex excitability due to changes in the efficacy of cortical synapses? *Clin. Neurophysiol.*, 112: 2138–2145.

Triggs, W.J., McCoy, K.J., Greer, R. et al. (1999). Effects of left frontal transcranial magnetic stimulation on depressed mood, cognition, and corticomotor threshold. *Biol. Psychiatry*, 45: 1440–1446.

Wassermann, E.M. & Lisanby, S.H. (2001). Therapeutic application of repetitive transcranial magnetic stimulation: a review. *Clin. Neurophysiol.*, 112: 1367–1377.

Wassermann, E.M., Grafman, J., Berry, C. et al. (1996). Use and safety of a new repetitive transcranial magnetic stimulator. *Electroencephalogr. Clin. Neurophysiol.*, 101: 412–417.

Wu, T., Sommer, M., Tergau, F. & Paulus, W. (2000). Lasting influence of repetitive transcranial magnetic stimulation on intracortical excitability in human subjects. *Neurosci. Lett.*, 287, 37–40.

Yang, T.T., Gallen, C.C., Ramachandran, V.S., Cobb, S., Schwartz, B.J. & Bloom, F.E. (1994). Noninvasive detection of cerebral plasticity in adult human somatosensory cortex. *Neuroreport*, 5: 701–704.

Yaroslavsky, Y., Grisaru, N., Chudakov, B. & Belmaker, R.H. (1999). Is TMS therapeutic in mania as well as in depression? *Electroencephalogr. Clin. Neurophysiol. Suppl.*, **51**: 299–303.

Ziemann, U., Corwell, B. & Cohen, L.G. (1998a). Modulation of plasticity in human motor cortex after forearm ischemic nerve block. *J. Neurosci.*, **18**: 1115–1123.

Ziemann, U., Hallett, M. & Cohen, L.G. (1998b). Mechanisms of deafferentation-induced plasticity in human motor cortex. *J. Neurosci.*, **18**: 7000–7007.

Index

Note: page numbers in *italics* refer to figures and tables. Illustrations in the Plate Section are identified by 'Fig. number (Plate)'